Central Nervous System Malignancies

Guest Editors

JILL LACY, MD
JOACHIM M. BAEHRING, MD, DSc

HEMATOLOGY/ONCOLOGY CLINICS OF NORTH AMERICA

www.hemonc.theclinics.com

Consulting Editors
GEORGE P. CANELLOS, MD
NANCY BERLINER, MD

August 2012 • Volume 26 • Number 4

SAUNDERS an imprint of ELSEVIER, Inc.

W.B. SAUNDERS COMPANY
A Division of Elsevier Inc.

1600 John F. Kennedy Blvd. • Suite 1800 • Philadelphia, PA 19103-2899

http://www.theclinics.com

HEMATOLOGY/ONCOLOGY CLINICS OF NORTH AMERICA Volume 26, Number 4
August 2012 ISSN 0889-8588, ISBN 13: 978-1-4557-4940-9

Editor: Patrick Manley
Developmental Editor: Donald Mumford

Hematology/Oncology Clinics (ISSN 0889-8588) is published bimonthly by Elsevier Inc., 360 Park Avenue South, New York, NY 10010-1710. Months of issue are February, April, June, August, October, and December. Business and Editorial Offices: 1600 John F. Kennedy Blvd., Ste. 1800, Philadelphia, PA 19103–2899. Customer Service Office: 3251 Riverport Lane, Maryland Heights, MO 63043. Periodicals postage paid at New York, NY and at additional mailing offices. Subscription prices are $353.00 per year (domestic individuals), $576.00 per year (domestic institutions), $173.00 per year (domestic students/residents), $401.00 per year (Canadian individuals), $705.00 per year (Canadian institutions) $477.00 per year (international individuals), $705.00 per year (international institutions), and $233.00 per year (international and Canadian students/residents). International air speed delivery is included in all *Clinics* subscription prices. All prices are subject to change without notice. **POSTMASTER:** Send address changes to *Hematology/Oncology Clinics of North America*, Elsevier Health Sciences Division, Subscription Customer Service, 3251 Riverport Lane, Maryland Heights, MO 63043. Customer Service (orders, claims, online, change of address): Elsevier Health Sciences Division, Subscription Customer Service, 3251 Riverport Lane, Maryland Heights, MO 63043. Tel: 1-800-654-2452 (U.S. and Canada); 314-447-8871 (outside U.S. and Canada). Fax: 314-447-8029. E-mail: journalscustomerservice-usa@elsevier.com (for print support); journalsonlinesupport-usa@elsevier.com (for online support).

Reprints. For copies of 100 or more, of articles in this publication, please contact the Commercial Reprints Department, Elsevier Inc., 360 Park Avenue South, New York, New York 10010-1710; Tel.: 212-633-3813, Fax: 212-462-1935, E-mail: reprints@elsevier.com.

Hematology/Oncology Clinics of North America is covered in *MEDLINE/PubMed (Index Medicus), EMBASE/ Excerpta Medica, and BIOSIS.*

Printed in the United States of America.

Transferred to Digital Printing, 2012

Contributors

CONSULTING EDITORS

GEORGE P. CANELLOS, MD
William Rosenberg Professor of Medicine, Department of Medical Oncology, Dana-Farber Cancer Institute, Boston, Massachusetts

NANCY BERLINER, MD
Chief, Division of Hematology, Brigham and Women's Hospital; Professor of Medicine, Harvard Medical School, Boston, Massachusetts

GUEST EDITORS

JILL LACY, MD
Associate Professor of Medicine, Section of Medical Oncology, Department of Medicine, Yale University School of Medicine, New Haven, Connecticut

JOACHIM M. BAEHRING, MD, DSc
Associate Professor of Neurology, Neurosurgery and Medicine, Yale University School of Medicine, Director, Yale Brain Tumor Center, New Haven, Connecticut

AUTHORS

KEVIN ANTON, MD, PhD
Department of Pharmacology, Cancer Institute of New Jersey, Robert Wood Johnson Medical School, University of Medicine and Dentistry of New Jersey, New Brunswick, New Jersey

JOACHIM M. BAEHRING, MD, DSc
Associate Professor of Neurology, Neurosurgery and Medicine, Yale University School of Medicine, Director, Yale Brain Tumor Center, New Haven, Connecticut

TRACY T. BATCHELOR, MD, MPH
Professor of Neurology, Stephen E. and Catherine Pappas Center for Neuro-Oncology, Division of Hematology and Oncology, Department of Neurology, Massachusetts General Hospital Cancer Center; Department of Radiation Oncology, Massachusetts General Hospital, Harvard Medical School, Boston, Massachusetts

KEVIN P. BECKER, MD, PhD
Department of Neurology, Yale University School of Medicine, New Haven, Connecticut

NICHOLAS A. BLONDIN, MD
Department of Neurology, Yale University School of Medicine, New Haven, Connecticut

PRISCILLA K. BRASTIANOS, MD
Fellow in Medical Oncology, Stephen E. and Catherine Pappas Center for Neuro-Oncology, Division of Hematology and Oncology, Department of Neurology, Massachusetts General Hospital Cancer Center; Department of Medical Oncology, Dana-Farber/Brigham and Women's Cancer Center, Harvard Medical School, Boston, Massachusetts

MARC C. CHAMBERLAIN, MD
Division of Neuro-Oncology, Department of Neurology and Neurological Surgery, University of Washington, Fred Hutchinson Cancer Research Center, Seattle Cancer Care Alliance, Seattle, Washington

VERONICA L.S. CHIANG, MD
Associate Professor, Director, Stereotactic Radiosurgery; Medical Director, Yale-New Haven Hospital Gamma Knife Center, Department of Neurosurgery, Yale University School of Medicine, New Haven, Connecticut

JOHN W. HENSON, MD
Ben and Catherine Ivy Foundation, Swedish Neuroscience Institute, Swedish Medical Center; Associate Chief Medical Director, Swedish Neuroscience Institute, Seattle, Washington

JÜRGEN HONEGGER, MD
Department of Neurosurgery, University of Tuebingen, Tuebingen, Germany

ANITA HUTTNER, MD
Assistant Professor, Department of Pathology, Yale University School of Medicine, New Haven, Connecticut

EUGENE HWANG, MD
The Brain Tumor Institute; Assistant Professor of Pediatrics, Division of Hematology and Oncology, Center for Cancer and Blood Disorders, Children's National Medical Center; School of Medicine and Health Sciences, The George Washington University, Washington, DC

BART P. KEOGH, MD, PhD
Chief of Radiology, Swedish Medical Center; Swedish Neuroscience Institute, Cherry Hill Campus, Swedish Medical Center, Seattle; Neuroradiology Section, Radia Inc., PS, Everett, Washington

JONATHAN P.S. KNISELY, MD
Associate Professor, Chief, Division of Radiosurgery and Stereotactic Program, Co-Director for Radiosurgery and Stereotactic Radiation Therapy, Department of Radiation Medicine, Hofstra North Shore-LIJ School of Medicine, North Shore University Hospital, Manhasset, New York

JILL LACY, MD
Associate Professor of Medicine, Section of Medical Oncology, Department of Medicine, Yale University School of Medicine, New Haven, Connecticut

TINA MAYER, MD
Departments of Medical Oncology, and Medicine, Cancer Institute of New Jersey, Robert Wood Johnson Medical School, University of Medicine and Dentistry of New Jersey, New Brunswick, New Jersey

SACIT BULENT OMAY, MD
Resident, Department of Neurosurgery, Yale University School of Medicine, New Haven, Connecticut

ROGER J. PACKER, MD
The Brain Tumor Institute, Children's National Medical Center; School of Medicine and Health Sciences, The George Washington University; Professor of Pediatrics, Center for Neuroscience and Behavioral Medicine, Division of Neurology, Children's National Medical Center, Washington, DC

TORAL R. PATEL, MD
Resident, Department of Neurosurgery, Yale University School of Medicine, New Haven, Connecticut

JOSEPH M. PIEPMEIER, MD
Nixdorff-German Professor of Neurosurgery, Vice-Chair of Clinical Affairs, Neurosurgery, Section Chief, Director, Surgical Neuro-Oncology, Department of Neurosurgery, Yale University School of Medicine, New Haven, Connecticut

FLORIAN ROSER, MD
Department of Neurosurgery, University of Tuebingen, Tuebingen, Germany

HAMID SAADATI, MD
Fellow, Section of Medical Oncology, Department of Medicine, Yale University School of Medicine, New Haven, Connecticut

AYMAN SAMKARI, MD
The Brain Tumor Institute; Pediatric Neuro-Oncology Fellow, Division of Hematology and Oncology, Center for Cancer and Blood Disorders, Children's National Medical Center; School of Medicine and Health Sciences, The George Washington University, Washington, DC

MARTIN U. SCHUHMANN, MD
Department of Neurosurgery, University of Tuebingen, Tuebingen, Germany

MARCOS S. TATAGIBA, MD
Department of Neurosurgery, University of Tuebingen, Tuebingen, Germany

JAMES B. YU, MD
Assistant Professor, Department of Therapeutic Radiology, Yale University School of Medicine, New Haven, Connecticut

Contents

> Contemporary neuropathology plays a key role in the multidisciplinary management of brain tumor patients, in part due to increased supplementation of histopathological assessments by molecular diagnostic tests involving brain tumor tissue. Several molecular tests have become routine for clinical practice, and not only contribute to a refinement of tumor classification, but also aid in improved prediction of prognosis and in development of a tailored approach to therapy. This review provides an overview of classification and grading of brain tumors, particularly neuroepithelial tumors, and describes genetic/epigenetic changes that have gained clinical significance for molecular diagnostic testing.

> The clinical manifestations of intracranial tumors are usually referable to the anatomic area of the brain involved or adjacent structures. Some anatomic regions may allow a tumor to reach substantial size while remaining clinically silent. In contrast, small lesions in critical areas are more likely to present early. The initial diagnosis of intracranial tumors is most efficiently made by imaging. This article discusses the clinicoanatomic features and imaging characteristics of brain tumors, including the use of dynamic susceptibility-weighted, T1 dynamic, diffusion, functional, and diffusion tensor imaging.

> In the United States, approximately 65,000 people are diagnosed with primary brain tumors each year, with an incidence of 19.3 cases per 100,000 person-years. These numbers represent a wide spectrum of disease, from benign to malignant, and prognosis varies widely based on disease. Treatment of primary brain tumors most often uses a combination of surgery and radiation. However, over the past several generations, technological advancements have significantly altered the treatment paradigm. This article reviews the current role of neurosurgery and radiation therapy in the management of primary brain tumors.

> The diverse medical and neurologic complications of central nervous system (CNS) neoplasms or their treatment cause significant morbidity and mortality. Thus, their recognition and appropriate management by all members of the interdisciplinary team engaged in the care of patients with brain tumors is essential in optimizing quality of life and extending survival. Recognition of the acute, early delayed, and late complications of brain irradiation is essential to optimize management and mitigate their clinical impact.

Gliomas

> Low-grade gliomas are uncommon tumors whose optimal management remains to be determined. Although well-designed clinical trials have been mounted to address certain aspects of postoperative radiotherapeutic management, additional studies are required to refine management based on tumor-specific and patient-specific variables. There is mounting evidence that the relative completeness of surgical resection can improve survival, and the molecular and histopathologic characterization of the glioma requires adequate samples for analysis. Current imaging and operative techniques can direct surgical resection, and the same imaging techniques can help monitor patients postoperatively and predict prognosis.

> The optimal treatment of anaplastic gliomas is controversial. Options for treatment include radiation, chemotherapy or a combination of modalities. This article describes how treatment algorithms for anaplastic gliomas have evolved and interprets the results of recent studies. The available evidence indicates that patients can be treated with either chemotherapy or radiation as initial therapy, with use of the other treatment modality at relapse. Whether subpopulations exist for whom one treatment modality is superior to the other at initial diagnosis must be studied prospectively.

> Glioblastoma multiforme is the most common primary malignant tumor of the central nervous system. Despite new insights into glioblastoma pathophysiology, the prognosis for patients diagnosed with this highly aggressive tumor remains bleak. Current treatment regimens combine surgical resection and chemoradiotherapy, providing an increase in median overall survival from 12.1 to 14.6 months. Ongoing preclinical and clinical studies evaluating the efficacy of novel therapies provide hope for increasing survival benefit. This article reviews the advancements in glioblastoma treatment in newly diagnosed and recurrent glioblastoma, including

novel therapies such as antiangiogenic agents, mammalian target of rapamycin inhibitors, poly(ADP-ribose) polymerase-1 inhibitors, and immunotherapies.

Nonglioma Primary Brain Tumors

Metastases

the most morbid of central nervous system metastases. The disease is challenging to treat for a variety of reasons, including challenges in making a diagnosis of neoplastic meningitis and lack of standardized treatment due to the paucity of clinical trials addressing treatment of neoplastic meningitis.

HEMATOLOGY/ONCOLOGY
CLINICS OF NORTH AMERICA

DOWNLOAD
Free App!

Review Articles
THE CLINICS

NOW AVAILABLE FOR YOUR iPhone and iPad

Preface

Central Nervous System Malignancies

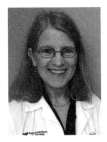 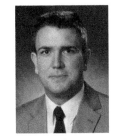

Jill Lacy, MD   Joachim M. Baehring, MD, DSc
Guest Editors

The last two decades have seen unprecedented changes in the field of Neuro-Oncology. A new classification system for primary nervous system neoplasms has been established by the World Health Organization. Technological advances have led to our ability to diagnose brain tumors earlier and to treat them more effectively and with reduced morbidity using multimodality approaches incorporating surgery, radiation, and chemotherapy. Our rapidly evolving understanding of the molecular and genetic mechanisms leading to brain cancer now provides powerful prognostic and predictive information that drives therapeutic decisions and is stimulating novel treatment strategies.

This special issue of *Hematology/Oncology Clinics of North America* provides an up-to-date and concise review of the molecular pathogenesis, novel diagnostic strategies, current standards of care, and novel therapies of primary brain tumors and CNS metastases. The issue comprises contributions from experts from the multiple disciplines relevant to Neuro-Oncology and provides a reflection of their personal experiences and interpretation of published studies.

We thank everyone who has helped in the preparation of this issue. Most importantly, we thank the contributing authors whose work provides the substance of this special issue. It has been a privilege working with them and reading their contributions

Hematol Oncol Clin N Am 26 (2012) xiii–xiv
http://dx.doi.org/10.1016/j.hoc.2012.06.001
0889-8588/12/$ – see front matter © 2012 Elsevier Inc. All rights reserved.

"first hand." We are grateful to the staff at the editorial office, whose efforts assured timely completion.

Jill Lacy, MD
Department of Medicine
Section of Medical Oncology
Yale University School of Medicine
333 Cedar Street
New Haven, CT 06510, USA

Joachim M. Baehring, MD, DSc
Departments of Neurology, Neurosurgery, and Medicine
Yale University School of Medicine
Yale Brain Tumor Center
15 York Street
New Haven, CT 06510, USA

E-mail addresses:
jill.lacy@yale.edu (J. Lacy)
joachim.baehring@yale.edu (J.M. Baehring)

Overview of Primary Brain Tumors
Pathologic Classification, Epidemiology, Molecular Biology, and Prognostic Markers

Anita Huttner, MD

KEYWORDS

- Neuroepithelial tumors • WHO classification • Pathology • Genetics

KEY POINTS

- Contemporary neuropathology plays a key role in the multidisciplinary management of brain tumor patients.
- The histopathologic characterization and grading of brain tumors is increasingly supplemented by molecular diagnostic tests involving brain tumor tissue.
- Several molecular tests have become routine for clinical practice and not only contribute to a refinement of the standard classification scheme but also aid in improved prediction of prognosis and in the development of a tailored approach to clinical therapy.

INTRODUCTION

Primary brain tumors in adults are rare and constitute fewer than 2% of all malignant neoplasms.[1,2] In children, however, they form the second most common type of tumor, after leukemias. Of all intracranial tumors, neuroepithelial tumors are the most common neoplasms, representing more than 60% of central nervous system (CNS)–derived lesions. Other lesions are meningothelial tumors (30%), tumors arising from cranial and spinal nerves (7%–8%), CNS lymphomas (4%), and germ cell neoplasms (approximately 1%).[1,2] The classification system of the World Health Organization (WHO) lists more than 120 different tumor types and subtypes for the CNS (**Table 1**).[3,4] This review focuses on some of the main groups of neuroepithelial tumors, in particular glial neoplasms and embryonal tumors. Detailed discussion of neuronal, glioneuronal, pineal, and other tumor entities is beyond the scope of this article, especially because there is only limited molecular information available, which

Disclosures: Anita Huttner has no relationship with any commercial company that has a direct financial interest in the subject matter or the materials discussed in the article or with any company making a competing product.
Department of Pathology, Yale University School of Medicine, 310 Cedar Street, BML 167, New Haven, CT 06510, USA
E-mail address: anita.huttner@yale.edu

Hematol Oncol Clin N Am 26 (2012) 715–732
doi:10.1016/j.hoc.2012.05.004
0889-8588/12/$ – see front matter © 2012 Elsevier Inc. All rights reserved.

Table 1
Neuroepithelial tumors

	WHO Grade			
	I	II	III	IV
Astrocytic Tumors				
Pilocytic astrocytoma	x			
Pilomyxoid astrocytoma		x		
Subependymal giant cell astrocytoma	x			
Pleomorphic xanthoastrocytoma		x		

Diffuse astrocytoma
  Variants
  Fibrillary astrocytoma
  Gemistocytic astrocytoma
  Protoplasmic astrocytoma
		x		

Anaplastic astrocytoma			x	

Glioblastoma
  Variants
  Giant cell glioblastoma
  Gliosarcoma
				x

Oligodendroglial Tumors				
Oligodendroglioma		x		
Anaplastic oligodendroglioma			x	
Oligoastrocytic Tumors				
Oligoastrocytoma		x		
Anaplastic oligoastrocytoma			x	
Ependymal Tumors				
Subependymoma	x			
Myxopapillary ependymoma	x			

Ependymoma
  Variants
  Cellular ependymoma
  Papillary ependymoma
  Clear cell ependymoma
  Tanycytic ependymoma
		x		

Anaplastic ependymoma			x	
Choroid Plexus Tumors				
Choroid plexus papilloma	x			
Atypical choroid plexus papilloma		x		
Choroid plexus carcinoma			x	
Embryonal Tumors				

Medulloblastoma
  Variants
  Desmoplastic/nodular medulloblastoma
  Medulloblastoma with extensive
  nodularity
  Anaplastic medullolastoma
  Large cell medulloblastoma
				x

(continued on next page)

	WHO Grade			
	I	II	III	IV
CNS PNET				x
Variants				
CNS neuroblastoma				
CNS ganglioneuroblastoma				
Medulloepithelioma				
Ependymomoblastoma				
Atypical teratoid/rhabdoid tumor				x
Neuronal and mixed Neuronal-glial Tumors				
Gangliocytoma	x			
Ganglioglioma	x			
Anaplastic ganglioglioma			x	
Desmoplastic infantile astrocytoma and ganglioglioma	x			
Dysembryoplastic neuroepithelial tumor	x			
Central neurocytoma		x		
Extraventricular neurocytoma		x		
Cerebellar liponeurocytoma		x		
Paraganglioma of the spinal canal	x			
Papillary glioneuronal tumor	x			
Rosette-forming tumor of the fourth ventricle	x			
Other Neuroepithelial Tumors				
Chordoid glioma of the third ventricle		x		
Angiocentric glioma	x			

Table 1
(continued)

contributes to clinical management. This review is divided into 2 sections: section I describes the WHO classification, grading, epidemiology, and pathology of tumors, and section II focuses on molecular biology and prognostic markers, particularly of gliomas.

SECTION I: PATHOLOGIC CLASSIFICATION, EPIDEMIOLOGY, AND MORPHOLOGY OF NEUROEPITHELIAL TUMORS
WHO Classification and Grading of Tumors

Brain tumors are classified according to international standards, which are established by the WHO.[4] The WHO classification of CNS tumors is based on consensus criteria developed by an international working group of pathologists and geneticists and forms a comprehensive worldwide standard for tumor definition. The most recent update was published in 2007 (4th edition) and led to an integration of several new histologic subtypes and a revision and expansion of molecular genetic data.[3,4]

Brain tumors are primarily classified according to their histopathologic appearance, which is based on the characterization of constituent cell types and growth patterns. Although the cellular origin of many tumors is still under investigation, the histologic classification relies on morphologic similarities of tumor cells with their presumed non-neoplastic counterpart, in addition to the presence of certain architectural patterns. The WHO subdivides the large group of neuroepithelial neoplasms into a variety of histologic tumor types, such as glial (astrocytomas, oligodendrogliomas, and ependymomas), neuronal, mixed glial-neuronal, embryonal, pineal, choroid plexus derived and others (see **Table 1**). Many molecular profiles have been incorporated and contribute to the subclassification of tumor entities.

The WHO classification also has devised a grading scheme, which can be considered a malignancy scale[3,4] that is used to predict the biologic behavior of neoplasms, therapeutic response, and clinical outcome. It is mainly based on histologic criteria, such as cell density, infiltrative nature, nuclear pleomorphism, mitoses, vascular proliferation, and necrosis. The grading of tumors follows a 4-tiered system and is designed to add a numeric value to the histologic grade (see **Table 1**), which ranges from I (benign) to IV (malignant). Grade I is assigned to tumors that are circumscribed, show a low proliferative potential, rarely progress to malignancy, and are likely cured with surgical resection alone. Grade II tumors have a low proliferative potential but tend to be infiltrative in nature and often recur. Many of these lesions progress to a higher grade of malignancy over time. Grade III lesions show histologic evidence of malignancy, such as nuclear atypia and high proliferative activity. These lesions cannot be cured with surgery alone and require adjuvant radiation and/or chemotherapy. Grade IV is reserved for frankly malignant tumors with an aggressive preoperative and postoperative course. Histologically, these lesions demonstrate pronounced nuclear atypia, high mitotic activity, vascular proliferation, and a tendency to necrose.

The WHO histologic grade, however, is only one of many factors that aid in predicting response to therapy and outcome. Additional, clinically important attributes are a patient's age and neurologic performance status, tumor location, and extent of surgical resection as well as radiologic aspects, such as tumor contrast enhancement. Molecular genetic alterations and proliferation indices play another major role. Combinations of these factors are used to provide an estimate of prognosis and outcome for each tumor entity. On average, patients with WHO grade II tumors tend to survive for greater than 5 years,[5] whereas the survival time of patient's with grade III lesions is reduced to 2 to 3 years. WHO grade IV tumors are in general rapidly fatal if untreated (survival <1 year), and survival rates are greatly influenced by effective adjuvant treatment regimens.

Astrocytic Tumors

Astrocytomas are a morphologically heterogeneous group of neoplasms and defined as tumors with predominantly astrocytic differentiation. They are divided into approximately 2 main groups: (1) diffuse astrocytic lesions, which are more common and biologically related, and (2) circumscribed astrocytic lesions, which are less frequent and biologically unrelated. Diffuse astrocytic tumors are further subdivided according to their degree of malignancy and range from WHO grade II (diffuse astrocytomas and variants), to WHO grade III (anaplastic astrocytomas), to WHO grade IV (glioblastoma and variants). The more circumscribed astrocytic tumors include pilocytic astrocytoma (WHO grade I), pleomorphic xanthoastrocytoma (WHO grade II), subependymal giant cell astrocytoma (WHO grade I), and pilomyxoid astrocytoma, a recently added variant, which is considered WHO grade II.[4] These circumscribed tumors have an indolent course and rarely progress to malignancy.

Diffuse astrocytomas

Diffusely infiltrating astrocytic tumors are the most common primary neoplasms in adults and constitute more than 60% of all brain tumors. The incidence of astrocytomas differs somewhat regionally, but recent estimates suggest an incidence rate of 0.4 per 100,000 people for grade II astrocytomas and an incidence rate of 3.2 per 100,000 people for glioblastoma.[1] The histologic grade shows a direct correlation with the age at presentation, whereby WHO grade II tumors present in younger adults in their fourth or fifth decades, whereas glioblastomas (WHO grade IV) peak in the elderly (mean age at diagnosis 61 years). Men seem more affected than women with a male-to-female ratio of 1.5:1.0 for all astrocytic tumors (except pilocytic astrocytoma).[1]

WHO grade II diffuse astrocytomas are morphologically heterogeneous and characterized by a high degree of cellular differentiation, slow growth, low mitotic activity, and diffuse infiltration and spread into adjacent brain structures (**Fig. 1**). Tumor cells express glial fibrillary acidic protein (GFAP), a protein typically found in astrocytomas. WHO grade II diffuse astrocytomas can be found at any site in the CNS but preferentially in the cerebral hemispheres, particularly in the subcortical and deep white matter of frontotemporal lobes. Although these lesions are rare in children, the main site in pediatric patients is the brainstem (so-called brainstem glioma). Three major variants of WHO grade II diffuse astrocytomas can be distinguished morphologically, and these comprise the fibrillary, gemistocytic, and protoplasmic variants. These subtypes, however, often coexist and a clear subclassification is not possible.

Anaplastic astrocytomas (WHO grade III) are defined as diffuse astrocytomas with focal or dispersed anaplasia. They may arise from low-grade astrocytomas but are also frequently diagnosed at first biopsy, without indication of a less malignant precursor lesion. These tumors are grossly more discernible because they are more cellular and form a more readily identifiable tumor mass. The infiltrative nature tends to create an overall increase of tissue volume without inducing a destructive effect. In comparison to low-grade tumors, these neoplasms are microscopically remarkable for increased cellularity and enlarged, irregular hyperchromatic nuclei (see **Fig. 1**). Capillaries are lined by a single layer of endothelium, and frank vascular proliferation and necrosis are not present. Immunoreactivity for GFAP is less consistent than for grade II lesions. In contrast to low-grade astrocytomas, these lesions display increased mitotic activity with a proliferative fraction (Ki-67/MIB-1 labeling) of 5% to 10%.

Glioblastomas (WHO grade IV) are the most malignant tumors within the spectrum of diffuse astrocytoma and account for approximately 12% to 15% of all intracranial neoplasms and up to 60% of all astrocytic tumors. They affect mainly adults with a peak incidence between 40 and 70 years. Fewer than 10% of glioblastomas arise from a lesion of lower malignancy grade (secondary glioblastoma) and manifest in younger patients (mean age of 45 years). Most are found de novo (primary glioblastoma) after a short clinical history and are seen in older individuals (mean age 62 years).[1–3] The majority of tumors are located within the cerebral hemispheres;

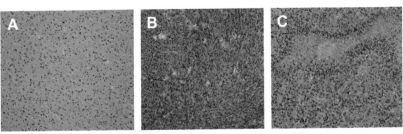

Fig. 1. Histologic features of diffuse astrocytomas (hematoxylin-eosin–stained sections). (*A*) WHO grade II diffuse astrocytoma with low cellularity and mild nuclear pleomorphism; (*B*) anaplastic sstrocytoma, WHO grade III, shows hypercellularity and anaplastic nuclei; (*C*) glioblastoma, WHO grade IV, shows tumor cells with pleomorphic cells and pseudopalisading necrosis.

they often infiltrate deep nuclei and spread along white matter tracts to the contralateral hemisphere. Brainstem involvement is rare and mainly present in children. Other sites, such as spinal cord or cerebellum, are infrequently involved. Microscopically, glioblastomas are heterogeneous. They show a high degree of cellularity, pleomorphism, and mitotic activity in addition to microvascular proliferation and necrosis (see **Fig. 1**). The latter two features are the cardinal diagnostic features of glioblastomas and help distinguish them from grade III astrocytomas. Three distinct glioblastoma variants have been described, which are gliosarcoma, giant cell glioblastoma, and small cell glioblastoma.

Gliosarcomas are defined as glioblastoma intermixed with a sarcomatous component and represent approximately 2% of all glioblastomas. The clinical features are similar to those of classic glioblastomas. Critical diagnostic parameters are a biphasic growth pattern with areas of glial and mesenchymal differentiation. Molecular changes are variable but similar to those occurring in glioblastoma; however, tumor histogenesis is controversial.

Giant cell glioblastomas are remarkable for the presence and predominance of markedly bizarre, multinucleated giant cells, within an abundant stromal reticulin network. In spite of their unusual appearance, the consistent expression of GFAP in conjunction with genetic profiling confirmed its astrocytic nature.

Small cell glioblastoma is characterized by a predominance of small, anaplastic cells that resemble those in a primitive neuroectodermal tumor (PNET). The distinction is made via immunohistochemistry, because these tumors lack expression of synaptophysin that is typical of PNET. The small cell phenotype seems to correlate with the presence of EGFR amplification. Although typical glioblastoma features are not present, overall survival times are less than 1 year.

Circumscribed astrocytic lesions

Pilocytic astrocytomas are slowly growing, well circumscribed glial tumors with preferential growth in midline CNS structures. More than 75% of these tumors are seen in children and adolescents within the ages of 8 to 13 years. These tumors represent approximately 6% of all intracranial tumors and occur at an incidence of less than 1 case per 100,000 individuals per year.[1–3] In infancy it is one of the most frequent brain tumors. The cerebellum is the most commonly affected site, with preferential involvement of the cerebellar hemispheres. The optic nerve and chiasm are second in frequency, followed by the cerebral cortical hemispheres, brainstem, infundibulum, hypothalamus, and spinal cord. In the brainstem, these lesions tend to occur mainly in the dorsal regions and pontomedullary junction, contrasting diffusely infiltrative astrocytomas, which grow typically in the ventral pons. The histopathology can show a variety of patterns and pose great diagnostic challenges. PAs typically demonstrate a biphasic pattern in which fibrillated, compact areas are intermingled with loosely structured, microcystic, and mucinous regions within the tumor tissue. The predominant cell type is an elongated, unipolar or bipolar cell with thin hair-like (Greek *pilos* [hair]) processes, which is immunoreactive for GFAP. The histogenetic origin of these tumors is still enigmatic. Characteristic of PAs is the presence of Rosenthal fibers and eosinophilic granular bodies. These are bright eosinophilic, either carrot-shaped or round structures, and considered amorphous degradation products associated with intermediate filaments. Mitoses are in general absent or infrequent, and the proliferative index (Ki-67/Mib-1) is less than 1%, although it can be focally slightly elevated. PAs have a tendency to invade leptomeninges or subarachnoid space. In contrast to diffusely infiltrating astrocytomas, PAs do not have an intrinsic tendency to progress to a higher grade and are considered a benign glial tumor. The survival rates range from close to 100% at 5 years to approximately 95% at 10 years with recurrence-free intervals of up to 20 years. The WHO assigned grade I to PAs, whereby the grading scheme developed for diffusely infiltrating astrocytomas does not apply. Rarely, these lesions show more aggressive biologic behavior characterized by significant proliferative activity; they are then considered WHO III tumors, equivalent to anaplastic astrocytomas.

Pilomyxoid astrocytoma is considered a variant of pilocytic astrocytoma and typically found in the hypothalamic/chiasmatic region. Histologically, pilomyxoid astrocytoma is composed of monomorphic, bipolar cells with angiocentric arrangements and a striking mucinous background. In contrast to pilocytic astrocytomas, these tumors do not display a biphasic cytoarchitecture; furthermore, they lack Rosenthal fibers or eosinophilic granular bodies and show a high mitotic rate. Infants and children (median age 10 months) are the main affected groups, and prognosis seems less favorable than for PAs. Local recurrences and spread through cerebrospinal fluid do occur more readily than with pilocytic astrocytomas; thus, the WHO assigned grade II to these tumors.

Pleomorphic xanthoastrocytomas are rare tumors, which account for fewer than 1% of glial neoplasms[1–3] and typically manifest in children and young adults, in whom they are associated with a longstanding history of seizures. The majority of these tumors are found in a superficial location, particularly in the temporal lobe, and there is a tendency to involve the overlying subarachnoid space. Characteristic histologic features are multinucleated and lipidized giant cells with bizarre nuclei, which tend to express GFAP, an astrocytic marker. A reticulin rich stromal background is a hallmark feature. These tumors show low proliferative activity. Macroscopically, they are well demarcated and only small portions seem to invade adjacent brain and perivascular spaces. These tumors have been assigned WHO grade II. Many pleomorphic xanthoastrocytomas show a benign clinical course, usually with long-term survival after tumor resection. Only few tumors undergo malignant transformation.

Subependymal giant cell astrocytomas are benign neuroepithelial tumors, which tend to develop in the context of tuberous sclerosis. These tumors typically manifest before age 30 years and are located within the walls of the lateral ventricles. Histologically, they are composed of large ganglioid cells with both astrocytic and neuronal differentiation. Their histogenesis, however, is largely unknown. It is hypothesized that they are related to and/or derived from hamartomatous lesions typically seen in tuberous sclerosis. Subependymal giant cell astrocytomas are designated WHO grade I. Symptomatic lesions are treated with resection and many studies have shown that these tumors have an almost uniformly favorable prognosis.

Oligodendroglial Tumors

Oligodendrogliomas form a group of diffusely infiltrative glial tumors with unique pathologic, clinical, and molecular characteristics. They are composed of neoplastic cells with features reminiscent of oligodendrocytes and often harbor deletions of the short arm of chromosome 1 (1p) and the long arm of chromosome 19 (19q).

Oligodendrogliomas account for approximately 5% to 6% of all glial neoplasms and for 2% to 3% of all primary brain tumors.[1,6] The annual estimated incidence rate lies in a range of 0.27 to 0.35 per 100,000 individuals. Although oligodendrogliomas can develop at any age, the majority of tumors arise in the fourth to fifth decade, and fewer than 2% of oligodendrogliomas are found in children younger than 14 years, with a slight male predominance.[1,7] Oligodendrogliomas can arise anywhere within the CNS, but the majority of tumors are found within the frontal and temporal lobes of the cerebral hemispheres. They are present to a lesser extent in other cortical regions and they are rare within the deep nuclei or spinal cord. Histologically, these tumors are composed of a monomorphous population of cells with round, regular nuclei, cytoplasmic clearing (on routinely formalin-fixed paraffin embedded sections), and growth in close proximity to fine branching vasculature (**Fig. 2**).

The WHO classification divides the spectrum of oligodendrogliomas into well-differentiated tumors, which are slow-growing neoplasms and histologically correspond to WHO grade II and anaplastic tumors, which are WHO grade III. Anaplastic oligodendrogliomas are characterized by a high degree of anaplasia, an increase in cellularity, nuclear pleomorphism, in addition to brisk mitotic activity, endothelial proliferation, and necrosis. In contrast to other gliomas, like astrocytomas and ependymomas, oligodendrogliomas show a more slowly progressive clinical course and demonstrate chemosensitivity. Their molecular signature is distinct and features codeletions of 1p and 19q. Classic oligodendroglial histology in conjunction with 1p/19q codeletions has been strongly linked to more favorable clinical behavior and is considered a defining constellation (discussed later).

Mixed Oligoastrocytomas

Oligoastrocytomas are defined as diffusely infiltrative glial neoplasms consisting of a mixture of 2 distinct neoplastic cell types, which morphologically resemble the tumor cells of diffuse astrocytomas as well as oligodendrogliomas. These 2 components coexist either side-by-side or in a diffusely intermingled fashion. Definitive criteria for identification and classification of these lesions, however, remain somewhat controversial. Oligoastrocytomas are graded as WHO grade II lesions and the acquisition of anaplastic features increase the grade to WHO grade III.

Ependymal Tumors

Ependymomas are defined as slowly growing glial neoplasms, which can arise anywhere along the walls of the cerebral ventricles or within the spinal canal. The group of ependymal tumors comprises classic ependymoma (plus variants), anaplastic ependymoma (malignant variant), and the benign variants, subependymoma and myxopapillary ependymoma.

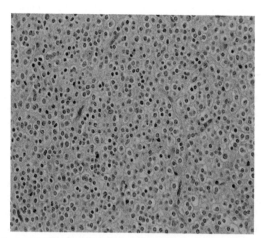

Fig. 2. Histologic features of an oligodendroglioma (WHO grade II). Tumor cell nuclei are round to oval and show typical cytoplasmic clearing (fried-egg appearance).

Ependymomas account for approximately 5% to 6% of all gliomas and for 2.5% of all primary intracranial neoplasms in adults.[1,2] In children younger than 14 years, these tumors play a significant role and form approximately 7% to 8% of all primary intracranial neoplasms, with an adjusted annual incidence rate of 5 to 6 per 1 million individuals. Overall, ependymomas are the third most common pediatric tumor after astrocytomas and medulloblastomas. Ependymomas can develop at any age; however, there are 2 distinct incidence peaks, the first one in children before the age of 14 years and the second one in adults between 35 and 45 years. These tumors can arise anywhere along the ventricular system within brain and spinal canal, but approximately 60% of lesions are located in the fourth ventricle, particularly in pediatric patients. In the spinal cord it is the most common type of glial neoplasm affecting adults. Male are in general slightly more affected than female.

Morphologically, classic ependymomas are composed of a monotonous population of cells, which tend to form characteristic rosette-like structures, so-called perivascular pseudorosettes, and ependymal rosettes that have been recognized as diagnostic hallmark features (**Fig. 3**). Recent studies suggest that they might arise from radial glial cells.[8]

The WHO classification separates ependymal tumors into 3 grades, wherein subependymoma and myxopapillary ependymoma correspond to WHO grade I, classic ependymoma and related variants (cellular, papillary, clear cell, and tanycytic ependymoma) correspond to WHO grade II, and anaplastic ependymomas are WHO grade III.

Anaplastic ependymomas are the malignant variant of classic ependymomas, characterized by high cell density, high mitotic activity, microvascular proliferation, and necrosis. Anaplastic ependymomas are associated with rapid disease progression and unfavorable outcome.

Myxopapillary ependymoma is a distinct type of low-grade ependymoma, which is almost exclusively located in the conus medullaris, cauda equina, and filum terminale. These lesions are circumscribed and composed of small cuboidal cells surrounding well-vascularized, acellular cores of connective tissue, which frequently undergo hyaline and mucoid degeneration, leading to a distinctive histologic appearance. Myxopapillary ependymomas are slow-growing tumors with an indolent clinical course and favorable outcome after surgical resection, thus the WHO assigned grade I.

Subependymomas are benign neoplasms, typically located within the ventricular wall and composed of clusters of uniform small tumor cells. These are embedded in a densely fibrillar glial matrix with microcystic degeneration. Subependymomas correspond to WHO grade I.

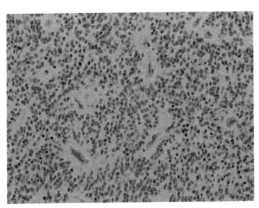

Fig. 3. Histologic appearance of a classic ependymoma (WHO grade II). Relative uniformity of tumor cells, which form perivascular pseudorosettes.

Embryonal Tumors

Embryonal tumors of the CNS are primitive neuroectodermal tumors (PNETs), which are composed of undifferentiated small cells with high nuclear-to-cytoplasmic ratio and a lack of distinctive architectural features (**Fig. 4**). This tumor group includes medulloblastoma (and variants), CNS PNETs, atypical teratoid/rhabdoid tumor, CNS neuroblastoma, CNS ganglioneuroblastoma, medulloepithelioma, and ependymo-blastoma.[1–3] The basis for grouping these lesions relates to their biologic tendency to differentiate into glial and neuronal lineages.

Medulloblastomas are the by far most common embryonal tumors, accounting for approximately 90%. They form the most frequent brain tumor in children aside from pilocytic astrocytomas, amounting to approximately 20% of pediatric brain tumors. The incidence rate in children is as high as 7 per 1 million compared with 1.8 per million in the general population. Most medulloblastomas present between the ages of 3 years and 10 years, and only approximately 20% occur in adolescence. There is a strong male predominance, especially in childhood. The majority of these tumors arise in the cerebellum, with predominant growth in the cerebellar vermis. Involvement of cerebellar hemispheres is more common in adolescence. Several vari-ants have been described by the 2007 WHO classification,[1–3] mainly based on morphologic criteria. These are the classic medulloblastoma, large cell/anaplastic medulloblastoma, nodular desmoplastic medulloblastoma, and medulloblastoma with extensive nodularity. The subclassification of medulloblastomas according to morphologic criteria is clinically important because histopathologic characteristics are used to stratify patients into low-risk and high-risk groups, which corresponds to clinical outcome studies. It was shown that patients with the nodular desmoplastic

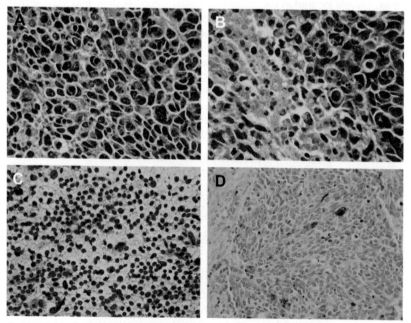

Fig. 4. Histologic features of medulloblastoma (WHO grade IV). (*A*) Highly pleomorphic tumor cells without pattern. (*B*) Foci of micronecrosis are intermixed. (*C*) Smear preparation demonstrating high degree of pleomorphism. (*D*) Synaptophysin staining with scant patchy positivity, typical of medulloblastoma.

variants have the best outcome, whereas those with large cell/anaplastic medulloblastomas have the worst outcome.[9–11] Recent approaches using advanced genomics, such as transcriptional profiling, however, might enhance the current standards of histologic subclassification through molecular subgrouping, to allow for improved drug target choices.[12]

Embryonal tumors outside the cerebellum, but with histologic features similar to medulloblastoma, have been termed *CNS PNET*. This heterogeneous group of non-cerebellar medulloblastoma-like lesions is largely united by the presence of poorly differentiated, immature small cells with a tendency to differentiate along glial, neuronal, and other lineages. Overall, CNS PNETs are uncommon and account for less than 1% of all primary brain tumors.[3] They are mainly found in a supratentorial location and less frequently in the spinal cord or suprasellar region. Tumors with predominantly neuronal differentiation are called *cerebral neuroblastoma*, or *ganglioneuroblastoma* if ganglion cells are present. Features of neural tube formation led to the term *medulloepithelioma*; tumors with ependymoblastic rosettes are labeled *ependymoblastomas*. This large group is in flux, however, and further subclassifications will depend on the integration of molecular data.

Atypical teratoid/rhabdoid tumors are highly aggressive lesions, which predominantly manifest in young children, with an estimated incidence of 1% to 2% of pediatric brain tumors.[13] Microscopically, they are characterized by the presence of rhabdoid cells and variable proportions of immature cells that show divergent differentiation along epithelial, mesenchymal, neuronal, and glial lineages.[3] These tumors were found associated with mutation or inactivation of the *INI1/hSNF5* gene at 22q11 in almost all cases.[14,15]

In general, the biologic behavior of embryonal tumors is highly aggressive with a tendency to recur and disseminate throughout the neuraxis. Thus, the WHO designated grade IV to all these lesions. A combination of chemotherapy and radiation in addition to surgical resection shows variable success and relative cure for only some cases.

SECTION II: MOLECULAR BIOLOGY AND PROGNOSTIC MARKERS

The past decade led to significant progress in the discovery and clinical implementation of molecular markers, which aid in the assessment and management of brain tumor patients. Molecular signatures of tumors play roles as diagnostic, prognostic, and predictive markers and influence the clinical decision making process. A dynamic classification of tumors is critical for the continuous integration of newly established molecular tools. This review focuses on various genetic and epigenetic changes that have been integrated into daily practice and gained significance for molecular diagnostic testing. These are 1p/19q deletions for oligodendrogliomas, O^6-methylguanine-DNA methyltransferase (MGMT) promoter hypermethylation, isocitrate dehydrogenase (IDH)-1 gene mutations, and epidermal growth factor receptor (EGFR) alterations.

Molecular Biology of Glial Neoplasms

As described previously, the WHO classification is the primary means for projecting tumor malignancy and prognosis of glial neoplasms, and histopathologic assessments have thus far been the gold standard. Accurate typing and grading of gliomas is challenging, however, because many diagnostic criteria leave room for subjectivity, and interobserver variability is considerable. Furthermore, glial neoplasms in the same histologic grade and with similar morphologic features often differ significantly in their clinical course and response to treatment, indicating that morphologic criteria alone are insufficient to predict clinical outcome. Thus, great effort is placed on identifying additional molecular genetic tools, which enhance current pathologic classification schemes and support greater prognostic and predictive accuracy.

Glial neoplasms develop as a result of genetic alterations that continuously accumulate with tumor progression. The past 10 to 15 years have led to significant progress in understanding of genetic alterations in various types and grades of malignancy of these lesions. To briefly summarize, more than 50% of WHO grade II diffuse astrocytomas harbor mutations of the tumor suppressor gene TP53 (located at 17p13.1) and show loss of heterozygosity on chromosome arm 17p in addition to gains on the long arm of chromosome 7. Oligodendroglial tumors, however, are remarkable for the combined loss of 1p and 19q. The recent discovery of mutations of the IDH1 gene in low-grade gliomas, in particular WHO grade II astrocytic, oligodendroglial, oligoastrocytic gliomas, and WHO grade III astrocytic tumors is pointing toward a potentially common initiating event within this diverse group of tumors. WHO grade III astrocytomas generally show further progression-related molecular changes, which involve, for example, chromosomal deletions (chr 6, 11p, and 22q), tumor suppressor gene alterations (CDKN2A, CDKN2B, and p14 ARF), gene amplifications (CDK4/CDK6), or inactivating mutations (RB1 gene). WHO grade IV glioblastomas overall demonstrate complex chromosomal and genetic alterations, which inactivate a variety of tumor suppressor genes and activate proto-oncogenes. Most glioblastomas present de novo (primary glioblastomas) in elderly patients and show a distinct pattern of genetic alterations, such as EGFR amplification and PTEN mutations, but not IDH1 mutations. This contrasts the less common secondary glioblastomas, which arise from pre-existing lower-grade gliomas[16] and harbor frequent mutations in the TP53 and IDH1 genes but lack EGFR amplification.[16–18] Despite these differences, the Cancer Genome Atlas Research Network[19] was able to demonstrate that the majority of genetic alterations in both primary and secondary glioblastomas can be attributed to a common set of functional pathways.

Prognostic Markers

Codeletion of 1p/19q

The combined deletion of 1p and 19q is the hallmark molecular signature of oligodendrogliomas. Mechanistically, this codeletion results from of an unbalanced centromeric translocation and leads to loss of entire chromosomal arms t(1;19)(q10;p10). The frequency of 1p/19q codeletions has been estimated at 80% to 90% in WHO grade II oligodendrogliomas and 50% to 70% in WHO grade III oligodendrogliomas.[4] In spite of a strong association between 1p/19q loss and classic oligodendroglioma morphology, morphology alone cannot predict the 1p/19q status.[20] The chromosomal regions of 1p and 19q have been mapped in great detail; however, no definitive candidates genes have been identified that could explain the tumorigenic effect. Although the genes on 1p/19q remain enigmatic, many correlations have been established demonstrating that many tumors with 1p/19q codeletions also show IDH1/IDH2 mutations[21]; however, 1p/19q loss seems to be absent in cases with tumor protein p53 (TP53) mutations or EGFR amplifications.[22] The combined loss of 1p/19q is also found in mixed glial tumors (oligoastrocytomas) but is rare in nonglial malignancies.[23]

Codeletions of 1p/19q in oligodendrogliomas were first described in 1994; a few years later, clinical observations made clear that a high proportion of oligodendrogliomas with 1p/19q loss demonstrated a favorable response to chemotherapeutic agents in addition to substantially improved survival times.[24,25] In contrast, patients with 1p/19q deleted tumors who undergo tumor resection alone without receiving any adjuvant chemotherapy or radiation do not show longer progression free survival,[26] suggesting that 1p/19q loss characterizes a group of tumors with greater sensitivity to genotoxic agents. These findings have been replicated many times over the past decade and extended to the use of chemotherapeutic drugs, such as temozolamide and radiation therapy.[27,28] Due to the well-accepted prognostic significance of 1p/19q loss in conjunction with adjuvant chemotherapy, many institutions have established molecular tests to detect this chromosomal aberration. The molecular mechanisms, however, that underlie the association between 1p/19q loss, chemosensitivity, and favorable prognosis remain to be elucidated.

Isocitrate dehydrogenase 1 mutations
Somatic mutations in the gene encoding human cytosolic NADPH-dependent IDH1, a citric acid cycle component, have been implicated in the tumor biology of gliomas. Recent genome-wide analyses identified mutations in codon 132 of the IDH1 gene,[29] an evolutionarily conserved residue that is located in the substrate-binding site of IDH1. Similar mutations were seen at lower frequency at corresponding codons of the IDH2 gene. Overall, it is, however, still largely unclear how these mutations contribute to oncogenesis. One hypothesis postulates that mutated IDH1 converts α-ketoglutarate to 2-hydroxyglutarate,[21] which invariably blocks a variety of enzymes, thereby contributing to tumor development.

Many studies established that IDH1 mutations are present at high frequency in secondary glioblastomas that originate from prior lower-grade gliomas (approximately 85%). In contrast, these mutations rarely occur in primary or de novo glioblastomas (<1%), which are found in the absence of lower-grade precursor lesion. IDH1 mutations were further identified in the majority of diffuse low-grade (WHO grade II) and anaplastic (WHO grade III) astrocytomas (approximately 70%–80%), oligodendrogliomas (80%), anaplastic oligodendrogliomas (85%), and mixed oligoastrocytomas (100%).[21] The IDH1 mutation frequency seems similar for WHO grade II and WHO grade III tumors. The mutation rate in pilocytic astrocytomas (WHO grade I), ependymal tumors, or other less-common glial tumors is low or absent.[30] It was further demonstrated that IDH1 mutations do not exist in reactive conditions related to cerebral ischemia or infarctions, viral infections, or radiation change.[31] These findings are of particular diagnostic value because they enable the distinction of reactive gliosis from low-grade diffuse astrocytoma, a diagnostically challenging task, especially in the context of small biopsy samples.

It is of clinical importance that IDH1 and IDH2 mutations were found associated with a favorable prognosis and overall prolonged survival time independent of treatment. The survival of patients with the mutant form of IDH1 in astrocytomas or oligodendrogliomas (WHO grade II-III) and glioblastoma is longer than that of their IDH1 wild-type counterparts. Patients with IDH1-mutated glioblastomas (WHO grade IV) show better survival than patients with wild-type anaplastic astrocytomas (WHO grade III).[26] The IDH status, however, does not predict treatment specific responses of patients with glioma.[32]

In 2010, an antibody was developed, which is able to specifically recognize the mutant IDH1-R132H protein, which represents the majority (90%) of IDH mutations in gliomas.[33] The widespread use of this antibody led to rapid accumulation of data and correlation with clinical outcome.[34] In daily clinical practice, the detection of IDH1 mutations might prove a significant component in the neuropathologic armamentarium, especially in the context of small and diagnostically challenging biopsy samples.

MGMT methylation status
The gene encoding O^6-methylguanine-DNA methyltransferase (MGMT) at 10q26 has become one of the most widely studied molecular markers in neurooncology. The

MGMT is a suicide DNA repair enzyme that protects cells against damage from ionizing radiation and alkylating agents.[35] Alkylating chemotherapeutic drugs, like temozolamide,[36] have been used for years in the treatment of patients with glioblastoma. Mechanistically, these drugs methylate the O^6 position of the DNA nucleotide guanine, which consequently triggers cell death. MGMT is constitutively expressed in cells and part of an inherent DNA repair mechanism that can counteract the effects of alkylating agents. It catalyzes DNA repair by transferring this methyl group from the O^6 position of the DNA nucleotide guanine to a cysteine residue of the MGMT protein, acting against the cytotoxic effects of chemotherapy.[35]

A significant proportion of glioblastomas have been found to express decreased levels of MGMT, which makes these tumors more susceptible to the effects of alkylating agents. The primary mechanism by which MGMT expression is downregulated is via methylation of the promoter of the MGMT gene, an epigenetic regulatory mechanism, which consequently leads to down-regulation of mRNA transcription and protein translation. As a consequence, glioblastoma cells with MGMT promoter (hyper) methylation respond better to temozolamide, because they lack the ability to efficiently repair the damage introduced by alkylation.

Many studies found an association between MGMT promoter hypermethylation and response of malignant gliomas to alkylating agents. In the European Organisation for Research and Treatment of Cancer/National Cancer Institute of Canada trial,[36] Hegi and colleagues found that patients with hypermethylated MGMT promoters who were treated with temozolamide and radiation showed significantly increased survival times compared with patients whose tumors were hypomethylated. When treated with radiation alone, there was no significant extension of survival times, emphasizing a predictive role for MGMT hypermethylation and a favorable response to chemotherapy. The MGMT promoter methylation status is at the moment viewed as one of the most significant predictors of clinical outcome and response to treatment with temozolamide.[37] Analyses by Gorlia and colleagues[38] go as far as to suggest a stratification of all patients according to MGMT status as soon as they are enrolled in glioblastoma trials that use alkylating agents. A retrospective analysis could show that MGMT promoter methylation patterns can change between initial tumor diagnosis and later recurrence, particularly in MGMT methylated cases.[39] This implies that MGMT methylation is only of prognostic value for the initial assessment and it is not predictive of outcome for recurrences.[39] Furthermore, MGMT promoter methylation seems frequent in low-grade and anaplastic gliomas (up to 90%),[40] which show 1p/19q codeletion. Treatment with temozolamide correlated positively with longer progression-free survival in those patients.[40] In the absence of alternative treatments, temozolamide is often applied as first-line agent, even without a methylated MGMT promoter, because these patients seem to benefit from this drug.

Role of EGFR Pathway Aberrations

Malignant glial neoplasms, in particular glioblastomas, have been found to upregulate several growth factors and their receptors. The EGFR gene at 7p12 has been described as the most frequently amplified and overexpressed gene in approximately 60% of glioblastomas and has been associated with shorter survival times.[41] Furthermore, approximately one-half of glioblastomas that overexpress wild-type EGFR also express EGFR mutant alleles, such as the EGFR variant III (EGFRvIII), which constitutes an 801-bp in-frame deletion of exons 2 to 7 and leads to a truncated receptor protein that lacks the ligand-binding domain.[42,43] This mutation ultimately leads to a constitutively activated EGFR-phosphoinositide 3-kinase pathway and seems to be unique to glial cells.[36]

The identification of EGFR amplifications and mutations, especially EGFRvIII, has been associated with poorer prognosis and in general is considered indicative of high-grade malignancy.[44] The prognostic value of this information is somewhat ambiguous, however, because several studies produced contradictory results. The EGFRvIII mutation, might be helpful in the identification of a subgroup of tumors with more malignant behavior than suggested by their histopathology alone.[45] Furthermore, gene expression profiling approaches for glioblastomas with EGFR amplifications enabled a subclassification of morphologically indistinguishable tumors based on their gene expression signatures.[46,47]

Although EGFR pathway aberrations represent attractive therapeutic targets for molecular inhibition, the clinical benefits thus far have been disappointing. Attempts to have an impact on tumor growth with the use of EGFR inhibitors, such as erlotinib and gefitinib, failed despite sufficient bioavailability and activity to dephosphorylate the EGFR in the tumor tissue.[48] The overall progression-free survival was not prolonged and only a subset of patients showed some response. Additional missense mutations have been identified in exons that encode extracellular EGFR domains, which seem to drive oncogenesis in vitro and potentially could convey sensitivity to small molecule tyrosine kinase inhibitors.[49]

In general, a network of complex and redundant signal transduction pathways that bridge cell surface–bound EGFRs with its oncogenic effects in the nucleus likely prevents simplistic therapeutic approaches from being successful. In addition, glioblastoma cells often show activation of multiple growth factor pathways, suggesting that a panel of targeting drugs might be necessary to interfere with tumor growth. At this stage, assessments of EGFR signaling pathways for glioblastomas is academically interesting but clinically not indicated due to a lack of standard drug regimens that specifically target these pathways.

REFERENCES

1. CBTRUS. CBTRUS Statistical Report: primary brain and central nervous system tumors diagnosed in the United States in 2004–2008. Hinsdale (IL): Central Brain Tumor Registry of the United States; 2012.
2. Kohler BA, Ward E, McCarthy BJ, et al. Annual report to the nation on the status of cancer, 1975-2007, featuring tumors of the brain and other nervous system. J Natl Cancer Inst 2011;103:714–36.
3. Louis DN, Ohgaki H, Wiestler OD, et al. The 2007 WHO classification of tumours of the central nervous system. Acta Neuropathol 2007;114:97–109.
4. WHO classification of tumors of the central nervous system. 3rd edition. Lyon (France): IARC Press; 2007.
5. Okamoto Y, Di Patre PL, Burkhard C, et al. Population-based study on incidence, survival rates, and genetic alterations of low-grade diffuse astrocytomas and oligodendrogliomas. Acta Neuropathol 2004;108:49–56.
6. Ohgaki H, Kleihues P. Population-based studies on incidence, survival rates, and genetic alterations in astrocytic and oligodendroglial gliomas. J Neuropathol Exp Neurol 2005;64:479–89.
7. Lebrun C, Fontaine D, Ramaioli A, et al. Long-term outcome of oligodendrogliomas. Neurology 2004;62:1783–7.
8. Taylor MD, Poppleton H, Fuller C, et al. Radial glia cells are candidate stem cells of ependymoma. Cancer Cell 2005;8:323–35.

9. Rutkowski S, von Hoff K, Emser A, et al. Survival and prognostic factors of early childhood medulloblastoma: an international meta-analysis. J Clin Oncol 2010; 28:4961–8.

10. Rutkowski S, Cohen B, Finlay J, et al. Medulloblastoma in young children. Pediatr Blood Cancer 2010;54:635–7.

11. Massimino M, Giangaspero F, Garrè ML, et al. Childhood medulloblastoma. Crit Rev Oncol Hematol 2011;79:65–83.

12. Taylor MD, Northcott PA, Korshunov A, et al. Molecular subgroups of medulloblastoma: the current consensus. Acta Neuropathol 2012;123:465–72.

13. Woehrer A, Slavc I, Waldhoer T, et al. Incidence of atypical teratoid/rhabdoid tumors in children: a population-based study by the Austrian Brain Tumor Registry, 1996-2006. Cancer 2010;116:5725–32.

14. Biegel JA, Zhou JY, Rorke LB, et al. Germ-line and acquired mutations of INI1 in atypical teratoid and rhabdoid tumors. Cancer Res 1999;59:74–9.

15. Versteege I, Sévenet N, Lange J, et al. Truncating mutations of hSNF5/INI1 in aggressive paediatric cancer. Nature 1998;394:203–6.

16. Ohgaki H, Kleihues P. Genetic pathways to primary and secondary glioblastoma. Am J Pathol 2007;170:1445–53.

17. Verhaak RG, Hoadley KA, Purdom E, et al. Integrated genomic analysis identifies clinically relevant subtypes of glioblastoma characterized by abnormalities in PDGFRA, IDH1, EGFR, and NF1. Cancer Cell 2010;17:98–110.

18. Toedt G, Barbus S, Wolter M, et al. Molecular signatures classify astrocytic gliomas by IDH1 mutation status. Int J Cancer 2011;128:1095–103.

19. Comprehensive genomic characterization defines human glioblastoma genes and core pathways. Nature 2008;455:1061–8.

20. Scheie D, Cvancarova M, Mørk S, et al. Can morphology predict 1p/19q loss in oligodendroglial tumours? Histopathology 2008;53:578–87.

21. Yan H, Parsons DW, Jin G, et al. IDH1 and IDH2 mutations in gliomas. N Engl J Med 2009;360:765–73.

22. Idbaih A, Marie Y, Lucchesi C, et al. BAC array CGH distinguishes mutually exclusive alterations that define clinicogenetic subtypes of gliomas. Int J Cancer 2008; 122:1778–86.

23. Aldape K, Burger PC, Perry A. Clinicopathologic aspects of 1p/19q loss and the diagnosis of oligodendroglioma. Arch Pathol Lab Med 2007;131:242–51.

24. Cairncross JG, Ueki K, Zlatescu MC, et al. Specific genetic predictors of chemotherapeutic response and survival in patients with anaplastic oligodendrogliomas. J Natl Cancer Inst 1998;90:1473–9.

25. Reifenberger J, Reifenberger G, Liu L, et al. Molecular genetic analysis of oligodendroglial tumors shows preferential allelic deletions on 19q and 1p. Am J Pathol 1994;145:1175–90.

26. Weller M, Felsberg J, Hartmann C, et al. Molecular predictors of progression-free and overall survival in patients with newly diagnosed glioblastoma: a prospective translational study of the German Glioma Network. J Clin Oncol 2009;27: 5743–50.

27. Kouwenhoven MC, Kros JM, French PJ, et al. 1p/19q loss within oligodendroglioma is predictive for response to first line temozolomide but not to salvage treatment. Eur J Cancer 2006;42:2499–503.

28. Brandes AA, Tosoni A, Cavallo G, et al. Correlations between O6-methylguanine DNA methyltransferase promoter methylation status, 1p and 19q deletions, and response to temozolomide in anaplastic and recurrent oligodendroglioma: a prospective GICNO study. J Clin Oncol 2006;24:4746–53.

29. Parsons DW, Li M, Zhang X, et al. The genetic landscape of the childhood cancer medulloblastoma. Science 2011;331:435–9.
30. Watanabe T, Nobusawa S, Kleihues P, et al. IDH1 mutations are early events in the development of astrocytomas and oligodendrogliomas. Am J Pathol 2009; 174:1149–53.
31. Horbinski C, Kofler J, Kelly LM, et al. Diagnostic use of IDH1/2 mutation analysis in routine clinical testing of formalin-fixed, paraffin-embedded glioma tissues. J Neuropathol Exp Neurol 2009;68:1319–25.
32. van den Bent MJ, Dubbink HJ, Marie Y, et al. IDH1 and IDH2 mutations are prognostic but not predictive for outcome in anaplastic oligodendroglial tumors: a report of the European Organization for Research and Treatment of Cancer Brain Tumor Group. Clin Cancer Res 2010;16:1597–604.
33. Camelo-Piragua S, Jansen M, Ganguly A, et al. Mutant IDH1-specific immunohistochemistry distinguishes diffuse astrocytoma from astrocytosis. Acta Neuropathol 2010;119:509–11.
34. Horbinski C, Kofler J, Yeaney G, et al. Isocitrate dehydrogenase 1 analysis differentiates gangliogliomas from infiltrative gliomas. Brain Pathol 2011;21:564–74.
35. Esteller M, Garcia-Foncillas J, Andion E, et al. Inactivation of the DNA-repair gene MGMT and the clinical response of gliomas to alkylating agents. N Engl J Med 2000;343:1350–4.
36. Hegi ME, Diserens AC, Gorlia T, et al. MGMT gene silencing and benefit from temozolomide in glioblastoma. N Engl J Med 2005;352:997–1003.
37. Stupp R, Hegi ME, Mason WP, et al. Effects of radiotherapy with concomitant and adjuvant temozolomide versus radiotherapy alone on survival in glioblastoma in a randomised phase III study: 5-year analysis of the EORTC-NCIC trial. Lancet Oncol 2009;10:459–66.
38. Gorlia T, van den Bent MJ, Hegi ME, et al. Nomograms for predicting survival of patients with newly diagnosed glioblastoma: prognostic factor analysis of EORTC and NCIC trial 26981-22981/CE.3. Lancet Oncol 2008;9:29–38.
39. Brandes AA, Franceschi E, Tosoni A, et al. O(6)-methylguanine DNA-methyltransferase methylation status can change between first surgery for newly diagnosed glioblastoma and second surgery for recurrence: clinical implications. Neuro Oncol 2010;12:283–8.
40. Everhard S, Kaloshi G, Crinière E, et al. MGMT methylation: a marker of response to temozolomide in low-grade gliomas. Ann Neurol 2006;60:740–3.
41. Yip S, Iafrate AJ, Louis DN. Molecular diagnostic testing in malignant gliomas: a practical update on predictive markers. J Neuropathol Exp Neurol 2008;67:1–15.
42. Sugawa N, Ekstrand AJ, James CD, Collins VP. Identical splicing of aberrant epidermal growth factor receptor transcripts from amplified rearranged genes in human glioblastomas. Proc Natl Acad Sci U S A 1990;87:8602–6.
43. Jeuken J, Sijben A, Alenda C, et al. Robust detection of EGFR copy number changes and EGFR variant III: technical aspects and relevance for glioma diagnostics. Brain Pathol 2009;19:661–71.
44. Shinojima N, Tada K, Shiraishi S, et al. Prognostic value of epidermal growth factor receptor in patients with glioblastoma multiforme. Cancer Res 2003;63: 6962–70.
45. Pelloski CE, Ballman KV, Furth AF, et al. Epidermal growth factor receptor variant III status defines clinically distinct subtypes of glioblastoma. J Clin Oncol 2007; 25:2288–94.
46. Parsons DW, Jones S, Zhang X, et al. An integrated genomic analysis of human glioblastoma multiforme. Science 2008;321:1807–12.

47. Shai R, Shi T, Kremen TJ, et al. Gene expression profiling identifies molecular subtypes of gliomas. Oncogene 2003;22:4918–23.
48. Preusser M, Gelpi E, Rottenfusser A, et al. Epithelial growth factor receptor inhibitors for treatment of recurrent or progressive high grade glioma: an exploratory study. J Neurooncol 2008;89:211–8.
49. Lee JC, Vivanco I, Beroukhim R, et al. Epidermal growth factor receptor activation in glioblastoma through novel missense mutations in the extracellular domain. PLoS Med 2006;3:e485.

Clinical Manifestations and Diagnostic Imaging of Brain Tumors

Bart P. Keogh, MD, PhD[a,b],*, John W. Henson, MD[c]

KEYWORDS

- Brain tumors • Diagnosis • Imaging • Clinical manifestations

KEY POINTS

- The initial diagnosis of intracranial tumors is most reliably and efficiently made by imaging.
- Diffusion-weighted imaging and diffusion tensor imaging can be best understood as special cases of diffusion imaging.
- The implementation of perfusion (DSC) and T1 dynamic imaging (DCE) requires careful consideration of technical aspects, both in image acquisition and post-processing.
- Distinguishing between early recurrence/pseudoprogression, recurrent tumor/delayed treatment effect, and true response/pseudoresponse has become increasingly complex because of the effects of antiangiogenic therapy on conventional (in particular) postcontrast imaging

INTRODUCTION

The clinical manifestations of intracranial tumors are myriad and most often referable to the anatomic area of the brain involved or adjacent structures. Some anatomic regions, particularly right frontal, may allow a tumor to reach substantial size while remaining clinically silent. In contrast, small lesions in critical areas (eg, cerebral aqueduct or primary motor cortex) are more likely to present early.

The initial diagnosis of intracranial tumors is most reliably and efficiently made by imaging. Particularly in the acute setting, noncontrast computed tomography (CT) is often the first imaging modality used. In virtually all instances, the identification of an abnormality on noncontrast CT (or in the setting of persistent clinical symptoms) is followed by magnetic resonance imaging (MRI) before and after contrast administration (usually a gadolinium chelate). The use of contrast-enhanced CT scan is, in many centers, restricted to those patients who cannot safely be placed in the magnet.

[a] Swedish Neuroscience Institute, Swedish Medical Center, 550 17th Avenue, Suite 500, Seattle, WA 98122, USA; [b] Neuroradiology Section, Radia Inc., PS, 728 134th Street, SW # 120, Everett, WA 98204, USA; [c] Ben and Catherine Ivy Foundation, Swedish Neuroscience Institute, Swedish Medical Center, 550 17th Avenue, Suite 500, Seattle, WA 98122, USA
* Corresponding author. MRI Suite, 1600 East Jefferson Street, Seattle, WA 98122.
E-mail address: Bart.Keogh@swedish.org

Hematol Oncol Clin N Am 26 (2012) 733–755
doi:10.1016/j.hoc.2012.05.002
0889-8588/12/$ – see front matter © 2012 Published by Elsevier Inc.

hemonc.theclinics.com

The value of MRI in defining the preoperative diagnosis, precise anatomic localization for operative planning, detection of response to therapy, discernment of tumor progression, and recognition of treatment-related side effect is based on both the high spatial resolution (<1 mm^3) and the large range of tissue characteristics that may be measured.[1]

This article discusses both the clinicoanatomic features and imaging characteristics of brain tumors, including the use of dynamic susceptibility-weighted, T1 dynamic, diffusion, functional, and diffusion tensor imaging.

IMAGING TECHNIQUES

Because imaging is central to the diagnosis and management of intracranial tumors, this article summarizes the predominant imaging techniques used.

CT

The first CT scanner available for patient care was released in 1974 and is largely credited to the work of Ambrose and Hounsfield[2] and Cormack.[3] CT takes advantage of differences in electron density between tissues to produce contrast. Current clinical CT scanners are capable of submillimeter in-plane resolution at acquisition times on the order of 90 seconds for noncontrast brain studies.

The rapidity and ease of CT imaging has fueled the growth in use.[4] The sensitivity and specificity of CT in comparison with MRI varies with specific disease process, but, in general is understood to provide considerably less information than MRI in the setting of infection,[5] tumor,[6] and across a spectrum of neurologic disorders.[7]

MRI

MRI evolved from nuclear magnetic resonance spectroscopy (NMR), for which Bloch and Purcell were awarded the Nobel Prize in 1952 for "their development of new methods for nuclear magnetic precision measurements and discoveries in connection therewith." The first paper describing the use of these physical properties for imaging was by Lauterbur in 1973.[8]

In brief, clinical MRI produces images in which the pixel intensity is proportional to proton density and influenced by the local magnetic environment. Although a comprehensive discussion of the various pulse sequences that allow image acquisition is beyond the scope of this article, the essentials necessary to understand the biologic substrate being measured by each technique are discussed.

Anatomic Imaging

Anatomic imaging by MRI can be most simply understood in terms of the predominant image contrast, which may originate from spin-lattice (T1) relaxation, spin-spin (T2) relaxation, or susceptibility (T2*). In general, T1-weighted images provide high anatomic resolution and, with contrast administration, an assessment of blood-brain barrier integrity (also called enhancement). T2 imaging is most useful for identifying fluid and edema. T2* is most widely used for identifying blood and the detection of variations in local magnetic environment. This characteristic makes T2* sequences useful for blood flow imaging (ie, functional and perfusion MRI, discussed later).

In addition to preoperative evaluation, MRI has been introduced into operating suites to permit real-time imaging during operation.[9] Studies have shown improvement in extent of tumor resection with the use of intraoperative MRI,[10] but lengthened survival has not been shown. Improving the extent of resection in patients with low-grade gliomas may provide the strongest rationale for intraoperative MRI,[9] with the usefulness in high-grade lesions not clearly shown.[11]

Spectroscopy

Proton magnetic resonance spectroscopy (1H-MRS) is used to quantify metabolites (choline [Chol], creatine [Cr], lactate [Lac] and N-acetyl aspartate [NAA] are the most widely interpreted) within tumor and adjacent tissue. The levels of these metabolites (and their ratios) provides information about the underlying metabolic state.

Choline signal is most often compared with Cr as an internal control, a ratio of greater than 3:1 is consistent with a neoplastic process. Increase of the choline signal is thought to be a consequence of increased synthesis and turnover of membrane phospholipids, and correlates with cell density in gliomas.[12] Anaplastic astrocytomas often give higher choline concentrations than does glioblastoma multiforme (GBM), likely because of the presence of necrotic tissue in the latter. **Fig. 1** shows an example of increased Cho/Cr and Cho/NAA ratios in this high-grade glioma.

Functional MRI

Functional MRI (fMRI) takes advantage of small variations in T2*-weighted imaging signal, as result of neuronal activity, to identify areas of the brain associated with specific tasks (eg, motor and language). The underlying physical substrate measured is predominantly the changing ratio of oxyhemoglobin/deoxyhemoglobin caused by neurovascular coupling. Measured signal variation is compared with the known functional paradigm producing a statistical map of areas most closely associated (by signal variation) with the task. The resultant images may be imported into the surgical navigation system for intraoperative use.

The relationship between fMRI, intraoperative mapping, and Wada testing has been studied extensively. Both Wada and intraoperative cortical stimulation identify those

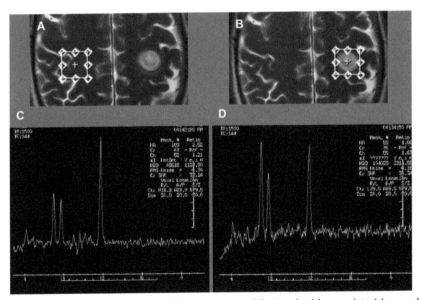

Fig. 1. High-grade glioma. Control (*A*) versus tumor (*B*). Voxel with associated long echo time spectra (*C* and *D*), shows increased Cho/NAA and Cho/Cr in this high-grade glioma.

areas where inhibition (either electrical or pharmaceutical) blocks the behavior being mapped. fMRI is different in that it identifies areas associated with performance of the action, rather than abrogating it. fMRI depends on the nature of the paradigm(s) used,[13] field strength,[14] patient attention, and decisions made at the time of interpretation with respect to what level of statistical significance is judged correct.

Despite fundamental differences between fMRI and more invasive approaches, outcomes based on fMRI language lateralization after anterior temporal lobe surgery in patients with epilepsy have been reported as superior to Wada testing[15] and have a high concordance with Wada.[16] fMRI has also been reported to accurately localize primary motor cortex.[17–19] Both expressive and receptive language may be mapped **(Fig. 2)**.

Dynamic Susceptibility-Weighted MRI

Dynamic susceptibility contrast (DSC) imaging is also often referred to as perfusion imaging and has been widely used in stroke care. DSC involves the rapid acquisition of sequential images at a given location(s) as the contrast bolus moves through the brain: the first pass. From the first pass curve, several physical quantities may be derived, including cerebral blood volume (CBV), cerebral blood flow (CBF), and mean transit time (MTT).

The application of DSC to tumor imaging is a more complex undertaking than its use in stroke, which is generally well implemented by any time derivative (eg, MTT[20]). Of the metrics derived from DSC, CBV has proved to be the most useful in evaluating tumors and treatment effect. The histopathologic substrate reflected in CBV seems to be microvascular density.[21] CBV values are most often normalized to contralateral tissue (nCBV); in many cases, normal white matter is used.

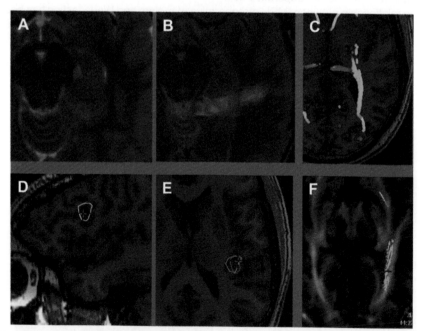

Fig. 2. Left temporal ganglioma (*A*) after resection (*B*) with preoperative fiber tracking for the optic radiations (*C* and *F*) and preoperative expressive (*D*) and receptive language (*E*) localization using fMRI.

Essential considerations in the application of DSC in tumor imaging include leakage correction (mathematical or by contrast preload),[22] arterial deconvolution (vs simpler mathematical techniques), choice of pharmacokinetic model,[23,24] the time course and dosing used for preload,[25] and consistent choice of the index tissue for normalization.

Application of DSC to tumor imaging has been shown to be accurate in distinguishing low-grade from high-grade tumors,[21,26–28] with CBV as the most useful metric. In both histologically low-grade and high-grade tumors, nCBV seems to provide additional stratification, identifying both low-grade and high-grade tumors that behave more aggressively.[23,29,30] Low-grade oligodendrogliomas may have increased rCBV without the same implications of aggressive behavior caused by the increased capillary density in all grades of this histopathologic subset.[26]

DSC may also aid in distinguishing high-grade glioma from metastatic disease. High-grade glioma tends to infiltrate the adjacent white matter, increasing the nCBV value, whereas, in metastatic disease, the adjacent edema is bland (**Figs. 3 and 4**).

Dynamic Contrast-Enhanced MRI

Although DSC uses T2*-weighted imaging sequences to indirectly measure capillary density and size, dynamic contrast-enhanced (DCE) imaging measures the rate of T1 signal change with contrast enhancement to approximate capillary permeability and related parameters. CBV may also be measured using DCE techniques.[31]

As with DSC, several metrics may be derived from DCE images, notably extracellular volume (V_e) and permeability (K_{trans}). Both K_{trans} and V_e are good predictors of tumor grade,[32–34] with correct classification of 92% or more of tumor using discriminant analysis. That DCE imaging is T1 weighted, rather than T2* weighted, has technical benefits compared with DSC imaging: there is less artifact associated with hemorrhage. Our current standard of practice is to perform both: the DCE first (this also preloads contrast), followed by DSC.

Diffusion-Weighted Imaging and Diffusion Tensor Imaging

Diffusion-weighted imaging (DWI) and diffusion tensor imaging (DTI) can be best understood as special cases of diffusion imaging (DI). In brief, DI takes advantage of variation in signal intensity after the application magnetic gradient fields vectors, identical in direction but opposite in magnitude. Using this kind of approach, images based on the diffusibility of water may be produced. In the brain, the major limitation to water motion is cell membranes, so DI provides a measure of cell intactness and density; this limited application of DI is usually referred to as DWI and has broad application, particularly in

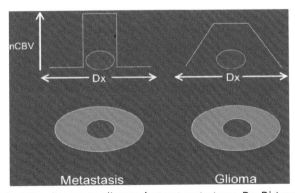

Fig. 3. Increase in CBV adjacent to gliomas, but not metastases. Dx, Distance.

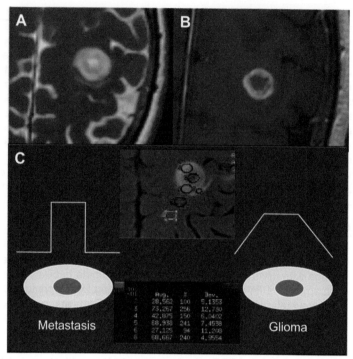

Fig. 4. High grade glioma in the left precentral gyrus (*A* and *B*) shows elevated nCBV in the adjacent vasogenic edema (*C*). Metastasis tend to have low nCBV values in adjacent edema (*C*).

stroke.[35] When many directions are used, white matter (ie, neuronal axonal membranes) tracts may be identified because of their effect on water motion (DTI).

In oncologic applications, DWI is of particular value in identifying lymphoma,[36] which tends to be densely packed, allowing differentiation from adjacent tissue. DWI may also be used for grading of gliomas[37] and abscess.[38,39]

Because of greater fine-structure definition, DTI may be of value in differentiating primary and metastatic tumors.[40,41] A lower rate of diffusion and more isotropic movement are seen in the white matter surrounding primary tumors, presumably because of the presence of infiltrating tumor, compared with the diffusion features of vasogenic edema surrounding a brain metastasis.[42] In densely cellular tumors, there is restriction in the diffusion of water, whereas areas of necrosis or less densely cellular tumor have increased levels of diffusion. Some data also suggest[43] that DTI metrics (planar anisotropy, in particular) may predict tumor aggressiveness, presumably because of the degree of adjacent white matter infiltration.

In preoperative planning, DTI can provide maps of white matter fiber tracts (tractography) in brain adjacent to tumors.[44] By elucidating the anatomic relationship of motor and sensory pathway to tumor tissue, DTI has been reported to reduce surgical morbidity.[45,46] **Fig. 2** shows an example in which a posterior mesial temporal tumor is defined relative to the optic radiations.

GLIAL PRIMARY TUMORS
Low-Grade Diffuse Fibrillary Astrocytomas (World Health Organization Grade II)

The average age at diagnosis of a low-grade astrocytoma is 34 years, although the range of ages is wide.[47] Astrocytomas of low-grade histopathology become progressively less common with increasing age, such that, by age 45 years, a nonenhancing mass lesion is more likely to be high grade than low grade.[48] There is an inverse correlation between increasing age at diagnosis and the time to progression from low to high grade.[49]

Low-grade diffuse fibrillary astrocytomas (LGA; World Health Organization [WHO] grade II) show moderate increase in cell density, which is seen as an expansile region of hyperintense T2-weighted (T2W) signal. There is little, if any, vasogenic edema or enhancement. The presence of enhancement within the mass suggests the presence of high-grade histology. However, the absence of gadolinium enhancement is not reliable evidence of low-grade histology, because one-third of nonenhancing lesions have anaplastic histology at biopsy.[48] Cysts seen on imaging often correlate with the presence of gemistocytes, which is a cell type that implies a tendency to aggressive behavior.

Calcification may be seen, but is less common than with oligodendroglioma. Magnetic resonance spectroscopy (MRS) shows a normal or mildly increased choline/creatine ratio and mildly decreased NAA. There is no evidence of restricted diffusion, and relative cerebral blood volume (rCBV) maps do not show increased CBV. These imaging findings reflect the histopathologic findings of mildly increased cellularity and infiltration of tumor cells into surrounding brain without significant vascular endothelial proliferation, mitotic activity, or necrosis.[50]

An approach based on multiparametric, discriminant analysis using values derived from both DCE and DSC (nCBV, K_{trans}, and V_e) has shown great accuracy in differentiating low-grade from high-grade lesions, correctly classifying 89% of high-grade and 100% of low-grade tumors in a sample of 76 patients.[32]

Patients with low-grade gliomas usually undergo maximal possible tumor resection but then do not receive adjuvant treatment with irradiation or chemotherapy unless there are tumor-related symptoms that limit quality of life (eg, intractable seizures) or there is evidence of rapid tumor growth. Thus, the rationale behind serial imaging surveillance in these patients is the early detection of tumor progression.

Low-grade gliomas often show progression as gradual enlargement of the region of nonenhancing hyperintense T2W signal surrounding the resection cavity. Mandonnet and colleagues[51] found that, in untreated low-grade oligodendrogliomas, there is approximately a 4-mm annual increase in cross-sectional diameter of the tumor. Thus, it is of great importance to compare each new MRI study with prior studies from as long a period as possible to detect the presence of gradual interval growth, which could escape detection if comparison is limited to the most recent prior examination.

Patients with low-grade gliomas may receive treatment when their tumors show growth or when there are symptoms, such as poorly controlled seizures, that might benefit from therapy. Treatment may consist of involved field irradiation or chemotherapy without irradiation. In these patients, response of the tumor may consist of shrinkage of the lesion or stabilization of size, with or without decrease in target symptoms (eg, decrease in seizure frequency). Clinical experience indicates that stabilization is the most common form of response. When shrinkage does occur, it is usually minor in degree and is often apparent only after 1 year or more following initiation of therapy; this is true for both LGA and low-grade oligodendrogliomas and compares with the more rapid responses seen in anaplastic oligodendrogliomas with a loss of the heterozygosity of the short arm of chromosome 1, in which best response is often seen after only 3 months of therapy.

Low-grade adult gliomas have a well-known tendency to become more histologically anaplastic and clinically aggressive over time, evolving toward GBM.[52–54] This evolution is called anaplastic progression and results from a stepwise accumulation of molecular genetic alterations within tumor cells. Although the numbers are difficult to determine, approximately 50% of LGA undergo radiographically detectable anaplastic progression, with the remainder of LGA showing gradual growth as low-grade lesions.[54]

GBM arising within a known LGA is termed secondary GBM. In contrast, patients whose GBM are diagnosed after a short interval of symptoms and in whom there is no known prior LGA are said to have de novo, or primary, GBM. There are several important distinctions between these 2 types of GBM. De novo tumors typically arise in older adults, and overexpress epidermal growth factor receptor (EGFR) without alterations in TP53. Patients with secondary GBM tend to be younger at the time of diagnosis, inactivate TP53, and do not overexpress EGFR.

In the case of anaplastic progression within low-grade gliomas, a new focus of rapidly growing, contrast-enhancing tumor appears within an existing, nonenhancing mass. The interval from initial diagnosis to anaplastic progression is strongly age dependent.[49] These patients are treated aggressively with irradiation and chemotherapy at the time progression is recognized. The imaging considerations regarding treatment responses in these patients are the same as those described later for high-grade gliomas.

A small group of patients are found to have incidental low-grade gliomas during imaging for some unrelated reason. Shah and colleagues[55] conducted a retrospective review of the available literature, finding no clear evidence for improved outcome with surgical treatment versus serial observation.

Anaplastic Astrocytoma and GBM

High-grade gliomas represent approximately 15% to 20% of all primary intracranial tumors.[56] Anaplastic astrocytoma (AA) and GBM (see **Fig. 1**) constitute high-grade diffuse fibrillary astrocytomas, and are characterized by high cell density, mitotic figures, and vascular endothelial proliferation. Necrosis is a defining feature of GBM. Multifocality is seen in one-third of cases.[57]

Compared with LGA, there is more mass effect, and areas of hemorrhage may produce heterogeneous signal on T1-weighted (T1W) and T2W imaging. Dense cellularity may produce relative hypointensity on T2W images as well as restricted diffusion. Enhancement with gadolinium may be homogeneous or heterogeneous. Irregular peripheral enhancement implies the presence of necrosis, and thus suggests GBM. Smooth linear enhancement around a centrally hypointense area can be seen with cysts in the absence of necrosis. A combination of vasogenic edema and infiltrating tumor cells usually produces extensive surrounding areas of hyperintense T2W signal within the white matter surrounding the enhancing portion of the tumor.[58,59] High-grade gliomas occasionally do not show enhancement after administration of gadolinium. The peak age incidence is 41 years for AA and 53 years for GBM.[47]

It is often the standard of care to image patients (including postcontrast sequences) after tumor resection to assess for the completeness of resection. The value of this practice in predicting progression-free survival has been shown by several groups[60–62] showing a direct correlation between extent of resection as determined by postoperative MRI and time to progression.

Patients who are diagnosed with high-grade gliomas (ie, WHO grade III and IV) are usually treated in the postoperative setting with a combination of involved field irradiation and concurrent temozolomide.[63] This has been associated with an increased risk of early treatment-related injury, referred to as pseudoprogression[64–66] (PP; discussed later). Increasingly, anaplastic oligodendrogliomas with loss of 1p are treated initially with chemotherapy alone, reserving irradiation until there is evidence of tumor progression.

In terms of response, high-grade tumors may show shrinkage, stability, or progression during these treatments. Shrinkage is common only with anaplastic oligodendrogliomas that have a deletion of 1p, and then best response is often seen within 3 months of initiation of therapy. Shrinkage may occur in the size of nodular enhancing disease and in the area of hyperintense T2W signal. Tumor cysts often do not change in size even when the surrounding tumor is shrinking. It has been reported that the change in CBV from baseline may predict high-grade glioma response to conventional therapy.[67]

Stability in the size of the tumor is a more common outcome with treatment, especially with astrocytomas. This fact has lead to the use of progression-free survival, or the duration of stable disease, as a common end point in clinical trials for high-grade gliomas.

Most high-grade gliomas show progressive enlargement within months of diagnosis. Progression most often is declared when there is enlargement of 1 or more enhancing nodules within the tumor, or appearance of a new nodular area of enhancement either locally at the tumor margin or distantly elsewhere in the brain. Increases in size of a tumor cyst and the appearance of hemorrhage when there is stability of the remainder of the lesion does not qualify as tumor progression.

Low-Grade Oligodendroglioma

Low-grade oligodendroglioma (LGO; **Fig. 5**) is a tumor of low to moderate cell density that usually has more well-defined margins with adjacent normal brain than do astrocytomas. There is abundant proliferation of capillaries, and absence of necrosis. These tumors show prominent involvement of cortex in addition to white matter, they often show microscopic spread into the subarachnoid space, and frequently calcify. The frontal and temporal lobes are the most common location.

These tumors are T1W hypointense, T2W hyperintense mass lesions that usually have well-defined margins, and expand cortex prominently.[68] Calcification may be seen as hyperdense foci on CT and variable signal intensity on MRI. Areas of contrast enhancement result from abnormal blood-brain barrier formation within tumor capillaries and is not as strong an indicator of a high grade as this finding is with astrocytomas. Cyst formation may occur. These tumors may show gradual enlargement over

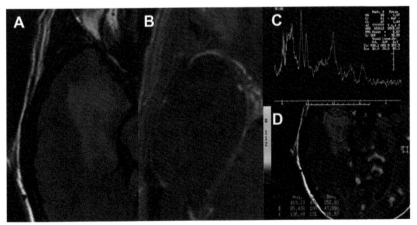

Fig. 5. LGO showing increase in T2 signal (A) but absent enhancement (B) with increase in Cho (C) and nCBV of 4.9 (D).

several years and, for this reason, it is important to compare each new examination with a baseline study from initial diagnosis, in addition to the most recent prior study. These tumors often have higher nCBV than would be expected.[26]

Treatment of LGOs remains incompletely determined, but the available data suggest that there does not seem to be an overall survival benefit to postoperative radiotherapy after surgical intervention (although there is decrease in progression-free survival[69]). Surgical intervention does seem to improve survival and quality of life.[70,71]

Anaplastic oligodendrogliomas

Anaplastic oligodendrogliomas (AOs) usually have more contrast enhancement than LGO and may have areas of necrosis. The frontal and temporal lobes are common locations.[72] The mass lesion is seen as a T1W hypointense, T2W hyperintense lesion that may be well circumscribed, and typically expands cortex in addition to involvement of white matter. Cystic areas and calcification are common.

Extensive infiltration, absence of a prominent pattern of ring-enhancement, and frontal and temporal lobe location are imaging findings that correlate with the loss of 1p or combined loss of 1p and 19q.[73]

AOs are unique among the gliomas, because they exhibit marked shrinkage in size during chemotherapy in 75% of cases with a sensitivity to nitrosourea-based chemotherapy.[74] Tumors that show this prominent response to chemotherapy have deletion of the short arm of chromosome or codeletion of the short arm of chromosome 1 and long arm of the chromosome 19.[75] These tumors can also show a benign natural history, compared with AAs and those anaplastic oligodendrogliomas that have maintained heterozygosity of 1p and 19q.

Ganglioglioma

Large dysplastic neurons and neoplastic astrocytic cells are present in gangliogliomas. The tumor is designated anaplastic ganglioglioma when the glial component seems to have more aggressive features. Tumors with predominantly neuronal features are called gangliocytomas. Cystic changes (see **Fig. 2**) and calcification are common. The tumors may be diagnosed in childhood or adulthood. Although they can be found in any intra-axial location, the most common location is in the temporal lobes.[47] These lesions are solid or cystic on imaging and often show nodular areas of contrast enhancement.[76] Calcification may be seen on CT.

Brainstem Glioma

There are 3 main types of brainstem gliomas of childhood. Diffuse pontine astrocytomas are the most common and have the poorest prognosis. They show diffuse enlargement of the pons, indistinct margins, and no enhancement, cystic change, or calcification. Astrocytomas of the cervicomedullary junction are less common, and are seen as nonenhancing, well-circumscribed lesions, often with an exophytic component. These tumors are less aggressive than the pontine type. Tectal astrocytomas are the rarest of the 3, and are nonenhancing lesions enlarging the tectal plate, often expanding into the supracerebellar cistern. Hydrocephalus may occur and is usually the cause of the patient's symptoms. This tumor is the least aggressive type of brainstem glioma.[47]

Brainstem gliomas in adults are characterized as low-grade diffuse lesions, and high-grade lesions.[77] The former present in young adults, are usually in the pons or medulla, and show no enhancement. High-grade lesions occur throughout the brainstem in older patients, and show contrast enhancement. Patients with the latter type have a poor prognosis.

Juvenile Cerebellar Pilocytic Astrocytoma

Juvenile cerebellar pilocytic astrocytoma (JPA) arises as a well-circumscribed cystic mass lesion with a mural nodule within the posterior fossa in children. These tumors do not show aggressive growth or brain invasion and complete surgical resection is often curative.[47] The lesions are well demarcated, hypointense on T1W images, and hyperintense on T2W images.[68] The cystic component may follow cerebrospinal fluid (CSF) signal or show evidence of increased protein with signal differing from CSF. A nodule or mass lesion showing dense, homogenous enhancement is almost always present Occasional tumors are solid without a cystic component. Hemorrhage and calcification may be seen, but are not common. Despite robust enhancement, these tumors[78] usually have low nCBV values (pilocytic astrocytoma, nCBV, **Fig. 6**).

NONGLIAL PRIMARY TUMORS
Primary Central Nervous System Lymphoma

Primary central nervous system lymphomas (PCNSL) are non-Hodgkin B-cell lymphomas that arise in the brain and eye (intraocular lymphoma). PCNSL has become more common in the past decades, at least in part because of an increase in cases in immunocompetent patients of older age. Peak age incidence is in the sixth and seventh decades. Synchronous systemic (ie, extra-central nervous system [CNS]) sites of disease are uncommon and suggest CNS metastasis rather than a primary neoplasm. The tumor arises as a mass of densely packed neoplastic lymphocytes without necrosis. Deep cerebral and periventricular structures are favored, and the lesions are multifocal in 25% of cases.[47]

Because of high cell density, these masses are often hyperdense on CT and hypo-intense on T2W images, and show restricted diffusion; moreover, they show dense homogeneous enhancement with gadolinium, and have extensive surrounding vaso-genic edema.[79] Choline is a prominent characteristic on MRS, with markedly diminished apparent diffusion coefficient (ADC) in lymphomatous tissue (**Fig. 7**).

Marked shrinkage of PCNSL lesions may occur within 1 to 2 days after administration of glucocorticoids such as dexamethasone. Glucocorticoids are sometimes initiated on an urgent basis because of concern about the presence of significant vasogenic edema, and therefore the radiological picture of a rapidly disappearing brain mass in this setting is consistent with a diagnosis of PCNSL. Biopsy in this situation is usually nondiagnostic, showing mainly inflammatory cells and cellular debris. Once glucocorticoids are discontinued, the tumor typically regrows rapidly over

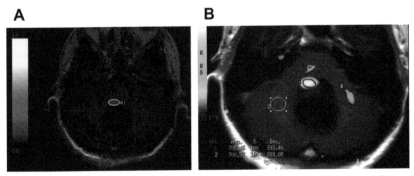

A **B**

Fig. 6. Pilocytic astrocytoma, showing peripheral enhancing nodule with increased K$_{trans}$ (*A*) but low nCBV (*B*).

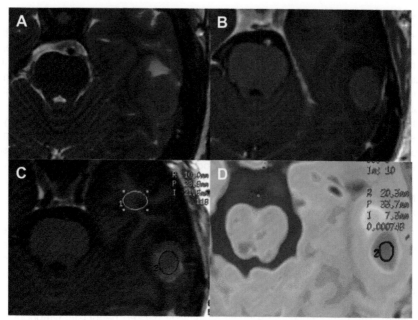

Fig. 7. Chloroma (myeloid sarcoma), showing intermediate T2 signal (*A*), enhancement (*B*), with nCBV measuring 0.8 relative to white matter (*C*, regions of interest 1 and 2) and diminished apparent diffusion coefficient (*D*, region of interest 2).

a period of several weeks. Glucocorticoids can usually be delayed, with or without the assistance of mannitol, until immediately following an urgent, diagnostic brain biopsy, and thus when PCNSL is suspected on neuroimaging grounds, withholding glucocorticoids can expedite early diagnosis and appropriate therapy.

PCNSL is also unique among brain tumors in that a complete response, as detected by resolution of contrast-enhancing tumor on MRI, is seen in one-half of cases with treatment. Because leptomeningeal dissemination is common, gadolinium-enhanced imaging of the spine is required. The ocular component requires a slit-lamp examination, because it cannot be seen with imaging.

Meningioma

Meningiomas arise along the leptomeninges, and therefore may occur at any point along the neuraxis. Meningiomas are also occasionally seen within the trigone of a lateral ventricle, where they originate from meningothelial cells in the choroid plexus, or along the optic nerve sheath.[47] The ventricular location is a feature of neurofibromatosis type 2. These tumors are isointense to brain on T1W and T2W images and show strong, homogeneous enhancement unless there is dense calcification, in which case the enhancement may appear heterogeneous. A dural tail may be seen, which consists of tapering of the enhancing mass lesion along the dura adjacent to the mass. However, dural tails are a nonspecific characteristic of many dural-based tumors other than meningiomas. Calcification is common. Mass effect on adjacent brain is often seen, and vasogenic cerebral edema may be extensive.[80] Evidence of brain invasion suggests the presence of a malignant meningioma. Sellar or cavernous sinus region meningiomas invade the cavernous sinuses, encase the adjacent internal carotid arteries, and extend into the sella without associated sellar enlargement.

METASTATIC DISEASE

Although systemic cancers usually involve the central and peripheral nervous system through direct metastasis or by compression of neural tissue by metastatic disease, other mechanisms including ischemic stroke, venous thrombosis, side effects of therapy, infection, paraneoplastic neurologic syndromes, and metabolic derangements are not rare and often have important imaging manifestations.

SCLC has the highest incidence among all cancers of paraneoplastic neurologic syndromes, but clinically detected paraneoplastic neurologic syndromes are exceedingly rare. Imaging manifestations that are most relevant occur with paraneoplastic encephalomyelitis, in which MRI shows T2W hyperintensity in the medial temporal lobes and brainstem in about one-half of cases. Herpes simplex encephalitis is an important differential diagnosis with this radiologic picture.

Primary tumors of lung, breast, melanoma, carcinoma of unknown primary (CUP), and colon give rise to most cases of brain metastasis. However, lung cancer is the tumor most likely to produce early metastasis, whereas most patients with breast and melanoma primaries have known cancer at the time the brain lesions are detected. About 80% of brain metastases occur supratentorially, with 15% in the cerebellum and 5% in brainstem structures, a distribution based on relative distribution of blood flow.[81,82] Pelvic malignancies, such as gastrointestinal, ovarian, and uterine cancers, and breast cancer may have a predilection to metastasize to the posterior fossa.[82] Multiple metastatic lesions are seen in 60% to 75% of all cases as determined by gadolinium-enhanced MR imaging.[83,84] Small cell lung cancer and melanoma are the primaries that are most likely to produce multiple metastasis. Significant surrounding vasogenic edema is often seen with metastasis, but this is not a universal finding, particularly with lesions less than 10 mm in diameter.

Metastases are typically hypodense to isodense on noncontrast CT but hyperdense metastases can indicate the presence of intratumoral hemorrhage, high cell density (seen with lymphoma, germinoma, and small cell lung cancer), melanin, calcification, or mucinous adenocarcinoma. Tumors most likely to have spontaneous hemorrhage are melanoma, choriocarcinoma, renal cell carcinoma, and thyroid carcinoma. The presence of calcification in a brain metastasis implies an indolent lesion.[85]

Most metastases enhance intensely. Enhancement can be of ring configuration or, especially with smaller lesions, homogeneous. Central nonenhancing areas are characteristic of necrotic or cystic lesions. The more densely cellular (ie, homogeneously enhancing) component may show relative hypointensity to brain on T2W images and may have restricted diffusion relative to adjacent brain, but hyperintensity is more common, especially in the cystic or necrotic portions and in the surrounding vasogenic edema.

There are occasionally unusual imaging features with brain metastasis, and these can be useful in the differential diagnosis of a newly detected mass. Hemorrhagic metastases show variable signal intensities depending on the stage of hemorrhage, with the most remarkable feature being intrinsic T1W hyperintensity. Evolution of signal intensity is slower with tumoral hemorrhage than with spontaneous hemorrhage. T2W hypointensity can be seen in some tumors because of hemorrhage, dense cellularity (such as metastatic lymphomas, small cell lung cancer), mucinous adenocarcinomas (especially of gastrointestinal, ovarian, and occasionally breast primaries), and rare instances of dystrophic calcification in metastasis.[86]

Approximately 50% of melanotic melanoma metastases are hyperintense on T1 images before the administration of gadolinium.[87] Melanin can also lead to T1 shortening,[88,89] and melanoma metastases have a propensity for hemorrhage, with blood products also producing T1 shortening. Gradient echo (T2*) images can increase the sensitivity of lesion detection in melanoma.[87] T2* sequences are valuable in patients with known melanoma who are undergoing CNS staging and in patients with suspected metastasis in whom the primary is not known.

In patients with a newly detected mass or in a patient with a distant history of cancer or an indolent primary, many diagnostic possibilities must be entertained. Primary brain tumors, abscesses, demyelinating lesions, subacute infarcts, and resolving hematomas can be difficult to distinguish from brain metastasis.

Leptomeningeal metastases (LM) are less common than brain metastases. Breast carcinoma, lung carcinoma, melanoma, lymphoma, and leukemia are the most common underlying primaries. Gadolinium-enhanced MRI is the most sensitive imaging technique for LM, and multifocal enhancement of the leptomeninges is the most common finding. Meningeal metastases may invade the underlying parenchyma and be associated with parenchymal T2W hyperintensity, swelling, and contrast enhancement. T2/fluid-attenuated inversion recovery imaging may show hyperintensity in the subarachnoid spaces. Dural metastases are nodular enhancing extra-axial lesions that do not extend into sulci along the subarachnoid pathways.

Neuro-oncologists often give particular emphasis to imaging evidence of diagnosis of LM when patients are unable to undergo lumbar puncture or in the common situation in which CSF cytopathologic findings are nondiagnostic. Nodular enhancement along the cauda equina may be particularly helpful in this situation, and, in addition to symptomatic areas, the neuraxis should be imaged with MRI after the administration of gadolinium.

Radionuclide cisternography can be helpful to assess the patency of the CSF flow before instillation of intrathecal chemotherapy.[90]

RECURRENT GLIOMA

Distinguishing between early recurrence/pseudoprogression (ER/PP), recurrent tumor (RT)/delayed treatment effect (DTE), and true response (TR)/pseudoresponse (PR) has become increasingly complex because of the effects of antiangiogenic therapy on conventional (in particular) postcontrast imaging. This issue is critical for patient care, and is most often resolved by serial MRI and biopsy, potentially missing an earlier opportunity to change therapy and adding additional invasive procedures.

Recent work has focused on the use of MRI, in particular DSC and DCE, to distinguish between ER/PP, TR/PR, and RT/DTE. Differences in identified threshold values for recurrent disease (discussed later) is likely related to substantial variability in technique. Preloading of contrast, numerical methods of leakage correction, use of arterial deconvolution, and multiple other parameters alter measured values. When implementing these methodologies into clinical practice, careful attention to the technical aspects and quality control with radiopathologic follow-up is essential.

ER/PP

Enhancement of T1 signal after gadolinium-based contrast agent administration is commonly seen after radiation therapy and can be difficult to distinguish from RT. The underlying histopathology and mechanism of PP, predominantly blood-brain barrier breakdown, seems to be distinct from DTEs/radiation necrosis.[91,92] Both processes are histologically distinct from TR, in which there are viable tumor cells and often microvascular proliferation.[93] ER occurs most commonly in patients with high-grade tumors in whom complete resection has not been possible.

The landmark demonstration of improved survival with surgical intervention followed by concurrent temozolamide and radiotherapy[63] has set the standard of care for high-grade gliomas. However, this has also greatly increased the incidence of therapy-related imaging findings of PP that are anatomically indistinguishable[66,94–96] from ER. Both processes are characterized by increased enhancement on postgadolinium sequences and T2 signal, generally within 2 to 6 months after starting radiation and chemotherapy. Moreover, each process accounts for approximately 50% of early postoperative enhancement, sometimes leaving the appropriate clinical response in doubt.[64,97–99] However, ER and PP are clinically distinct, with resolution of symptoms and eventual radiologic resolution[66] occurring with PP (**Fig. 8**). Methylguanine methyltransferase promoter methylation status seems to predict the likelihood of PP,[100,101] increasing the likelihood from approximately 30% to 40% to approximately 70% to 90%.

In general DSC-based and DCE-based approaches have focused on the average value of the given parameter within enhancing tissue or abnormal white matter. In most cases, higher average nCBV of enhancing tissue ($>2.6^{102}$; $>1.47^{103}$) is associated with ER, and low values indicate PP ($\leq0.6^{102}$; $\leq1.47^{103}$), as shown in **Fig. 8**. The substantial variation between groups is likely accounted for by technical aspects of image acquisition, inviting the creation of a standard. A voxel-wise approach[94] with coregistration between the initial postoperative scan and subsequent studies has shown substantial differences between PP and ER groups in fractional nCBV change, although inherent in this approach is the potential for coregistration error.

RT/DTE

The typical time course for radiation-induced enhancement is 6 to 24 months after radiation therapy and is commonly in the 12 month range, but can occur long after therapy.[104] DSC/DCE-based approaches to differentiating RT from DTE have also found CBV to be the most useful metric. As with distinguishing ER/PP, independent

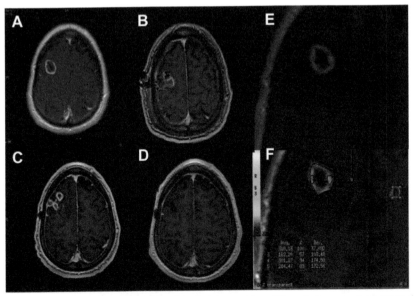

Fig. 8. PP in high-grade glioma (A) after total resection (B) and chemoradiotherapy (C). Complete resolution of enhancement is seen at 1 year (D), consistent with PP. Despite enhancement (E), nCBV values are less than 1.0 (F).

groups have found that high average nCBV values ($>0.71^{105}$; $>1.6^{106}$; $>1.8^{107}$; $>3.69^{108}$) predict RT, whereas low values indicate radiation effect. Despite the range of values, sensitivity and specificity tends to be high. The variability in absolute values again underscores the need for thoughtful implementation and standardized imaging/post-processing approaches.

MRS has also been used to distinguish progressive tumor from treatment effects.[109] A marked increase of choline (eg, $\geq$3:1 ratio of choline/creatine) in an enlarging lesion increases the confidence that the imaging finding represents RT.

A type of progressive disease not amenable to evaluation by perfusion imaging is evolving gliomatosis cerbri/infiltrating avascular tumor, which has been reported to have low nCBV values.[50]

TR/PR

Therapeutic options for recurrent high-grade glioma are limited, with bevacizumab (BZ), with or without irinotecan (IR), as the mainstay.[110] In considering the available data (predominantly phase 2), BZ and BV plus IR are associated with improvement in progression-free survival.[110,111] BZ has a substantial immediate effect on a subset of patients with recurrent disease; those patients who respond may be identified by near-immediate (<24 hours) decrease in nCBV values. A recent finding in nude rats suggests that, although clinical experience indicates response to therapy, and imaging shows less evidence of disease, this may come at the cost of increased tumor cell invasion into normal tissue.[112]

A pattern of response seen with BZ is loss of enhancement and decreased vasogenic-appearing edema, but with persistent tumor growth, termed PR. In our experience, this is associated with a nodular and salt-and-pepper appearance in the area of recurrence. Several recent papers have suggested that clinically relevant response to antioangiogenic therapy is best determined by DSC and CBV measurements, rather than conventional postcontrast imaging in response to both BZ[113]

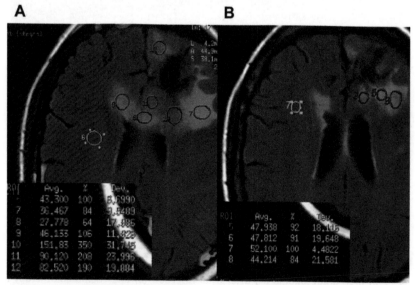

Fig. 9. TR to BZ therapy, showing marked diminution in nCBV values before therapy (A) compared with after therapy (B).

and cediranib.[114,115] An example of imaging response with marked diminution in nCBV is shown in **Fig. 9**. High B-value diffusion imaging has recently been reported to help identify PR in 10 patients. Those patients showing greater DWI signal had poorer survival.[116] Marked elevation in diffusion signal and decrease in ADC has also been reported after BZ treatment[117,118] and preceding tumor recurrence[101] in particular after BZ treatment.[119]

REFERENCES

1. Al-Okaili RN, Krejza J, Woo JH, et al. Intraaxial brain masses: MR imaging–based diagnostic strategy—initial experience. Radiology 2007;243(2):539. Radiological Society of North America. Available at: http://radiology.rsna.org/content/243/2/539.short. Accessed January 15, 2012.
2. Ambrose J, Hounsfield G. Computerized transverse axial tomography. Br J Radiol 1973;46(542):148–9.
3. Cormack AM. Recollections of my work with computer assisted tomography. Mol Cell Biochem 1980;32(2):59–61.
4. Broder J, Warshauer DM. Increasing utilization of computed tomography in the adult emergency department, 2000-2005. Emerg Radiol 2006;13(1):25–30.
5. Wilson AJ, Sayer RA, Edwards SG, et al. A comparison of computed tomography and magnetic resonance brain imaging in HIV-positive patients with neurological symptoms. Int J STD AIDS 2010;21(3):198–201.
6. Brant-Zawadzki M, Badami JP, Mills CM, et al. Primary intracranial tumor imaging: a comparison of magnetic resonance and CT. Radiology 1984;150(2):435–40.
7. Orrison WW, Stimac GK, Stevens EA, et al. Comparison of CT, low-field-strength MR imaging, and high-field-strength MR imaging. Work in progress. Radiology 1991;181(1):121–7.
8. Lauterbur PC. Image formation by induced local interactions: examples employing nuclear magnetic resonance. Nature 1973;242:190–1.
9. Albayrak B, Samdani AF, Black P M. Intra-operative magnetic resonance imaging in neurosurgery. Acta neurochirurgica 2004;146(6):543–56 [discussion 557].
10. Knauth M, Wirtz CR, Tronnier VM, et al. Intraoperative MR imaging increases the extent of tumor resection in patients with high-grade gliomas. AJNR. American journal of neuroradiology 1999;20(9):1642–6.
11. Kubben PL, Ter Meulen KJ, Schijns OE, et al. Intraoperative MRI-guided resection of glioblastoma multiforme: a systematic review. Lancet Oncol 2011;12(11):1062–70.
12. Croteau D, Scarpace L, Hearshen D, et al. Correlation between magnetic resonance spectroscopy imaging and image-guided biopsies: semiquantitative and qualitative histopathological analyses of patients with untreated glioma. Neurosurgery 2001;49(4):823–9.
13. Harrington GS, Buonocore MH, Farias ST. Intrasubject reproducibility of functional MR imaging activation in language tasks. AJNR Am J Neuroradiol 2006;27(4):938–44.
14. Norris DG. Principles of magnetic resonance assessment of brain function. J Magn Reson Imaging 2006;23(6):794–807.
15. Binder JR. Functional MRI is a valid noninvasive alternative to Wada testing. Epilepsy Behav 2011;20(2):214–22.
16. Medina LS, Bernal B, Ruiz J. Role of functional MR in determining language dominance in epilepsy and nonepilepsy populations: a Bayesian analysis. Radiology 2007;242(1):94–100.

17. Bizzi A, Blasi V, Falini A, et al. Presurgical functional MR imaging of language and motor functions: validation with intraoperative electrocortical mapping. Radiology 2008;248(2):579–89.
18. Hirsch J, Ruge MI, Kim KH, et al. An integrated functional magnetic resonance imaging procedure for preoperative mapping of cortical areas associated with tactile, motor, language, and visual functions. Neurosurgery 2000;47(3):711–21 [discussion: 721–2].
19. Ruge MI, Victor J, Hosain S, et al. Concordance between functional magnetic resonance imaging and intraoperative language mapping. Stereotact Funct Neurosurg 1999;72(2–4):95–102.
20. Kane I, Carpenter T, Chappell F, et al. Comparison of 10 different magnetic resonance perfusion imaging processing methods in acute ischemic stroke: effect on lesion size, proportion of patients with diffusion/perfusion mismatch, clinical scores, and radiologic outcomes. Stroke 2007;38(12):3158–64.
21. Knopp EA, Cha S, Johnson G, et al. Glial neoplasms: dynamic contrast-enhanced T2*-weighted MR imaging. Radiology 1999;211(3):791–8.
22. Paulson ES, Schmainda KM. Comparison of dynamic susceptibility-weighted contrast enhanced MR methods: recommendations for measuring relative cerebral blood volume in tumors. Radiology 2008;249(2):601–13 Radiological Society of North America. Available at: http://radiology.rsna.org/content/249/2/601.short. Accessed January 15, 2012.
23. Law M, Young R, Babb J, et al. Comparing perfusion metrics obtained from a single compartment versus pharmacokinetic modeling methods using dynamic susceptibility contrast-enhanced perfusion MR imaging with glioma grade. AJNR Am J Neuroradiol 2006;27(9):1975–82.
24. Law M, Oh S, Johnson G, et al. Perfusion magnetic resonance imaging predicts patient outcome as an adjunct to histopathology: a second reference standard in the surgical and nonsurgical treatment of low-grade gliomas. Neurosurgery 2006;58(6):1099–107.
25. Hu LS, Baxter LC, Pinnaduwage DS, et al. Optimized preload leakage-correction methods to improve the diagnostic accuracy of dynamic susceptibility-weighted contrast-enhanced perfusion MR imaging in posttreatment gliomas. AJNR Am J Neuroradiol 2010;31(1):40–8.
26. Lev MH, Ozsunar Y, Henson JW, et al. Glial tumor grading and outcome prediction using dynamic spin-echo MR susceptibility mapping compared with conventional contrast-enhanced MR: confounding effect of elevated rCBV of oligodendrogliomas [corrected]. AJNR Am J Neuroradiol 2004;25(2):214–21.
27. Sugahara T, Korogi Y, Kochi M, et al. Correlation of MR imaging-determined cerebral blood volume maps with histologic and angiographic determination of vascularity of gliomas. AJR Am J Roentgenol 1998;171(6):1479–86.
28. Whitmore RG, Krejza J, Kapoor GS, et al. Prediction of oligodendroglial tumor subtype and grade using perfusion weighted magnetic resonance imaging. J Neurosurg 2007;107(3):600–9.
29. Law M, Yang S, Wang H, et al. Glioma grading: sensitivity, specificity, and predictive values of perfusion MR imaging and proton MR spectroscopic imaging compared with conventional MR imaging. AJNR Am J Neuroradiol 2003;24(10):1989–98.
30. Law M, Young RJ, Babb JS, et al. Gliomas: predicting time to progression or survival with cerebral blood volume measurements at dynamic susceptibility-weighted contrast-enhanced perfusion MR imaging. Radiology 2008;

247(2):490–8. Radiological Society of North America. Available at: http://radiology.rsna.org/content/247/2/490.short. Accessed January 15, 2012.

31. Larsson HB, Courivaud F, Rostrup E, et al. Measurement of brain perfusion, blood volume, and blood-brain barrier permeability, using dynamic contrast-enhanced T(1)-weighted MRI at 3 tesla. Magn Reson Med 2009;62(5):1270–81.

32. Awasthi R, Rathore RK, Soni P, et al. Discriminant analysis to classify glioma grading using dynamic contrast-enhanced MRI and immunohistochemical markers. Neuroradiology 2012;54(3):205–13.

33. Patankar TF, Haroon HA, Mills SJ, et al. Is volume transfer coefficient (K(trans)) related to histologic grade in human gliomas? AJNR Am J Neuroradiol 2005; 26(10):2455–65.

34. Xyda A, Haberland U, Klotz E, et al. Brain volume perfusion CT performed with 128-detector row CT system in patients with cerebral gliomas: a feasibility study. Eur Radiol 2011;21(9):1811–9.

35. Schaefer PW, Grant PE, Gonzalez RG. Diffusion-weighted MR imaging of the brain. Radiology 2000;217(2):331–45.

36. Chang L, Ernst T. MR spectroscopy and diffusion-weighted MR imaging in focal brain lesions in AIDS. Neuroimaging Clin North Am 1997;7(3):409–26.

37. Hilario A, Ramos A, Perez-Nuñez A, et al. The added value of apparent diffusion coefficient to cerebral blood volume in the preoperative grading of diffuse gliomas. AJNR Am J Neuroradiol 2012;33(4):701–7.

38. Reiche W, Schuchardt V, Hagen T, et al. Differential diagnosis of intracranial ring enhancing cystic mass lesions–role of diffusion-weighted imaging (DWI) and diffusion-tensor imaging (DTI). Clin Neurol Neurosurg 2010;112(3):218–25.

39. Toh CH, Wei KC, Ng SH, et al. Differentiation of brain abscesses from necrotic glioblastomas and cystic metastatic brain tumors with diffusion tensor imaging. AJNR Am J Neuroradiol 2011;32(9):1646–51.

40. Byrnes TJ, Barrick TR, Bell BA, et al. Diffusion tensor imaging discriminates between glioblastoma and cerebral metastases in vivo. NMR Biomed 2011; 24(1):54–60.

41. Lu S, Ahn D, Johnson G, et al. Peritumoral diffusion tensor imaging of high-grade gliomas and metastatic brain tumors. AJNR Am J Neuroradiol 2003; 24(5):937–41.

42. Provenzale JM, McGraw P, Mhatre P, et al. Peritumoral brain regions in gliomas and meningiomas: investigation with isotropic diffusion-weighted MR imaging and diffusion-tensor MR imaging. Radiology 2004;232(2):451–60.

43. Saksena S, Jain R, Narang J, et al. Predicting survival in glioblastomas using diffusion tensor imaging metrics. J Magn Reson Imaging 2010;32(4):788–95.

44. Berman JI, Berger MS, Mukherjee P, et al. Diffusion-tensor imaging-guided tracking of fibers of the pyramidal tract combined with intraoperative cortical stimulation mapping in patients with gliomas. Journal of Neurosurgery 2004; 101(1):66–72.

45. Kuhnt D, Bauer MH, Becker A, et al. Intraoperative visualization of fiber tracking based reconstruction of language pathways in glioma surgery. Neurosurgery 2012;70(4):911–9 [discussion 919-20].

46. Wu JS, Zhou LF, Tang WJ, et al. Clinical evaluation and follow-up outcome of diffusion tensor imaging-based functional neuronavigation: a prospective, controlled study in patients with gliomas involving pyramidal tracts. Neurosurgery 2007; 61(5):935–48 [discussion: 948–9].

47. Kleihues P, Cavenee W. Tumours of the nervous system. WHO classification. Oxford: Oxford University Press; 2000.

48. Barker FG, Chang SM, Huhn SL, et al. Age and the risk of anaplasia in magnetic resonance-nonenhancing supratentorial cerebral tumors. Cancer 1997;80(5): 936–41.

49. Shafqat S, Hedley-Whyte ET, Henson JW. Age-dependent rate of anaplastic transformation in low-grade astrocytoma. Neurology 1999;52(4):867–9.

50. Yang S, Wetzel S, Law M, et al. Dynamic contrast-enhanced T2*-weighted MR imaging of gliomatosis cerebri. AJNR Am J Neuroradiol 2002;23(3):350–5.

51. Mandonnet E, Delattre JY, Tanguy ML, et al. Continuous growth of mean tumor diameter in a subset of grade II gliomas. Ann Neurol 2003;53:524–8.

52. Recht LD, Lew R, Smith TW. Suspected low-grade glioma: is deferring treatment safe? Annals of neurology 1992;31(4):431–6.

53. Kleihues P, Soylemezoglu F, Schäuble B, et al. Histopathology, classification, and grading of gliomas. Glia 1995;15(3):211–21.

54. Recht LD, Bernstein M. Low-grade gliomas. Neurologic clinics 1995;13(4): 847–59.

55. Shah AH, Madhavan K, Heros D, et al. The management of incidental low-grade gliomas using magnetic resonance imaging: systematic review and optimal treatment paradigm. Neurosurg Focus 2011;31(6):1–9.

56. Hou LC, Veeravagu A, Hsu AR, et al. Recurrent glioblastoma multiforme: a review of natural history and management options. American Association of Neurological Surgeons. Neurosurg Focus 2006;20(4):E5.

57. Ulmer S, Mavrakis A, Barker FG, et al. Incidence of Multifocal Lesions in Malignant Glioma as Detected by MRI. Neurology 2006;66:A431.

58. Kelly P, Daumas-Duport C, Kispert D. Imaging-based stereotactic serial biopsies in untreated intracranial glial neoplasms. J Neurosurg 1987;66:865–74.

59. Burger PC, Heinz ER, Shibata T, et al. Topographic anatomy and CT correlations in the untreated glioblastoma multiforme. J Neurosurg 1988;68:698–704.

60. Jain R, Narang J, Schultz L, et al. Permeability estimates in histopathology-proved treatment-induced necrosis using perfusion CT: can these add to other perfusion parameters in differentiating from recurrent/progressive tumors? AJNR Am J Neuroradiol 2011;32(4):658–63.

61. Murakami R, Hirai T, Nakamura H, et al. Recurrence patterns of glioblastoma treated with postoperative radiation therapy: relationship between extent of resection and progression-free interval. Jpn J Radiol 2012;30(3):193–7.

62. Vidiri A, Carapella CM, Pace A, et al. Early post-operative MRI: correlation with progression-free survival and overall survival time in malignant gliomas. J Exp Clin Cancer Res 2006;25(2):177–82.

63. Stupp R, Mason WP, van den Bent MJ, et al. Radiotherapy plus concomitant and adjuvant temozolomide for glioblastoma. N Engl J Med 2005;352(10): 987–96.

64. Brandsma D, Stalpers L, Taal W, et al. Clinical features, mechanisms, and management of pseudoprogression in malignant gliomas. Lancet Oncol 2008; 9(5):453–61.

65. Chamberlain MC. Pseudoprogression in glioblastoma. J Clin Oncol 2008; 26(26):4359 [author reply: 4359–60].

66. Chamberlain MC, Glantz MJ, Chalmers L, et al. Early necrosis following concurrent Temodar and radiotherapy in patients with glioblastoma. J Neurooncol 2007;82(1):81–3.

67. Mangla R, Singh G, Ziegelitz D, et al. Changes in relative cerebral blood volume 1 month after radiation-temozolomide therapy can help predict overall survival in patients with glioblastoma. Radiology 2010;256(2):575–84.

68. Lee YY, Van Tassel P. Intracranial oligodendrogliomas: imaging findings in 35 untreated cases. AJNR Am J Neuroradiol 1989;10:119–27.

69. van den Bent MJ, Afra D, de Witte O, et al. Long-term efficacy of early versus delayed radiotherapy for low-grade astrocytoma and oligodendroglioma in adults: the EORTC 22845 randomised trial. Lancet 2005;366(9490):985–90.

70. Sanai N, Berger MS. Glioma extent of resection and its impact on patient outcome. Neurosurgery 2008;62(4):753–64 [discussion: 264–6].

71. Sanai N, Polley MY, Berger MS. Insular glioma resection: assessment of patient morbidity, survival, and tumor progression. J Neurosurg 2010;112(1):1–9.

72. Laigle-Donadey F, Martin-Duverneuil N, Lejeune J, et al. Correlations between molecular profile and radiologic pattern in oligodendroglial tumors. Neurology 2004;63(12):2360–2.

73. Megyesi JF, Kachur E, Lee DH, et al. Imaging correlates of molecular signatures in oligodendrogliomas. Clin Cancer Res 2004;10(13):4303–6.

74. Cairncross JG, Macdonald DR. Successful chemotherapy for recurrent malignant oligodendroglioma. Ann Neurol 1988;23(4):360–4.

75. Cairncross JG, Ueki K, Zlatescu MC, et al. Specific genetic predictors of chemo-therapeutic response and survival in patients with anaplastic oligodendroglio-mas. J Natl Cancer Inst 1998;90(19):1473–9.

76. Castillo M, Davis PC, Takei Y. Intracranial ganglioglioma: MR imaging, CT, and clinical findings in 18 patients. AJNR Am J Neuroradiol 1990;11:109–14.

77. Guillamo JS, Doz F, Delattre J-Y. Brainstem gliomas. Current Opin Neurol 2001; 14:711–5.

78. Bing F, Kremer S, Lamalle L, et al. Value of perfusion MRI in the study of pilocytic astrocytoma and hemangioblastoma: preliminary findings. J Neuroradiol 2009; 36(2):82–7.

79. Buhring U, Herrlinger U, Krings T, et al. MRI features of primary central nervous system lymphomas at presentation. Neurology 2001;57:393–6.

80. Nakano T, Asano K, Miura H, et al. Meningiomas with brain edema: radiological characteristics on MRI and review of the literature. Clin Imaging 2002;26:243–9.

81. Delattre JY, Krol G, Thaler HT, et al. Distribution of brain metastases. Arch Neurol 1988;45:741–4.

82. Posner JB. Management of brain metastases. Rev Neurol (paris) 1992;148: 477–87.

83. Sze G, Milano E, Johnson C. Detection of brain metastases: comparison of contrast-enhanced MR with unenhanced MR and enhanced CT. AJNR Am J Neuroradiol 1990;11:785–91.

84. Hutter A, Schwetye KE, Bierhals AJ, et al. Brain neoplasms: epidemiology, diag-nosis, and prospects for cost-effective imaging. Neuroimaging Clin North Am 2003;13:237–50.

85. Ohmoto Y, Nishizaki T, Kajiwara K, et al. Calcified metastatic brain tumor–two case reports. Neurol Med Chir (Tokyo) 2002;42:264–7.

86. Ricke J, Baum K, Hosten N. Calcified brain metastases from ovarian carcinoma. Neuroradiology 1996;38:460–1.

87. Gaviani P, Mullins ME, Braga TA, et al. Improved detection of metastatic mela-noma by T2*-weighted imaging. AJNR Am J Neuroradiol 2006;27:605–8.

88. Atlas SW, Braffman BH, LoBrutto R. Human malignant melanoma with varying melanin content in nude mice: MR imaging, histopathology, and electron para-magnetic resonance. J Comput Assist Tomogr 1990;14:547–54.

89. Enochs WS, Petherick P, Bogdanova A, et al. Paramagnetic metal scavenging by melanin: MR imaging. Radiology 1997;204:417–23.

90. Chamberlain MC, Kormanik PA. Prognostic significance of 111indium-DTPA CSF flow studies in leptomeningeal metastases. Neurology 1996;46:1674–7.
91. Li YQ, Chen P, Haimovitz-Friedman A, et al. Endothelial apoptosis initiates acute blood-brain barrier disruption after ionizing radiation. Cancer Res 2003;63(18): 5950–6.
92. Moore AH, Olschowka JA, Williams JP, et al. Radiation-induced edema is dependent on cyclooxygenase 2 activity in mouse brain. Radiat Res 2004; 161(2):153–60.
93. Pytel P, Lukas RV. Update on diagnostic practice: tumors of the nervous system. Arch Pathol Lab Med 2009;133(7):1062–77.
94. Tsien C, Galbán CJ, Chenevert TL, et al. Parametric response map as an imaging biomarker to distinguish progression from pseudoprogression in high-grade glioma. J Clin Oncol 2010;28(13):2293–9.
95. Young RJ, Gupta A, Shah AD, et al. Potential utility of conventional MRI signs in diagnosing pseudoprogression in glioblastoma. Neurology 2011;76(22): 1918–24.
96. Yung WK, Albright RE, Olson J, et al. A phase II study of temozolomide vs. procarbazine in patients with glioblastoma multiforme at first relapse. Br J Cancer 2000;83(5):588–93.
97. Hygino da Cruz LC, Rodriguez I, Domingues RC, et al. Pseudoprogression and pseudoresponse: imaging challenges in the assessment of posttreatment glioma. AJNR Am J Neuroradiol 2011;32(11):1978–85.
98. Taal W, Brandsma D, de Bruin HG, et al. Incidence of early pseudo-progression in a cohort of malignant glioma patients treated with chemoirradiation with temozolomide. Cancer 2008;113(2):405–10.
99. Topkan E, Topuk S, Oymak E, et al. Pseudoprogression in patients with glioblastoma multiforme after concurrent radiotherapy and temozolomide. Am J Clin Oncol 2011;00(00):1–6.
100. Brandes AA, Franceschi E, Tosoni A, et al. MGMT promoter methylation status can predict the incidence and outcome of pseudoprogression after concomitant radiochemotherapy in newly diagnosed glioblastoma patients. J Clin Oncol 2008;26(13):2192–7.
101. Gupta A, Omuro AMP, Shah AD, et al. Continuing the search for MR imaging biomarkers for MGMT promoter methylation status: conventional and perfusion MRI revisited. Neuroradiology 2011;11–3.
102. Sugahara T, Korogi Y, Tomiguchi S, et al. Posttherapeutic intraaxial brain tumor: the value of perfusion-sensitive contrast-enhanced MR imaging for differentiating tumor recurrence from nonneoplastic contrast-enhancing tissue. AJNR Am J Neuroradiol 2000;21(5):901–9.
103. Kong DS, Kim ST, Kim EH, et al. Diagnostic dilemma of pseudoprogression in the treatment of newly diagnosed glioblastomas: the role of assessing relative cerebral blood flow volume and oxygen-6-methylguanine-DNA methyltransferase promoter methylation status. AJNR Am J Neuroradiol 2011;32(2):382–7.
104. Giglio P, Gilbert MR. Cerebral radiation necrosis. Neurologist 2003;9(4):180–8.
105. Hu LS, Baxter LC, Smith KA, et al. Relative cerebral blood volume values to differentiate high-grade glioma recurrence from posttreatment radiation effect: direct correlation between image-guided tissue histopathology and localized dynamic susceptibility-weighted contrast-enhanced perfusion. AJNR Am J Neuroradiol 2009;30(3):552–8.
106. Barajas RF, Chang JS, Segal MR, et al. Differentiation of recurrent glioblastoma multiforme from radiation necrosis after external beam radiation therapy with

dynamic susceptibility-weighted contrast-enhanced perfusion MR imaging. Radiology 2009;253(2):486–96.
107. Gasparetto EL, Pawlak MA, Patel SH, et al. Posttreatment recurrence of malignant brain neoplasm: accuracy of relative cerebral blood volume fraction in discriminating low from high malignant histologic volume fraction. Radiology 2009;250(3):887–96.
108. Kim YH, Oh SW, Lim YJ, et al. Differentiating radiation necrosis from tumor recurrence in high-grade gliomas: assessing the efficacy of 18F-FDG PET, 11C-methionine PET and perfusion MRI. Clin Neurol Neurosurg 2010;112(9):758–65.
109. Rock JP, Scarpace L, Hearshen D, et al. Associations among magnetic resonance spectroscopy, apparent diffusion coefficients, and image-guided histopathology with special attention to radiation necrosis. Neurosurgery 2004; 54:1111–7 [discussion 1117-9].
110. Chamberlain MC. Bevacizumab for the treatment of recurrent glioblastoma. Clin Med Insights Oncol 2011;5:117–29.
111. Vredenburgh JJ, Desjardins A, Herndon JE, et al. Bevacizumab plus irinotecan in recurrent glioblastoma multiforme. J Clin Oncol 2007;25(30):4722–9.
112. Keunen O, Johansson M, Oudin A, et al. Anti-VEGF treatment reduces blood supply and increases tumor cell invasion in glioblastoma. Proc Natl Acad Sci U S A 2011;108(9):3749–54.
113. Sawlani RN, Raizer J, Horowitz SW, et al. Glioblastoma: a method for predicting response to antiangiogenic chemotherapy by using MR perfusion imaging–pilot study. Radiology 2010;255(2):622–8.
114. Emblem KE, Bjornerud A, Mouridsen K, et al. T(1)- and T(2)(*)-dominant extravasation correction in DSC-MRI: part II-predicting patient outcome after a single dose of cediranib in recurrent glioblastoma patients. J Cereb Blood Flow Metab 2011;31(10):2054–64.
115. Sorensen AG, Batchelor TT, Zhang WT, et al. A "vascular normalization index" as potential mechanistic biomarker to predict survival after a single dose of cediranib in recurrent glioblastoma patients. Cancer Res 2009;69(13):5296–300.
116. Yamasaki F, Kurisu K, Aoki T, et al. Advantages of high b-value diffusion-weighted imaging to diagnose pseudo-responses in patients with recurrent glioma after bevacizumab treatment. Eur J Radiol 2011. DOI:10.1016/j.ejrad.2011.10.018.
117. Hattingen E, Jurcoane A, Bähr O, et al. Bevacizumab impairs oxidative energy metabolism and shows antitumoral effects in recurrent glioblastomas: a 31P/1H MRSI and quantitative magnetic resonance imaging study. Neuro Oncol 2011; 13(12):1349–63.
118. Rieger J, Bähr O, Müller K, et al. Bevacizumab-induced diffusion-restricted lesions in malignant glioma patients. J Neurooncol 2010;99(1):49–56.
119. Paldino MJ, Desjardins A, Friedman HS, et al. A change in the apparent diffusion coefficient after treatment with bevacizumab is associated with decreased survival in patients with recurrent glioblastoma multiforme. The British journal of radiology 2011. DOI:10.1259/bjr/24774491.

Role of Neurosurgery and Radiation Therapy in the Management of Brain Tumors

Toral R. Patel, MD[a], James B. Yu, MD[b], Joseph M. Piepmeier, MD[a],*

KEYWORDS

- Primary brain tumors • Treatment • Surgery • Radiation • Prognosis

KEY POINTS

- The basic goals of any intracranial tumor surgery are to safely obtain a tissue diagnosis and, when possible, to totally remove the tumor.
- Recent advances in imaging techniques (functional magnetic resonance imaging, diffusion tensor imaging, intraoperative magnetic resonance imaging) have helped to maximize extent of resection and preserve neurologic function.
- Radiation therapy seeks to open a therapeutic window between damage to the tumor and damage to normal brain.
- Improvements in targeting and treatment planning technologies have allowed for more conformal radiotherapy, with sparing of normal brain tissue.

INTRODUCTION

Management of primary brain tumors requires a multidisciplinary approach that includes input from both neurosurgeons and radiation oncologists. Over the past several decades, advances in surgical and radiation techniques have improved outcomes for patients with brain tumors. In this article, the role of neurosurgery and radiation therapy in the management of the most common primary brain tumors is described. General treatment principles, tumor-specific paradigms, and ongoing and future clinical trials are discussed.

NEUROSURGERY
Basic Surgical Principles

Surgical approach varies widely based on tumor type, location, and size. Surgical options are also heavily influenced by the patient's overall clinical status, including

Disclosures: None. Funding Sources: None. Conflict of Interest: None.
[a] Department of Neurosurgery, Yale University School of Medicine, PO Box 208082, New Haven, CT 06520, USA; [b] Department of Therapeutic Radiology, Yale University School of Medicine, PO Box 208040, New Haven, CT 06520, USA
* Corresponding author.
E-mail address: joseph.piepmeier@yale.edu

Hematol Oncol Clin N Am 26 (2012) 757–777
doi:10.1016/j.hoc.2012.04.001
0889-8588/12/$ – see front matter © 2012 Elsevier Inc. All rights reserved.

Karnofsky Performance Score, age, and the presence of medical comorbidities. The basic goals of any intracranial tumor surgery are to safely obtain a tissue diagnosis and, when possible, to totally remove the tumor. When a total removal is not possible, surgical intervention allows for decompression and relief of mass effect, with consequent improvement in neurologic status. Surgical resection can result in significant cytoreduction, thereby reducing tumor burden and enhancing the efficacy of adjuvant therapy.

Technological Advances

Current neurosurgical practice uses many technological advances to improve outcome. Central to this improvement are advancements in magnetic resonance imaging (MRI) technologies. Improved MRI allows for high-resolution delineation of critical anatomic, functional, and metabolic regions. Specifically, functional imaging with MRI (fMRI) has been used to identify primary cortical regions that subserve motor/sensory capacity, language, and vision (**Fig. 1**). In addition, diffusion tensor imaging (DTI) tractography can accurately delineate the corticospinal tract, arcuate fasciculus, or optic radiations (**Fig. 2**). This technology has significant implications for operative planning; more aggressive surgical resections can be accomplished and neurologic function preserved.

Advances in MRI have also translated to improvements in intraoperative stereotactic guidance. This allows the surgeon to precisely localize their operative position and facilitates both lesion resection and biopsy.

The development of intraoperative MRI (iMRI) has further increased the surgeon's operative options. Use of iMRI allows for correction of brain shifts, detection of residual tumor, and earlier identification of potential complications.

Tumor-specific Management: Surgery

High-grade gliomas

Malignant gliomas have an annual incidence of approximately 5 cases per 100,000 people. Amongst malignant gliomas approximately 60% to 70% are glioblastomas, 10% to 15% are anaplastic astrocytomas, and 10% are anaplastic oligodendrogliomas or oligoastrocystomas (**Fig. 3**).[1]

Irrespective of disease, the surgical goals for all malignant gliomas are the same: establishing a tissue diagnosis and cytoreduction and preserving or improving neurologic status. Although no prospective, randomized trials exist, dozens of studies have retrospectively examined the effect of extent of resection on survival for patients with malignant gliomas. Most of these studies have reported that greater extent of resection independently confers a survival benefit.[1–9]

Many malignant gliomas are located in eloquent regions of the brain, which are not easily amenable to surgical resection. However, advances in fMRI and DTI have improved the surgeon's ability to operate in these areas. By combining these imaging modalities with traditional intraoperative stimulation for cortical and subcortical mapping, extent of resection can be safely maximized.[3]

Recent improvements in technology have also aided the surgeon to achieve maximal surgical resection. Specifically, the use of 5-aminolevulinic acid (an agent that accumulates as fluorescent porphyrins in portions of the tumor that contain an impaired blood-brain barrier) has been shown to increase extent of resection.[10] In addition, the presence of residual tumor has decreased in cases that use iMRI.[11]

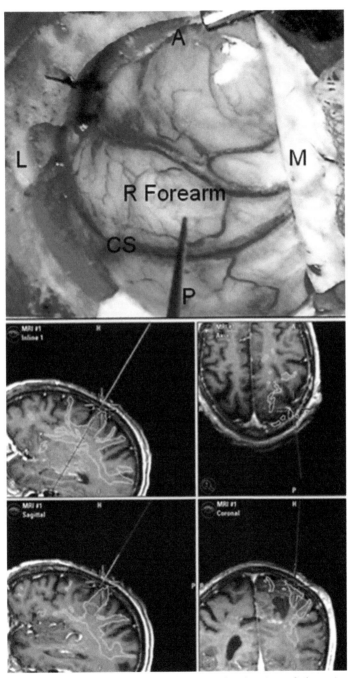

Fig. 1. (*Above*) Intraoperative image of stereotactic localization of the primary motor region for the forearm. (*Below*) Stereotactic image showing the probe seen in the operative image placed medial to the primary motor region for the hand (*orange region*). A, anterior; CS, central sulcus; L, lateral; M, medial; P, posterior.

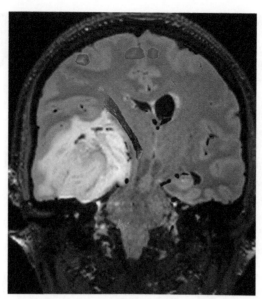

Fig. 2. Coronal MRI using diffusion tractography to show the corticospinal tract (*purple*) displaced by a large tumor (*white area*).

Thus, all patients with surgically accessible malignant gliomas should undergo maximal, safe surgical resection, and evolving technologies should be used as needed to achieve this goal. Adjuvant therapy consists of chemotherapy and radiation; the specifics of these treatments are based on tumor pathology.

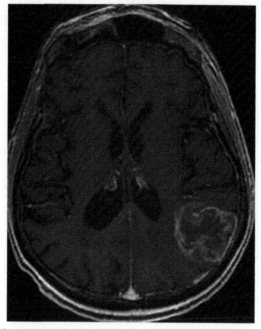

Fig. 3. T1-weighted contrast-enhanced MRI of a glioblastoma.

Low-grade gliomas

Low-grade gliomas (LGGs) encompass a heterogeneous group of World Health Organization (WHO) grade I and II gliomas and account for approximately 15% of all primary brain tumors.[12] The management of WHO grade I and II LGGs is different (**Fig. 4**).

Most WHO grade I lesions (pilocytic astrocytoma, subependymal giant cell astrocytoma, pleomorphic xanthoastrocytoma, subependymoma) are well demarcated from surrounding brain tissue and complete surgical resection is curative. Surgical resection is the gold standard; after resection, patients should be monitored with surveillance imaging.

WHO grade II lesions (diffuse astrocytomas, oligodendrogliomas, oligoastrocytomas) are molecularly distinct from grade I lesions and have a more invasive phenotype. However, they do not have the anaplastic features of a grade III lesion and in turn have a more favorable prognosis. Surgical resection is needed to ensure proper diagnosis and subsequent treatment. In addition, multiple studies have reported that extent of resection is associated with survival in patients with grade II LGGs.[3,12–15] Hence, the surgical goal for all patients with grade II LGGs is gross total resection; for those lesions located in eloquent areas of the brain, the technologies discussed earlier are often used to achieve this goal. Adjuvant therapy is determined based on histopathology and molecular markers.

Ependymomas

Ependymomas are glial-based tumors that arise from the ependymal lining of the ventricular system (**Fig. 5**). They are rare intracranial tumors and occur more commonly in children than adults. Most often, intracranial ependymomas are intimately associated with the ventricles, although ependymomas may occasionally occur at sites distant from the ventricular system.[16,17] Surgical resection is critical

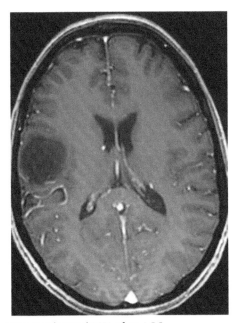

Fig. 4. T1-weighted contrast-enhanced MRI of an LGG.

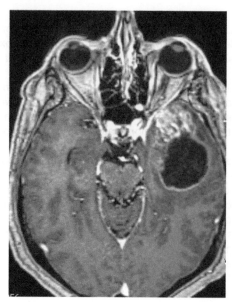

Fig. 5. T1-weighted contrast-enhanced MRI of an anaplastic ependymoma.

to treatment; several studies have reported that extent of resection is associated with progression-free and overall survival.[18–21] Thus, if complete resection is possible, this should be achieved. In addition, surgical resection can often restore normal cerebrospinal fluid (CSF) outflow in the case of an obstructing mass lesion, and this should be attempted. Given the propensity of this tumor to disseminate via CSF, staging of the entire neuroaxis is necessary to determine a comprehensive treatment plan. Need for adjuvant therapy is determined by tumor grade (WHO II vs III) and the presence of disseminated disease.

Pineal tumors

Pineal region tumors represent a heterogeneous group of lesions, ranging from benign to malignant. Overall, these are rare tumors, which occur more commonly in children than adults. Given their location deep within the brain, surgical resection of pineal region tumors is challenging (**Fig. 6**). Before the advent of microsurgical techniques, surgical mortality was upwards of 50%. In current practice, with the use of the operative microscope and improvements in neuroanesthesia, the operative mortality has been reduced to less than 5%.[22]

Surgical approach varies widely with disease; however, a few basic principles exist when addressing any pineal region tumor. First, these lesions often cause obstructive hydrocephalus secondary to compression of the aqueduct of Sylvius. To correct this condition, an endoscopic third ventriculostomy can be performed (preferably) or a ventriculoperitoneal shunt can be placed. Second, tissue diagnosis is required to direct further treatment; this can be achieved via endoscopic, stereotactic, or open biopsy. CSF and serum tumor markers can also be sent to aid in pathologic diagnosis. If test results show a pure germinoma, surgical resection is not required because these tumors can be effectively treated with radiation alone. For all other lesions (nongerminomatous germ cell tumors, gliomas, pineal-parenchymal tumors, dermoids/epidermoids, meningiomas), maximal, safe surgical resection should be achieved, followed

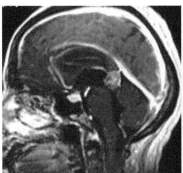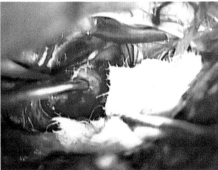

Fig. 6. (*Left*) T1-weighted contrast-enhanced MRI of a pineal region tumor. (*Right*) Intraoperative image of a dissector placed on a pineal region tumor. The vein of Galen is seen above the tumor.

by adjuvant therapy (chemotherapy/radiation) for malignant lesions and surveillance imaging for benign lesions.[22]

Primary central nervous system lymphoma
A rare variant of non-Hodgkin lymphoma, primary central nervous system lymphoma (PCNSL) can affect any part of the neuroaxis. In contrast to most primary brain tumors, PCNSL is more sensitive to chemotherapy, corticosteroids, and radiation.[23,24] Radiographically, PCNSL tends to present as an infiltrative, homogeneously enhancing lesion on MRI (**Fig. 7**). Nonetheless, PCNSL can have highly variable imaging features and is known to mimic the appearance of many other intracranial lesions. Because of its highly infiltrative nature, complete surgical resection is not feasible. Even large lesions with symptomatic mass effect respond well to medical therapies. Therefore, surgical involvement in disease management is limited to stereotactic biopsy, to establish a histopathologic diagnosis. In addition, if there is evidence of leptomeningeal spread and a desire to deliver intrathecal chemotherapy, surgical involvement may extend to placement of an Ommaya reservoir.

Meningiomas
Meningiomas are common, predominantly benign intracranial tumors that arise from arachnoid cap cells (**Fig. 8**). Surgical resection is the mainstay of treatment and is used for symptomatic lesions or those with rapid growth on surveillance imaging. Studies have shown that lesions greater than 2.5 cm in initial diameter and tumors with linear growth rates of more than 10% per year are most likely to cause progressive neurologic symptoms and require surgical intervention.[25,26] More than 90% of meningiomas are histologically benign WHO grade I lesions; the remainder are grade II (atypical) or grade III (anaplastic). For grade I lesions, complete surgical resection, when achieved, is curative. Adjuvant therapy (primarily radiotherapy) may be used for incompletely resected lesions, WHO grade II or III lesions, lesions that are not easily amenable to surgical resection, or patients who are poor surgical candidates.

Vestibular schwannomas
Vestibular schwannomas are benign lesions arising from Schwann cells that myelinate the vestibular portion of the eighth cranial nerve (**Fig. 9**). Because of their location in the cerebellopontine angle, surgical treatment of these lesions is technically challenging. Historically, surgery for vestibular schwannomas has been associated with

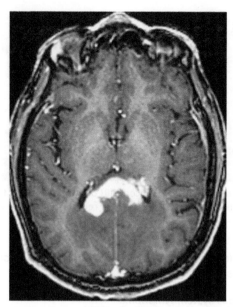

Fig. 7. T1-weighted contrast-enhanced MRI of a PCNSL of the splenium.

high rates of morbidity and mortality. However, advances in microsurgical techniques have significantly reduced this risk.[27] In current practice, surgical morbidity is most often related to CSF leak and postoperative cranial neuropathy (particular the facial nerve). Despite these risks, microsurgical resection is required for large lesions that exert mass effect on the brainstem. In addition, microsurgery is the most durable treatment strategy for vestibular schwannomas; less than 2% of patients require additional treatments at an average follow-up of 5 years.[27] Nonetheless, for small lesions without associated mass effect, radiotherapy (particularly stereotactic radiosurgery [SRS]) plays an increasingly importantly role in management, as discussed later.[27,28]

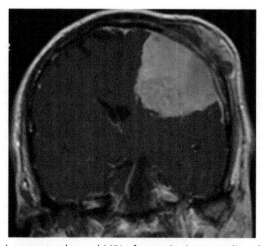

Fig. 8. T1-weighted contrast-enhanced MRI of a meningioma eroding through the skull.

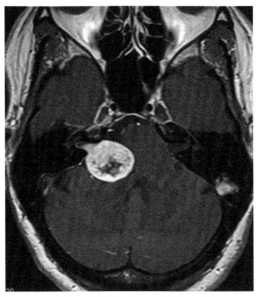

Fig. 9. T1-weighted contrast-enhanced MRI of a vestibular schwannoma.

Pituitary tumors

Most pituitary tumors are benign and are generally classified as nonsecreting or secreting (**Fig. 10**). Surgical resection is the primary treatment of all pituitary adenomas, with the exception of prolactin-secreting tumors, which respond well to medical management. Current surgical practice relies heavily on advancements in both the surgical endoscope and neuronavigation.[29,30] For secreting adenomas, large reviews have consistently reported hormonal-remission rates of more than 70% after surgical intervention. With respect to nonsecreting macroadenomas, if gross-total resection is achieved, surgical intervention is curative. Nonetheless, although surgery is required to reduce mass effect from large pituitary lesions (which often compress the optic chiasm), gross-total resection is not always possible. For example, if there is tumor infiltration of the cavernous sinus, it is not advisable to resect these portions of the tumor. In the event of residual tumor (based on either MRI or hormonal studies), SRS is commonly used. Early studies suggest that SRS provides adequate tumor control and hormonal stabilization; however, the long-term durability of this strategy is not yet known.[29]

Brain metastases

A complete discussion of brain metastases is beyond the scope of this review; however, there are a few well-established surgical principles (**Fig. 11**). In the 1990s, a series of pivotal studies by Patchell and colleagues[31,32] determined that patients with good functional status and solitary intracranial metastases should undergo surgical resection. In addition, surgery may be required to (1) alleviate mass effect from large, symptomatic lesions, (2) treat hydrocephalus via placement of a ventriculoperitoneal shunt, or (3) establish a tissue diagnosis if a primary cannot be found.

RADIATION THERAPY
Basics of Radiation Physics and Biology

In external beam radiation therapy, high-energy photons or electrons (or protons) are delivered to the brain while the head is immobilized using a patient-specific

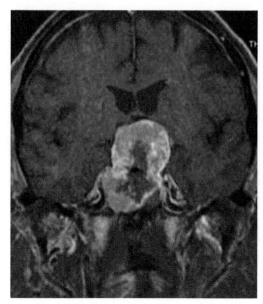

Fig. 10. T1-weighted contrast-enhanced MRI of a pituitary adenoma.

customized immobilization device. In standard practice, this procedure involves the use of a thermoplastic mask that has been shaped and conformed to the patient's face and is securely fastened to the treatment table, allowing for day-to-day reproducibility of positioning. Although the physical property of radiation beams has remained largely unchanged over the past decade, our ability to immobilize the patient, target

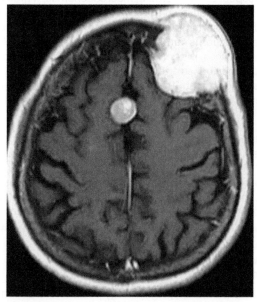

Fig. 11. T1-weighted contrast-enhanced MRI of 2 metastatic tumors.

the tumor, and shape the radiation dose has improved our ability to deliver treatment in a more customized and predictable fashion. Nonetheless, with modern photon therapy, there remains dose scattering and diffusion as the radiation beams interact with matter, and there also remains entry and exit dose, regardless of the number of overlapping beams of radiotherapy used. With photon radiotherapy, normal tissue in the path of entering or exiting radiotherapy beams are irradiated regardless of the precision of patient immobilization or accuracy of radiation dose calculation. In addition, normal brain is necessarily targeted because of tumor infiltration into normal brain itself.

High-energy photons or electrons (or protons) as delivered by modern radiotherapy cause double-strand DNA breaks in the cancer and normal tissue indiscriminately, in a dose-dependent and oxygen-dependent fashion. Hypoxic tumor is less likely to have DNA damage fixed by oxygen-free radicals, and therefore is considered more radioresistant.

Attempts to open a therapeutic window between damage to the tumor and damage to normal brain is based on 3 main principles: (1) spatial improvement in the irradiation of the tumor preferentially over adjacent normal tissue because of improvements in both radiation delivery and targeting, (2) selective radiosensitization of tumor cells over normal tissue, and (3) attempting to exploit radiobiology using optimal fractionation of treatment.

Attempting to more precisely deliver radiation to brain tumors has been the subject of intensive research. In recent years, improved shaping of radiation dose around the tumor using complex arrangements of radiation has led logically from using multiple static shaped beams of differing weight with three-dimensional (3D) computer-calculated dosimetry (3D conformal radiation) to using multiple beams with the beams themselves of varying intensity throughout the beam (intensity-modulated radiation therapy [IMRT]). IMRT potentially allows for more conformal treatment, with relative sparing of normal brain,[33] although careful 3D conformal radiotherapy can approximate IMRT for most intracranial tumors. IMRT techniques are now widely available in the United States. Tomotherapy and volumetric arc therapy are essentially variations on the IMRT theme, with IMRT now delivered in continuous arcs rather than static beam angles.

In addition to improved delivery of radiation, improved targeting of the tumor has occurred as a result of a concept known as image guidance. Image-guided radiation therapy (IGRT) involves the daily verification of patient setup and positioning. Because daily patient setup typically involves a tight-fitting aquaplast (CIVCO Medical Solutions, Kalona, IA, USA) mask, standard (non-IGRT) treatment typically allows for setup error of only 3 to 5 mm. Daily treatment setup verification performed with the patient lying on the treatment table using either orthogonal kilovoltage radiographs, or a CT scan using a CT scanner built into the radiation linear accelerator itself (a cone-beam CT) with resultant adjustment in patient positioning allows for treatment within a 2-mm to 3-mm tolerance. The use of orthogonal radiographs and specialized software integrated with a robotic couch allowing $6°$ of freedom in precise positioning of the patient and patient couch allows treatment error to be within 1 mm, allowing for more specialized treatment such as SRS either in a single session or multiple sessions.

Selective radiosensitization of cancer cells over normal tissue is another area in which radiation therapy has progressed in recent years. One example of a successful trial of radiosensitization is the Bonner cetuximab trial,[34] in which the addition of cetuximab to radiation therapy improved cancer outcomes and cure without a subsequent worsening of treatment toxicity. For intracranial disease, the use of temozolomide concurrent with radiotherapy is an example of radiosensitization of tumor cells to radiotherapy[35]; other trials involving radiosensitization are ongoing.

Proton and Heavy Particle Therapy

Protons and other particles with rest mass have a physical property called the Bragg peak, wherein the particle interacts with matter and penetrates to a depth more or less defined by its energy. In addition to having no exit dose, protons and other heavy particles have comparatively less entry dose, because of the preferential deposition of energy at the Bragg peak. Proton therapy and other heavy particle therapy have been suggested as being helpful in the treatment of spinal cord and brain tumors, by limiting overall dose deposited to normal surrounding tissue. Because of the relatively prohibitive cost of building and running a proton facility, proton and heavy particle therapy is not yet widely used in the United States. However, as technology is improved and proton machines are shrunk to fit a standard linear accelerator vault, it is likely that proton therapy will become more widely available throughout the United States.[36]

In anticipation of this availability, 2 heavy ion trials are under way in Germany. One phase I/II trial, the [Randomised Phase I/II Study to Evaluate Carbon Ion Radiotherapy Versus Fractionated Stereotactic Radiotherapy in Patients With Recurrent or Progressive Gliomas (NCT01166308; CINDERELLA)] trial, evaluates carbon ion radiotherapy compared with photon stereotactic radiotherapy for recurrent or progressive gliomas. This trial, after phase I dose escalation using carbon ion radiotherapy, will compare the phase I recommended dose level with fractionated stereotactic radiotherapy to the relatively standard low retreatment dose of 36 Gy in 2-Gy fractions.[37] The other trial, called the [Randomized Phase II Study Evaluating a Carbon Ion Boost Applied After Combined Radiochemotherapy With Temozolomide Versus a Proton Boost After Radiochemotherapy With Temozolomide in Patients With Primary Glioblastoma (NCT01165671; CLEOPATRA)] trial, will investigate the effect of carbon ion radiotherapy as a boost after conventional radiotherapy compared with proton boost, the idea being that carbon ions have an increase in relative biologic effectiveness compared with proton ions, and at the same time have the same sharp dose deposition that proton ions have.[38] These trials are perhaps of limited interest currently, but as proton therapy and heavy ion therapy become more affordable[36] and therefore more prevalent, these trials could be harbingers of future radiotherapy.

Tumor-specific Management: Radiation

High-grade gliomas: glioblastoma multiforme

The treatment of glioblastoma multiforme has taken a major step forward with the combination of temozolomide and radiation as adjuvant treatment. Although the initial report of the US National Cancer Institute/European Organisation for Research and Treatment of Cancer (EORTC) temozolomide plus radiotherapy trial[39] reported an improvement in median survival of only 2.5 months (from 12.1 months to 14.6 months), 9.8% of patients survived 5 years if temozolomide was used in combination with radiotherapy (compared with 1.9% without), indicating that there may exist a small population of long-term survivors in a disease that continues to be considered incurable.[40]

Relevant advances in radiotherapy for glioblastoma multiforme include improved targeting and more accurate treatment planning. Daily verification of patient position using either orthogonally paired radiograph images or CT scan that is integrated into the treatment machine itself has improved treatment accuracy and setup. More accurate treatment planning may also allow for shortening of treatment time by integrating the boost of dose typically given to the gross tumor (distinct from the surrounding edematous brain presumed to be microscopically infiltrated by tumor cells). This technique, called simultaneous integrated boost, has been shown to be safe in high-grade gliomas[41] and takes full advantage of current computational power in tailoring radiation dose distributions within the tumor itself.

Future investigation involves even more precise targeting of the tumor using SRS (in 1–5 fractions) or stereotactic radiotherapy (in 6–20+ fractions). Some investigators have recently suggested using relatively tight margins when treating with radiotherapy, significantly reducing the amount of normal tissue irradiated.[42] This relatively conformal technique does not seem to have an increased number of marginal failures, although it will likely need prospective comparison with standard treatment margins before it is widely accepted in the radiation oncology community.

High-grade gliomas: anaplastic astrocytoma
Prognosis for anaplastic astrocytomas is significantly better than glioblastoma, and because of this relative longevity, patients with anaplastic astrocytoma have a higher chance of experiencing late treatment-related toxicities.

Two major trials are under way investigating the optimal adjuvant treatment of anaplastic astrocytoma. North Central Cancer Treatment Group (NCCTG) N0577/ Radiation Therapy Oncology Group (RTOG) 1071 [Phase III Intergroup Study of Radiotherapy Versus Temozolomide Alone Versus Radiotherapy With Concomitant and Adjuvant Temozolomide for Patients With 1p/ 19q Codeleted Anaplastic Glioma (NCT00887146)] is a 3-arm randomized trial investigating radiotherapy versus temozolomide versus the combination of the two. The dose of radiotherapy will be radiobiologically lower than typically used for glioblastoma multiforme (59.4 Gy in 33 fractions), and the trial will also include anaplastic oligodendrogliomas and mixed anaplastic gliomas. The CATNON [Phase III Trial on Concurrent and Adjuvant Temozolomide Chemotherapy in Non-1p/19q Deleted Anaplastic Glioma (NCT00626990; CATNON)] trial (EORTC/RTOG 0834) will investigate patients with non-1p/19q codeleted anaplastic gliomas, and therefore will not have a temozolomide-alone arm (because noncodeleted tumors are less likely to respond to chemotherapy alone). Rather, this 4-arm trial will investigate radiation with or without temozolomide concurrently and will also investigate the benefit of giving or not giving maintenance temozolomide after radiotherapy ± temozolomide.

While these trials are being conducted, radiotherapy for anaplastic astrocytoma varies by institution. In our institution, treatment is individualized by patient, and based on functional status, signs and symptoms, age, and histologic aggressiveness.

High-grade gliomas: anaplastic oligodendroglioma
Current treatment of anaplastic oligodendroglioma typically involves surgical resection followed by chemotherapy and/or radiotherapy, either sequentially, or with 1 treatment saved for salvage. In previous randomized trials (RTOG 9402 and EORTC 26951) [Phase III Study of Adjuvant Procarbazine, CCNU and Vincristine Chemotherapy in Patients with highly Anaplastic Oligodendroglioma (NCT00002840)], chemotherapy after radiotherapy involved procarbazine, lomustine, and vincristine (PCV). These trials showed no difference in overall survival with the addition of PCV either sequentially or concurrently to radiotherapy, likely because of the high proportion of patients who received chemotherapy as salvage treatment. Nonetheless, PCV chemotherapy in combination with radiotherapy did delay progression of disease. However, whether a delay in progression was significant enough to justify the toxicity of PCV remains in question.[43] In current practice, the use or nonuse of PCV chemotherapy has become an outdated question, because more recent trials are now investigating the better-tolerated temozolomide in combination with radiotherapy as neoadjuvant treatment,[44] or as initial therapy, with radiotherapy reserved as salvage treatment.[45] For patients with 1p/19q loss of heterozygosity, chemotherapy response is high, and radiotherapy can likely be delayed until progression, without affecting

overall survival. NOA-04 [Randomized Phase III Study of Sequential Radiochemother-apy of Anaplastic Glioma With PCV or Temozolomide (NCT00717210; NOA-04)] showed no difference with either starting with radiotherapy or starting with chemo-therapy (PCV or temozolomide), allowing for salvage therapy on progression.[46] Patients with codeleted or noncodeleted 1p/19q anaplastic oligodendrogliomas also qualify for the NCCTG N0577/RTOG 1071 and CATNON trials, respectively.

LGGs

Radiotherapy for LGGs has benefited from improved conformality in radiation treat-ment delivery, and improved lesion visualization on MRI. Although the optimal timing of radiotherapy remains unclear, mounting evidence supports delaying radiotherapy until the time of progression. Because EORTC 22845 [Phase III Randomized Compar-ison of Early vs No or Late Radiotherapy in Adult Patients with Grade I/II Supratentorial Astrocytomas and Oligodendrogliomas (EORTC 22845)] found no difference in overall survival (but improved progression-free survival) with early radiotherapy,[47] and radio-therapy could be avoided altogether in 35% of patients, many clinicians delay radio-therapy until tumor progression and failure of systemic agents. Recent evidence indicates that patients treated with radiotherapy for LGGs (vs those who were not treated with radiotherapy) have a higher rate of significant neurocognitive side effects (53% vs 27%).[48]

Dose of radiotherapy for LGGs remains 45 to 50.4 Gy,[49,50] given the lack of evidence for improved outcomes with higher doses. This dose has been challenged, and a recent retrospective analysis questioned whether larger-volume tumors, or tumors with more residual disease, should receive more radiotherapy.[51] Nonetheless, in the absence of randomized evidence supporting higher doses of radiotherapy, the concept of escalating doses for large residual LGGs remains investigational and is not the standard of care.

Current trials (ECOG E3F05/RTOG 1072) [Phase III Study of Radiation Therapy With or Without Temozolomide for Symptomatic or Progressive Low-Grade Gliomas (NCT00978458)] are investigating whether the addition of temozolomide to fraction-ated radiotherapy improves progression-free survival and/or overall survival for patients with progressive or symptomatic LGGs.

Recurrent, previously irradiated gliomas

With increasing patient survival, gliomas often recur peripheral to a previously irradi-ated region of the brain. The high risk of radiation necrosis associated with retreatment of the brain must be weighed against the inevitable disease progression when salvage systemic therapies have failed. If feasible, surgery can confirm disease progression from pseudoprogression. Multiple case series regarding reirradiation via fractionated SRS have been published[52–54]; most investigators suggest doses of 36 to 46 Gy[55] in 2-Gy fractions,[56] although full-dose retreatment may be possible when the recurrent disease is peripheral to the previous tumor, or if 11 months or more have passed since the previous treatment. Treatment margins are typically tighter for retreatment, because the goal is to obtain local control and minimize the risk of radionecrosis. Nonetheless, radiation necrosis rates remains high given the substantial cumulative doses delivered.[57]

Ependymomas

The role of radiotherapy after gross total resection of low-grade intracranial ependy-momas is controversial; radiotherapy is typically reserved for adjuvant treatment after subtotal resection, if reoperation and gross total resection are not possible. For higher-grade intracranial ependymomas, radiotherapy is typically delivered to the gross tumor bed. Craniospinal irradiation is still delivered at some institutions, followed by a boost to any residual intracranial tumor.

Radiosurgery as a boost for recurrent intracranial disease has been investigated by the Pittsburgh group, among others.[58] Outcomes are modest, with a 5-year progression-free survival of 45.8%. Small-volume tumors and homogeneously enhancing tumors on MRI seemed to have the best outcomes, although these findings need to be validated by other institutions.

Germ cell tumors

Radiotherapy for germ cell tumors in adults still involves treatment of the gross disease and ventricular system.[59] Focal therapy that avoids ventricular irradiation is associated with an unacceptable rate of recurrent disease. In patients with, or at high risk for, disseminated disease, craniospinal irradiation, although toxic, remains a mainstay of treatment.

PCNSL

Treatment of PCNSL has traditionally involved radiotherapy with or without chemotherapy. However, recent investigations have focused on the use of high-dose chemotherapy as initial treatment, without radiotherapy. Various methods of chemotherapy delivery are being investigated, including intrathecal and intra-arterial administration, as well as high-dose intravenous therapy requiring stem cell support. Despite this escalation in chemotherapy intensity, most patients eventually need radiotherapy.[60,61] Therefore, some clinicians advocate treatment of all patients with whole-brain radiotherapy (WBRT) (to a dose of 45 Gy in 1.8-Gy fractions), with treatment portals modified depending on ocular involvement.[62] To determine whether or not patients who have had a complete response to systemic therapy need WBRT, patients should be enrolled in RTOG 1114 [Phase II Randomized Study of Rituximab, Methotrexate, Procarbazine, Vincristine, and Cytarabine With and Without Low-Dose Whole-Brain Radiotherapy for Primary Central Nervous System Lymphoma (NCT01399372)], which is a randomized phase II trial investigating rituximab, methotrexate, procarbazine, vincristine, and cytarabine with or without WBRT delivered to a low dose of 23.4 Gy. Progression-free survival is the primary outcome investigated in this trial, with overall survival a secondary outcome of interest.

Traditionally benign lesions: meningiomas, vestibular schwannomas, and pituitary tumors

Radiation is used for the treatment of benign lesions when (1) the likelihood and severity of future complications (from nontreatment) is greater than the risk of late radiation-induced complications and radiation-induced malignancy, (2) surgery is believed to be too dangerous for the patient because of tumor location or comorbidities, and (3) radiation has a reasonable chance of benefit. Weighing these 3 conditions is a matter of physician judgment; treatment recommendations preferably involve a multidisciplinary team of clinicians.

Because benign conditions such as WHO grade I meningiomas, vestibular schwannomas, and pituitary adenomas are usually well circumscribed with sharply defined margins, treatment techniques that use an equally sharp dose gradient at the desired treatment volume edge are used. These techniques typically involve treatment with stereotaxis, either with SRS or fractionated stereotactic radiotherapy. Radiosurgical treatment (typically a single fraction) is used if the tumor size and local neuroanatomy allow for it. A typical size limit for benign tumor treatment with SRS is in the order of 3 to 4 cm in the greatest dimension. Doses typically used for SRS treatment are usually less than that given for malignant tumors, because growth arrest of the tumor is all that is required, rather than ablation and death of all targeted cells.

SRS has shown 10-year local control rates in the order of 95% to 99%[63] for meningiomas and is similarly excellent for vestibular schwannomas.[64] For nonsecretory pituitary adenomas, control of tumor growth is an important outcome that is effectively managed by SRS 90% to 100% of the time.[65] However, obtaining normalization of hormone levels for secretory adenomas is more difficult, and often requires multimodal management with other medical disciplines. For these hormone-secreting tumors, single-treatment SRS is preferred over fractionated treatment because of a more rapid normalization in hormone levels after treatment.[66]

Fractionated radiotherapy is delivered when the tumor is too large for single-fraction SRS, or the lesion is too close to critical anatomic structures such as the optic chiasm or brainstem. For meningiomas, tumor control rates reported in the literature appear slightly worse than single-fraction radiotherapy.[67] However, this finding may be a function of selection (larger tumors are typically treated with fractionated treatment at centers in which SRS is available), in addition to radiobiology. For vestibular schwannomas, some investigators believe that fractionated radiotherapy is associated with improved hearing preservation compared with SRS,[68] but conflicting studies exist showing no difference between the two.[69,70] Hearing preservation with SRS is likely better when care is taken to avoid high dose to the cochlea[71,72] and/or vestibular canals.[73] For pituitary adenomas, SRS is generally preferred over fractionated treatment,[74] unless the tumor is immediately adjacent to the optic chiasm, or SRS is not available or otherwise not logistically possible.

Brain metastases

The mainstay of the treatment of intracranial metastatic disease has been WBRT. However, because medical oncologists are increasingly able to control systemic disease for prolonged periods, the approach to the treatment of brain metastases is turning toward balancing intracranial tumor control with preservation of neurocognition.

Patients with oligometastatic disease and good extracranial disease control are being increasingly treated with SRS. Three randomized trials[75–77] have investigated radiosurgery alone compared with radiosurgery followed by WBRT in patients with 1 to 3 metastases. These trials indicated no detriment to survival with the omission of WBRT, and 1 trial[75] reported an increase in survival for patients in whom WBRT was omitted. For patients with more metastases, treatment needs to be tailored to their survival and systemic therapy, in a multidisciplinary manner. If long-term survival is expected, aggressive radiosurgical treatment, in the interest of neuropreservation, should be considered.

Childhood tumors

A comprehensive update of childhood tumors and their treatment with radiotherapy is beyond the scope of this review. However, in general, advances in radiotherapy for pediatric intracranial tumors have centered around 3 main themes[78]: (1) the use of molecular subtyping to more accurately stratify tumor aggressiveness and the selection of treatments based on this stratification, (2) radiation and chemotherapy intensification for tumors that are traditionally believed to be treatment resistant, and (3) reduction of radiation dose and extent for patients with tumors that have a high likelihood of control, to reduce long-term toxicity, an especially important consideration in pediatric radiotherapy.

SUMMARY

Over the past several decades, technological advances have led to significant improvements in the treatment of primary brain tumors. Development of the operating microscope, neuroanesthesia, and robust MRI have revolutionized the practice of neurosurgery. Improved targeting and treatment planning technology has allowed for more conformal radiotherapy, with sparing of normal brain tissue.

Future research will exploit existing surgical technologies to deliver novel therapeutics.[79] The application of proton and heavy ion therapy will become more widespread, as these machines become miniaturized and more affordable. Improved understanding of the molecular basis of cancer and cancer treatment is paving the way for future therapy that will be defined not only by histopathology but also by the molecular signature of the tumor. Although many primary brain tumors have been historically incurable, given the enormity of ongoing research efforts, it is anticipated that the coming decades will bring significant improvements in the treatment of these diseases.

REFERENCES

1. Wen PY, Kesari S. Malignant gliomas in adults. N Engl J Med 2008;359:492–507.
2. Preusser M, de Ribaupierre S, Wohrer A, et al. Current concepts and management of glioblastoma. Ann Neurol 2011;70:9–21.
3. Sanai N, Berger MS. Intraoperative stimulation techniques for functional pathway preservation and glioma resection. Neurosurg Focus 2010;28:E1.
4. Laws ER, Parney IF, Huang W, et al. Survival following surgery and prognostic factors for recently diagnosed malignant glioma: data from the Glioma Outcomes Project. J Neurosurg 2003;99:467–73.
5. Stummer W, van den Bent MJ, Westphal M. Cytoreductive surgery of glioblastoma as the key to successful adjuvant therapies: new arguments in an old discussion. Acta Neurochir (Wien) 2011;153:1211–8.
6. Sanai N, Polley MY, McDermott MW, et al. An extent of resection threshold for newly diagnosed glioblastomas. J Neurosurg 2011;115:3–8.
7. Sawaya R. Extent of resection in malignant gliomas: a critical summary. J Neurooncol 1999;42:303–5.
8. Lacroix M, Abi-Said D, Fourney DR, et al. A multivariate analysis of 416 patients with glioblastoma multiforme: prognosis, extent of resection, and survival. J Neurosurg 2001;95:190–8.
9. Simpson JR, Horton J, Scott C, et al. Influence of location and extent of surgical resection on survival of patients with glioblastoma multiforme: results of three consecutive Radiation Therapy Oncology Group (RTOG) clinical trials. Int J Radiat Oncol Biol Phys 1993;26:239–44.
10. Stummer W, Pichlmeier U, Meinel T, et al. Fluorescence-guided surgery with 5-aminolevulinic acid for resection of malignant glioma: a randomised controlled multicentre phase III trial. Lancet Oncol 2006;7:392–401.
11. Senft C, Bink A, Franz K, et al. Intraoperative MRI guidance and extent of resection in glioma surgery: a randomised, controlled trial. Lancet Oncol 2011;12: 997–1003.
12. Pouratian N, Schiff D. Management of low-grade glioma. Curr Neurol Neurosci Rep 2010;10:224–31.
13. van den Bent MJ, Wefel JS, Schiff D, et al. Response assessment in neuro-oncology (a report of the RANO group): assessment of outcome in trials of diffuse low-grade gliomas. Lancet Oncol 2011;12:583–93.
14. Smith JS, Chang EF, Lamborn KR, et al. Role of extent of resection in the long-term outcome of low-grade hemispheric gliomas. J Clin Oncol 2008;26: 1338–45.

15. McGirt MJ, Chaichana KL, Attenello FJ, et al. Extent of surgical resection is independently associated with survival in patients with hemispheric infiltrating low-grade gliomas. Neurosurgery 2008;63:700–7 [author reply: 707–8].
16. Gilbert MR, Ruda R, Soffietti R. Ependymomas in adults. Curr Neurol Neurosci Rep 2010;10:240–7.
17. Niazi TN, Jensen EM, Jensen RL. WHO grade II and III supratentorial hemispheric ependymomas in adults: case series and review of treatment options. J Neurooncol 2009;91:323–8.
18. Metellus P, Barrie M, Figarella-Branger D, et al. Multicentric French study on adult intracranial ependymomas: prognostic factors analysis and therapeutic considerations from a cohort of 152 patients. Brain 2007;130:1338–49.
19. Kawabata Y, Takahashi JA, Arakawa Y, et al. Long-term outcome in patients harboring intracranial ependymoma. J Neurosurg 2005;103:31–7.
20. Schwartz TH, Kim S, Glick RS, et al. Supratentorial ependymomas in adult patients. Neurosurgery 1999;44:721–31.
21. Paulino AC, Wen BC, Buatti JM, et al. Intracranial ependymomas: an analysis of prognostic factors and patterns of failure. Am J Clin Oncol 2002;25:117–22.
22. Konovalov AN, Pitskhelauri DI. Principles of treatment of the pineal region tumors. Surg Neurol 2003;59:250–68.
23. Gerstner ER, Batchelor TT. Primary central nervous system lymphoma. Arch Neurol 2010;67:291–7.
24. Morris PG, Abrey LE. Therapeutic challenges in primary CNS lymphoma. Lancet Neurol 2009;8:581–92.
25. Oya S, Kim SH, Sade B, et al. The natural history of intracranial meningiomas. J Neurosurg 2011;114:1250–6.
26. Sughrue ME, Rutkowski MJ, Aranda D, et al. Treatment decision making based on the published natural history and growth rate of small meningiomas. J Neurosurg 2010;113:1036–42.
27. Arthurs BJ, Fairbanks RK, Demakas JJ, et al. A review of treatment modalities for vestibular schwannoma. Neurosurg Rev 2011;34:265–77 [discussion: 277–9].
28. Quant EC, Wen PY. Response assessment in neuro-oncology. Curr Oncol Rep 2011;13:50–6.
29. Winder MJ, Mayberg MR. Recent advances in pituitary tumor management. Curr Opin Endocrinol Diabetes Obes 2011;18:278–88.
30. Strychowsky J, Nayan S, Reddy K, et al. Purely endoscopic transsphenoidal surgery versus traditional microsurgery for resection of pituitary adenomas: systematic review. J Otolaryngol Head Neck Surg 2011;40:175–85.
31. Patchell RA, Tibbs PA, Walsh JW, et al. A randomized trial of surgery in the treatment of single metastases to the brain. N Engl J Med 1990;322:494–500.
32. Patchell RA, Tibbs PA, Regine WF, et al. Postoperative radiotherapy in the treatment of single metastases to the brain: a randomized trial. JAMA 1998;280:1485–9.
33. Amelio D, Lorentini S, Schwarz M, et al. Intensity-modulated radiation therapy in newly diagnosed glioblastoma: a systematic review on clinical and technical issues. Radiother Oncol 2010;97:361–9.
34. Bonner JA, Harari PM, Giralt J, et al. Radiotherapy plus cetuximab for squamous-cell carcinoma of the head and neck. N Engl J Med 2006;354:567–78.
35. van Nifterik KA, van den Berg J, Stalpers LJ, et al. Differential radiosensitizing potential of temozolomide in MGMT promoter methylated glioblastoma multiforme cell lines. Int J Radiat Oncol Biol Phys 2007;69:1246–53.
36. Martin M. Laser accelerated radiotherapy: is it on its way to the clinic? J Natl Cancer Inst 2009;101:450–1.

37. Combs SE, Burkholder I, Edler L, et al. Randomised phase I/II study to evaluate carbon ion radiotherapy versus fractionated stereotactic radiotherapy in patients with recurrent or progressive gliomas: the CINDERELLA trial. BMC Cancer 2010;10:533.

38. Combs SE, Kieser M, Rieken S, et al. Randomized phase II study evaluating a carbon ion boost applied after combined radiochemotherapy with temozolomide versus a proton boost after radiochemotherapy with temozolomide in patients with primary glioblastoma: the CLEOPATRA trial. BMC Cancer 2010;10:478.

39. Stupp R, Mason WP, van den Bent MJ, et al. Radiotherapy plus concomitant and adjuvant temozolomide for glioblastoma. N Engl J Med 2005;352:987–96.

40. Stupp R, Hegi ME, Mason WP, et al. Effects of radiotherapy with concomitant and adjuvant temozolomide versus radiotherapy alone on survival in glioblastoma in a randomised phase III study: 5-year analysis of the EORTC-NCIC trial. Lancet Oncol 2009;10:459–66.

41. Cho KH, Kim JY, Lee SH, et al. Simultaneous integrated boost intensity-modulated radiotherapy in patients with high-grade gliomas. Int J Radiat Oncol Biol Phys 2010;78:390–7.

42. McDonald MW, Shu HK, Curran WJ Jr, et al. Pattern of failure after limited margin radiotherapy and temozolomide for glioblastoma. Int J Radiat Oncol Biol Phys 2011;79:130–6.

43. Gilbert MR, Lang FF. Anaplastic oligodendroglial tumors: a tale of two trials. J Clin Oncol 2006;24:2689–90.

44. Vogelbaum MA, Berkey B, Peereboom D, et al. Phase II trial of preirradiation and concurrent temozolomide in patients with newly diagnosed anaplastic oligodendrogliomas and mixed anaplastic oligoastrocytomas: RTOG BR0131. Neuro Oncol 2009;11:167–75.

45. Gan HK, Rosenthal MA, Dowling A, et al. A phase II trial of primary temozolomide in patients with grade III oligodendroglial brain tumors. Neuro Oncol 2010;12:500–7.

46. Wick W, Hartmann C, Engel C, et al. NOA-04 randomized phase III trial of sequential radiochemotherapy of anaplastic glioma with procarbazine, lomustine, and vincristine or temozolomide. J Clin Oncol 2009;27:5874–80.

47. van den Bent MJ, Afra D, de Witte O, et al. Long-term efficacy of early versus delayed radiotherapy for low-grade astrocytoma and oligodendroglioma in adults: the EORTC 22845 randomised trial. Lancet 2005;366:985–90.

48. Douw L, Klein M, Fagel SS, et al. Cognitive and radiological effects of radiotherapy in patients with low-grade glioma: long-term follow-up. Lancet Neurol 2009;8:810–8.

49. Shaw E, Arusell R, Scheithauer B, et al. Prospective randomized trial of low- versus high-dose radiation therapy in adults with supratentorial low-grade glioma: initial report of a North Central Cancer Treatment Group/Radiation Therapy Oncology Group/Eastern Cooperative Oncology Group study. J Clin Oncol 2002;20:2267–76.

50. Kiebert GM, Curran D, Aaronson NK, et al. Quality of life after radiation therapy of cerebral low-grade gliomas of the adult: results of a randomised phase III trial on dose response (EORTC trial 22844). EORTC Radiotherapy Co-operative Group. Eur J Cancer 1998;34:1902–9.

51. Leighton C, Fisher B, Macdonald D, et al. The dose-volume interaction in adult supratentorial low-grade glioma: higher radiation dose is beneficial among patients with partial resection. J Neurooncol 2007;82:165–70.

52. Minniti G, Armosini V, Salvati M, et al. Fractionated stereotactic reirradiation and concurrent temozolomide in patients with recurrent glioblastoma. J Neurooncol 2011;103:683–91.

53. Torok JA, Wegner RE, Mintz AH, et al. Re-irradiation with radiosurgery for recurrent glioblastoma multiforme. Technol Cancer Res Treat 2011;10:253–8.

54. Fogh SE, Andrews DW, Glass J, et al. Hypofractionated stereotactic radiation therapy: an effective therapy for recurrent high-grade gliomas. J Clin Oncol 2010;28:3048–53.

55. Combs SE, Thilmann C, Edler L, et al. Efficacy of fractionated stereotactic reirradiation in recurrent gliomas: long-term results in 172 patients treated in a single institution. J Clin Oncol 2005;23:8863–9.

56. Nieder C, Astner ST, Mehta MP, et al. Improvement, clinical course, and quality of life after palliative radiotherapy for recurrent glioblastoma. Am J Clin Oncol 2008; 31:300–5.

57. Kong DS, Lee JI, Park K, et al. Efficacy of stereotactic radiosurgery as a salvage treatment for recurrent malignant gliomas. Cancer 2008;112:2046–51.

58. Kano H, Niranjan A, Kondziolka D, et al. Outcome predictors for intracranial ependymoma radiosurgery. Neurosurgery 2009;64:279–87 [discussion: 287–8].

59. Chen YW, Huang PI, Ho DM, et al. Change in treatment strategy for intracranial germinoma: long-term follow-up experience at a single institute. Cancer 2011. DOI: 10.1002/cncr.26564. [Epub ahead of print].

60. Montemurro M, Kiefer T, Schuler F, et al. Primary central nervous system lymphoma treated with high-dose methotrexate, high-dose busulfan/thiotepa, autologous stem-cell transplantation and response-adapted whole-brain radiotherapy: results of the multicenter Ostdeutsche Studiengruppe Hamato-Onkologie OSHO-53 phase II study. Ann Oncol 2007;18:665–71.

61. Colombat P, Lemevel A, Bertrand P, et al. High-dose chemotherapy with autologous stem cell transplantation as first-line therapy for primary CNS lymphoma in patients younger than 60 years: a multicenter phase II study of the GOELAMS group. Bone Marrow Transplant 2006;38:417–20.

62. Schultz CJ, Bovi J. Current management of primary central nervous system lymphoma. Int J Radiat Oncol Biol Phys 2010;76:666–78.

63. Kondziolka D, Madhok R, Lunsford LD, et al. Stereotactic radiosurgery for convexity meningiomas. J Neurosurg 2009;111:458–63.

64. Roos DE, Potter AE, Brophy BP. Stereotactic radiosurgery for acoustic neuromas: what happens long term? Int J Radiat Oncol Biol Phys 2012;82(4):1352–5.

65. Loeffler JS, Shih HA. Radiation therapy in the management of pituitary adenomas. J Clin Endocrinol Metab 2011;96(7):1992–2003.

66. Kong DS, Lee JI, Lim do H, et al. The efficacy of fractionated radiotherapy and stereotactic radiosurgery for pituitary adenomas: long-term results of 125 consecutive patients treated in a single institution. Cancer 2007;110:854–60.

67. Estall V, Treece SJ, Jena R, et al. Pattern of relapse after fractionated external beam radiotherapy for meningioma: experience from Addenbrooke's Hospital. Clin Oncol (R Coll Radiol) 2009;21:745–52.

68. Andrews DW, Suarez O, Goldman HW, et al. Stereotactic radiosurgery and fractionated stereotactic radiotherapy for the treatment of acoustic schwannomas: comparative observations of 125 patients treated at one institution. Int J Radiat Oncol Biol Phys 2001;50:1265–78.

69. Meijer OW, Vandertop WP, Baayen JC, et al. Single-fraction vs. fractionated linac-based stereotactic radiosurgery for vestibular schwannoma: a single-institution study. Int J Radiat Oncol Biol Phys 2003;56:1390–6.

70. Collen C, Ampe B, Gevaert T, et al. Single fraction versus fractionated linac-based stereotactic radiotherapy for vestibular schwannoma: a single-institution experience. Int J Radiat Oncol Biol Phys 2011;81:e503–9.

71. Timmer FC, Hanssens PE, van Haren AE, et al. Gamma knife radiosurgery for vestibular schwannomas: results of hearing preservation in relation to the cochlear radiation dose. Laryngoscope 2009;119:1076–81.
72. Kano H, Kondziolka D, Khan A, et al. Predictors of hearing preservation after stereotactic radiosurgery for acoustic neuroma. J Neurosurg 2009;111:863–73.
73. Gerosa M, Mesiano N, Longhi M, et al. Gamma Knife surgery in vestibular schwannomas: impact on the anterior and posterior labyrinth. J Neurosurg 2010;113(Suppl):128–35.
74. Pollock BE. Comparing radiation therapy and radiosurgery for pituitary adenoma patients. World Neurosurg 2011, in press.
75. Chang EL, Wefel JS, Hess KR, et al. Neurocognition in patients with brain metastases treated with radiosurgery or radiosurgery plus whole-brain irradiation: a randomised controlled trial. Lancet Oncol 2009;10:1037–44.
76. Aoyama H, Shirato H, Tago M, et al. Stereotactic radiosurgery plus whole-brain radiation therapy vs stereotactic radiosurgery alone for treatment of brain metastases: a randomized controlled trial. JAMA 2006;295:2483–91.
77. Kocher M, Soffietti R, Abacioglu U, et al. Adjuvant whole-brain radiotherapy versus observation after radiosurgery or surgical resection of one to three cerebral metastases: results of the EORTC 22952-26001 study. J Clin Oncol 2011; 29:134–41.
78. Pollack IF. Multidisciplinary management of childhood brain tumors: a review of outcomes, recent advances, and challenges. J Neurosurg Pediatr 2011;8:135–48.
79. Patel T, Zhou J, Piepmeier JM, et al. Polymeric nanoparticles for drug delivery to the central nervous system. Adv Drug Deliv Rev 2012;64(7):701–5.

Complications of Brain Tumors and Their Treatment

Jill Lacy, MD[a,*], Hamid Saadati, MD[a], James B. Yu, MD[b]

KEYWORDS

- Vasogenic edema • Corticosteroids • Venous thromboembolic disease • Seizures
- Antiepileptic drugs • Radiation-related toxicities • Pseudoprogression

KEY POINTS

- Recognition and appropriate treatment of complications of brain tumors, including vasogenic edema, venous thromboembolic disease, seizures, and the neurologic complications of radiation therapy, is essential to optimize quality of life and extend survival.
- Symptomatic peritumoral edema is treated with dexamethasone, tapered to the lowest dose that optimizes neurologic function, and seizures are treated with a newer antiepileptic drug (eg, levetiracetam) to minimize adverse effects and drug interactions; seizure prophylaxis is not indicated in patients who never had a seizure.
- Clinicians must maintain a high index of suspicion for pulmonary embolism or deep venous thrombosis in patients with brain tumors. Most patients with venous thromboembolism can be safely anticoagulated according to consensus guidelines for anticoagulation in patients with cancer, without undue risk of intracranial hemorrhage, obviating the need for inferior vena cava filtration devices.
- Complications of radiation therapy encompass diverse pathogenetic mechanisms and neurologic manifestations and are temporally defined as acute (during or shortly after), early delayed (weeks to 4 months), and late (more than 6 months) reactions.
- Symptomatic acute and early delayed radiation reactions are managed with corticosteroids; the early delayed reaction may mimic progression of disease (pseudoprogression), but is paradoxically associated with a favorable prognosis and should not lead to premature termination of effective therapy.

INTRODUCTION

Patients with central nervous system (CNS) neoplasms are at risk for an array of medical and neurologic complications of their disease or its treatment. These complications represent a significant cause of neurologic and systemic morbidity, and their recognition and appropriate management is essential in optimizing quality of life and

Disclosures: None.
[a] Section of Medical Oncology, Department of Medicine, Yale University School of Medicine, 333 Cedar Street, New Haven, CT 06510, USA; [b] Department of Therapeutic Radiology, Yale University School of Medicine, 333 Cedar Street, New Haven, CT 06510, USA
* Corresponding author.
E-mail address: jill.lacy@yale.edu

Hematol Oncol Clin N Am 26 (2012) 779–796
doi:10.1016/j.hoc.2012.04.007
0889-8588/12/$ – see front matter © 2012 Elsevier Inc. All rights reserved.

hemonc.theclinics.com

extending survival for patients with brain tumors. Peritumoral edema, seizures, and thromboembolic disease are among the most common complications related to the underlying neoplasm, whereas complications of treatment include radiation-related toxicities and the adverse effects of medications, including corticosteroids, antiepileptic drugs, and chemotherapy.

This article discusses the clinical features and management of the common or serious tumor- and treatment-related complications of CNS neoplasms, including peritumoral edema, thromboembolic disease, seizures, and radiation-related toxicities.

PERITUMORAL EDEMA
Pathophysiology

Cerebral edema is a significant cause of morbidity and mortality in patients with CNS neoplasms. The edema associated with primary and metastatic brain tumors is typically vasogenic, that is, due to increased vascular permeability associated with blood brain barrier (BBB) disruption, rather than cytoxic, that is, hypoxia induced by ischemia or trauma. BBB disruption allows passage of plasma fluid and proteins from the vascular compartment into brain parenchyma, resulting in edema and increased interstitial pressure within and around the tumor. Peritumoral edema correlates with histologic BBB abnormalities, including abnormal tight junctions, fenestrations, thickened basement membrane of the capillary endothelium, and diminished contact between pericytes and astrocytes.[1,2]

Although the precise mechanism of BBB disruption is not fully understood, the pro-angiogenic peptide, vascular endothelial growth factor (VEGF), plays a central role. VEGF is over expressed and secreted by glial tumors, metastatic tumors, and meningiomas.[3–7] In pre-clinical models, VEGF stimulates aberrant vascular proliferation and induces the histologic changes in capillary endothelium associated with BBB disruption.[4] Levels of tumor-associated VEGF expression correlate with the grade of glial tumors.[8] Thus, high-grade gliomas (anaplastic astrocytoma, oligodendroglioma, and glioblastoma) and metastatic lesions typically demonstrate peritumoral edema and enhancement on imaging, whereas low-grade gliomas do not.

Imaging

Radiographically, disruption of the BBB is associated with contrast enhancement and edema. The most widely used magnetic resonance imaging (MRI) sequences to assess vascular permeability are the post-contrast (gadolinium) T1 sequences, which demonstrate parenchymal enhancement in areas of brain where disrupted BBB does not exclude gadolinium. Edema is best visualized on the noncontrast T2 and fluid-attenuated inversion recovery (FLAIR) sequences. These sequences show hyperintensity in areas of edema that are typically much more extensive than the enhancing area, although hyperintensity may also reflect infiltrative nonenhancing tumor or post-treatment gliosis. Other MRI sequences (diffusion-weighted, dynamic contrast-enhanced) have been explored to distinguish vasogenic edema from infiltrative tumor but have not proven definitive.

Clinical Presentation

At initial diagnosis, most patients with high-grade gliomas or brain metastases present with symptoms related to vasogenic edema. Vasogenic edema exacerbates focal neurologic symptoms related to tumor mass and causes nonfocal symptoms of increased intracranial pressure, including headache, lethargy, and confusion. Patients may experience near syncope or syncope due to "plateau waves" caused by transient increases in intracranial pressure from activities associated with the Valsalva maneuver or upon standing. Progressive, extensive vasogenic edema can lead to herniation and death.

Over the course of their disease, patients with brain tumors often develop symptomatic exacerbations of vasogenic edema. Common causes of increasing edema are steroid withdrawal, radiation effects (discussed later in this article), or tumor progression. Repeat brain imaging usually shows increasing edema and/or contrast enhancement, although it is not possible to distinguish increasing edema caused by tumor progression and pseudoprogression.

Treatment

Corticosteroids have been used to treat vasogenic edema for over 5 decades and are the mainstay of management. On imaging studies, corticosteroids decrease capillary permeability as early as 6 hours and decrease water content of peritumoral brain tissue 48 to 72 hours after administration.[9,10] The mechanism of action of corticosteroids in stabilizing the BBB is uncertain. Pre-clinical studies suggest that corticosteroids downregulate VEGF and upregulate angiopoietin-1 production in glial tumors via the glucocorticoid receptor.[11,12]

Corticosteroids are indicated in all patients with symptomatic vasogenic edema. Although there is a paucity of controlled studies, clinical experience over decades has established practice principles guiding the use of corticosteroids as follows[13]: (1) Dexamethasone is preferred because of its relative lack of mineralocorticoid effects and long half-life compared with other corticosteroids, although other corticosteroids have similar efficacy in equipotent doses; (2) once maximum clinical benefit has been achieved with initial dosing, dexamethasone should be tapered slowly to the lowest dose needed to maintain optimum neurologic function; (3) patients must be closely monitored and treated for adverse effects; (4) asymptomatic patients do not require corticosteroids; (5) in the event of impending herniation from mass effect, emergent neurosurgical evaluation for surgical decompression or initiation of osmotherapy is indicated.

Dose, Duration, and Efficacy of Dexamethasone

Dexamethasone is often administered every 6 hours, although its half-life allows twice daily dosing. Intravenous dosing is not required, as oral absorption is excellent. Most patients receive an initial dose of 16 mg daily in divided doses. However, in patients with brain metastases not at risk for herniation, one randomized trial showed no advantage of 16 mg compared with 4 or 8 mg/d, with respect to improving Karnofsky performance status (KPS), whereas toxicities were substantially increased at the higher dose.[14] Thus, in patients with mild symptoms, an initial dose of 4 to 8 mg/d is appropriate; for moderate or severe symptoms, 16 mg/d is recommended.

Most patients with symptomatic vasogenic edema experience an improvement in neurologic symptoms and KPS within hours of initiation of dexamethasone, although maximum benefit is usually not seen for several days.[14] Once maximum clinical benefit is achieved, dexamethasone should be tapered to the lowest dose that optimizes neurologic function or discontinued, if tolerated. A slow taper is advised to avoid rebound edema, especially during radiotherapy. Decrements of no greater than 50% of the previous dose at intervals of no less than every 4 days are recommended. Because radiation may transiently increase vasogenic edema, continuation of dexamethasone during radiotherapy may be necessary.

Adverse Effects of Dexamethasone

The acute and chronic toxicities of corticosteroids are well known. In patients with brain tumors, acute and subacute toxic effects of dexamethasone are common and cause significant iatrogenic morbidity (**Table 1**). The incidence of toxic effects correlates with the height of the daily dose, duration of treatment, and cumulative total dose.[14-16] Thus, dexamethasone should be administered in the lowest possible daily dose for the shortest duration needed to optimize neurologic status.

In one large series of patients with brain metastases, the incidence of specific adverse effects of dexamethasone (16 mg/d for 7 or 28 days) was as follows: cushingoid facies 65%, proximal weakness 38%, peripheral edema 26%, hypertension 26%, gastrointestinal side effects 24%, mental status changes 21%, hyperglycemia 21%, and infectious complications 9%.[14]The incidence and severity of adverse effects in patients with high-grade gliomas is generally higher than that in patients with metastases because of the longer duration of treatment (mean 4–6 months compared with <2 months).[15] Complications of long-term corticosteroid use (eg, cataracts, glaucoma, osteopenia) are encountered infrequently because of the limited survival of patients with brain tumors requiring chronic dexamethasone.

Steroid-Induced Myopathy

Steroid myopathy is common in patients with brain tumors, causing significant debility in 10% to 40% of patients.[14,17] In adult patients with primary brain tumors treated with dexamethasone for 2 or more weeks, 10% developed myopathy at a median of 11 weeks (range 4–48 weeks).[17] The onset is subacute, over weeks, and usually not seen before 8 weeks of exposure. Myopathy can occur over a wide range of daily, continuous, and cumulative steroid dosing, although duration of treatment has the greatest impact on incidence. There is a positive correlation between myopathy and cushingoid body habitus and a negative correlation with concomitant use of phenytoin, possibly due to phenytoin-induced hepatic catabolism of dexamethasone.[17]

Steroid myopathy is characterized by nontender, bilateral proximal muscle weakness affecting legs more than arms, with preservation of normal sensation, bowel and bladder function, and deep tendon reflexes. This complication has a significant negative

Table 1		
Important side effects of corticosteroids in patients with brain tumors		
Systemic		**Neurologic**
Common, not serious		
Increased appetite		Insomnia
Weight gain		Tremor
Fluid retention		Emotional lability
Acne		Hiccups
Skin fragility, purpura		
Serious		
Myopathy		Delirium
Infections		Psychosis
Hyperglycemia, diabetes		
Hpokalemia		
Potentially life-threatening		
Pneumocystis pneumonia		Seizures (drug interactions)
GI bleeding		
GI perforation		

Abbreviation: GI, gastrointestinal.

impact on quality of life. All patients with steroid myopathy experience a decline in KPS, and 35% of previously ambulatory patients require assistance with ambulation.[17]

Treatment is challenging, as recovery requires withdrawal or dose attenuation of corticosteroids and may take months. Anecdotal reports suggest that nonfluorinated corticosteroids are less likely to cause myopathy than dexamethasone, and thus, transitioning to prednisone is an option if dexamethasone withdrawal is impossible. Physical therapy is advised, although there are no controlled studies evaluating its efficacy. In patients with progressive or recurrent tumor, the prognosis for recovery is poor, because of inability to taper dexamethasone and tumor-related decline in function.

Pneumocytis Jiorvecci (Carinii) Pneumonia

Pneumocytis jiorveci (carinii) pneumonia (PCP) is a potentially fatal complication of corticosteroid therapy. Although PCP is rare in patients with brain tumors (<2%), the mortality is high (33%–40%).[18,19] The risk of symptomatic PCP may be greatest as dexamethasone is tapered, but up to 50% of cases have occurred in patients on a stable steroid dose. Because lymphopenia is the major predisposing factor for PCP, the risk is particularly high in patients receiving dexamethasone while undergoing concurrent radiation and temozolomide.[20] Thus, all patients should receive PCP prophylaxis during chemoradiotherapy with temozolomide. In addition, PCP prophylaxis is recommended in patients receiving protracted dexamethasone treatment (>1–2 months) or who have persistent absolute lymphopenia (<500 cells/mm^3).

Gastrointestinal Effects

Corticosteroids do not substantially increase the risk of symptomatic gastritis or peptic ulcer disease unless other risk factors are present.[21] Thus, prophylactic therapy in patients on dexamethasone is restricted to those patients who are in the perioperative period, on high doses of dexamethasone (>16 mg/d), on concomitant nonsteroidal antiinflammatory drugs (NSAIDs), or with a history of gastritis or ulcer disease. When prophylaxis is indicated, proton pump inhibitors are recommended, as H2 receptor antagonists do not prevent NSAID-associated gastroduodenal disease.

Perforation of the bowel, especially of colonic diverticula, is a rare but potentially fatal complication in patients receiving corticosteroids.[22,23] Because steroids can mask the clinical signs of peritonitis, resulting in delays in diagnosis and intervention, bowel perforation must be considered in any patient on high dose or chronic steroids who presents with abdominal pain, fever of unknown origin, or unexplained leukocytosis.

Role of Bevacizumab

Given the central role of VEGF in BBB disruption and vasogenic edema, targeting the VEGF pathway represents a rational corticosteroid-sparing treatment strategy. In preclinical xenograft models of glioblastoma, VEGF pathway inhibitors decrease vascular permeability and normalize tumor vasculature in association with decreased edema.[24] The efficacy of this approach has been demonstrated in phase I/II studies in patients with recurrent glioblastoma treated with the VEGF inhibitor, bevacizumab, or the pan-VEGF receptor inhibitor, cedirinib.[25–29] These agents dramatically reduce contrast enhancement on T1 sequences and vasogenic edema on T2/FLAIR sequences in most patients, and favorable radiographic changes are associated with clinical benefit, including reduction in dexamethasone dosage. Bevacizumab is approved for treatment of progressive glioblastoma, and in this setting, it is an effective agent for management of peritumoral edema. However, in other clinical settings, the use of bevacizumab or other angiogenesis inhibitors for treatment of vasogenic edema remains investigational.

THROMBOEMBOLIC DISEASE

Venous thromboembolic disease is a widely recognized complication of malignancy, including primary and metastatic brain tumors. Historically, the risk of tumor-related intracranial hemorrhage (ICH) was considered a strong contraindication to the use of anticoagulation in patients with brain tumors. However, over the past 2 decades, clinical experience and retrospective studies have demonstrated that most patients with brain tumors are safely anticoagulated for venous thromboembolism (VTE), without increased risk of ICH. Thus, current treatment guidelines focus on identifying those patients who have an unacceptable risk of ICH, precluding anticoagulation, and treating all other patients according to consensus guidelines for management of VTE in malignancy.

Pathophysiology, Risk Factors, Incidence

Active malignancy is a recognized risk factor for VTE, and patients with malignant glial tumors have one of the highest rates of cancer-associated VTE, exceeded only by ovarian cancer. Hypercoagulability in patients with malignancy, including brain tumors, derives from complex alterations in homeostatic mechanisms of coagulation and fibrinolysis, related in part to tumor production of procoagulants and fibrinolytic inhibitors.[30] Glioma cells constitutively produce abundant procoagulants, most notably tissue factor and cancer procoagulant.[31,32] Biochemical evidence of activated coagulation, including elevated D-dimer levels, is often present in patients with glioma. In addition, aberrant fibrinolysis is apparent, with elevated circulating levels of plasminogen activator inhibitor-1, plasminogen, tissue plasminogen activator, and total fibrinolytic activity.[32]

The reported incidence of VTE in patients with malignant glioma is approximately 30%, and up to 20% of patients with brain metastases or primary CNS lymphoma develop symptomatic VTE.[31–34] The risk is highest in the post-operative period, but persists throughout the course of disease. Additional risk factors include paretic limb, glioblastoma histology, age more than 60 years, large tumor size, length of surgery, immobility, and administration of chemotherapy.[31–34]

Given the incidence of VTE in patients with brain tumors, clinicians must maintain a high degree of suspicion for pulmonary embolism or deep venous thrombosis in this setting. Subtle respiratory symptoms, unexplained tachycardia or fatigue, or lower extremity edema always warrant consideration of VTE in this high-risk patient population.

Contraindications to Anticoagulation

Although most patients with brain tumor who develop VTE can be safely anticoagulated, there are defined subsets of patients at high risk of ICH in whom anticoagulation is not advised. However, it is important to recognize that contraindications to anticoagulation are relative, and careful assessment of risks and benefits is imperative in decision making in all patients with life-threatening VTE.

Contraindication to anticoagulation in patients with brain tumors is related to the risk of spontaneous symptomatic intratumoral hemorrhage. This risk is low in gliomas and in metastases from most solid tumors (eg, breast, lung, gastrointestinal) (<5%). However, brain metastases from melanoma, choriocarcinoma, thyroid carcinoma, and renal carcinoma have a high risk of spontaneous hemorrhage (up to 70%), and thus, anticoagulation is contraindicated in these 4 diagnoses until the metastases have been definitively treated.[32] Other contraindications to anticoagulation unrelated to tumor type include prior history of ICH, bleeding diathesis including thrombopenia (usually <50,000), or ongoing life-threatening extracranial bleeding.

The incidence of VTE is particularly high in the post-operative period after craniotomy. The decision to anticoagulate is complicated by the uncertain risk of ICH in the post-operative period and must be made in consultation with neurosurgeons. Recent experience using continuous rather than bolus heparin indicates that anticoagulation does not increase the risk of ICH when initiated on post-op day 3 or 5.[35] Importantly, the risk of ICH is high when anticoagulation is initiated less than 48 hours after surgery or exceeds therapeutic levels. Blood products in the resection cavity is a common post-operative finding on imaging and does not necessary preclude initiation of anticoagulation for VTE.

Treatment and Secondary Prevention

In the absence of specific contraindications (as described earlier), VTE in patients with brain tumors should be treated with anticoagulants according to standard consensus guidelines for management of VTE in patients with cancer.[36–39] Multiple retrospective studies in patients with primary or metastatic brain tumors have shown that anticoagulation with warfarin or low-molecular-weight heparin (LMWH) is safe and not associated with an increased rate of ICH compared with patients without VTE.[40–42] Placement of an inferior vena cava filter is a suboptimal intervention because of the high rate of recurrent VTE after filter placement alone, exceeding 60% in one series,[41] and is appropriate only in patients in whom anticoagulation is contraindicated.

The need for neuroimaging to rule out occult brain metastases in patients with systemic cancer before initiation of anticoagulation is debated. In patients whose tumors are associated with a high risk of spontaneous hemorrhage (melanoma, renal, thyroid, choriocarcinoma), a pre-treatment noncontrast computed axial tomography scan or magnetic resonance imaging (MRI) is recommended, whereas the need for imaging with other diagnoses, in the absence of neurologic symptoms, is uncertain. In patients with known treated brain tumors (metastatic or primary), the need for a screening scan is also uncertain, in the absence of new neurologic symptoms.

Fixed dose of LMWH is the preferred agent for both initial therapy and long-term treatment.[36–39] The use of LMWH simplifies initial management and facilitates outpatient treatment in suitable patients. For long-term anticoagulation, LMWH is more effective than warfarin in reducing risk of recurrent VTE in patients with malignancy, albeit with no overall survival benefit, and the risk of hemorrhage with LMWH is the same or reduced compared with warfarin.[43,44] Based on these observations, LMWH is recommended for long-term anticoagulation of VTE in patients with brain tumors, although it has not been directly compared with warfarin specifically in this patient population. In addition to its superior efficacy, LMWH has the added advantage of absence of drug interactions or need for regular monitoring. In patients who do not tolerate daily injections, warfarin is an acceptable alternative, with the caveat that overanticoagulation may increase the risk of ICH. The optimum duration of anticoagulation after VTE is unresolved. However, because the risk of recurrent VTE after withdrawal of anticoagulation remains high in patients with active malignancy, indefinite anticoagulation is generally recommended in patients with brain tumors.

The use of bevacizumab in patients with primary or metastatic brain tumors has raised concerns about the safety of anticoagulants and concomitant bevacizumab. One series suggested no significant ICH in glioma patients treated with LMWH and bevacizumab.[45] However, until more data are available, bevacizumab should be used with caution in patients with brain tumors requiring anticoagulation.

Primary Prevention

Despite the high incidence of VTE in patients with malignant glioma, an extended course of prophylactic LMWH beyond the immediate post-operative period is not recommended. Long-term primary VTE prophylaxis with LMWH was evaluated in a placebo-controlled trial in patients with newly diagnosed malignant gliomas. Although there was a nonsignificant decrease in VTE incidence with LMWH, there was an increase in ICH events and no difference in overall survival.[46]

SEIZURES

Epilepsy is a common and potentially devastating complication of CNS neoplasms. Control of seizures is an important component of the interdisciplinary management of patients with brain tumors, and special challenges in these patients include interactions of antiepileptic drugs (AEDs) with chemotherapeutic agents and enhanced toxicities of AEDs.

Incidence, Risk Factors, Clinical Presentation

Approximately 25% of patients with brain tumors present with a seizure at diagnosis (range 14%–51%), and an additional 20% of patients will have seizures during the course of their disease (range 10%–45%).[47,48] The risk of seizures is related to the pathologic type and the anatomic location of the tumor.[47–52] Primary brain tumors are more epileptogenic than metastatic tumors, with a seizure incidence of approximately 60% versus 25%. In patients with primary brain tumors, seizures are more common in low-grade gliomas than in high-grade gliomas. In one large series, the prevalence of epilepsy was 85%, 69%, and 49% in low-grade gliomas, anaplastic gliomas, and glioblastomas, respectively.[49] In patients with metastases, risk of seizures is greatest in those with melanoma or hemorrhagic metastases.[51] Infratentorial tumors are rarely associated with epilepsy, whereas the risk of seizures is highest with cortical tumors, especially those located in the motor cortex or when there is involvement of leptomeninges.

Seizures in patients with brain tumors are typically localization-related, presenting as simple or complex seizures with or without secondary generalization. Although uncommon in patients with brain tumors, the risk of status epilepticus is greatest at the time of diagnosis or tumor progression.[53] Approximately 4% of patients with systemic cancers without brain metastases experience one or more seizures. Multiple factors in patients with malignancy can precipitate seizures or, alternatively, lower the seizure threshold from a known brain tumor, including metabolic derangements (hyponatremia, hypoglycemia), chemotherapy toxicities (intrathecal chemotherapy, vinca alkaloids, taxanes, busulfan), concomitant medications (antidepressants, neuroleptic agents, antibiotics), or infection.

Drug Treatment and Adverse Effects

All patients with a brain tumor who experience a seizure should be treated with an AED because of the high risk of recurrent seizures, according to treatment guidelines for symptomatic localization-related epilepsy.[54]

The enzyme-inducing AEDs that stimulate the hepatic cytochrome P450 (CYP) system (phenytoin, carbamazepine, and phenobarbital) should be avoided because of potential for clinically significant pharmacokinetic interactions, as many chemotherapeutic drugs and corticosteroids are metabolized by the CYP enzyme system. Thus, enzyme-inducing AEDs diminish antitumor efficacy of camptothecins, taxanes, vinca alkaloids, methotrexate, nitrosoureas, cyclophosphamide, procarbazine, thiotepa, and etoposide.[55] Conversely, some chemotherapeutics lower therapeutic levels of enzyme-inducing AEDs, increasing the risk of seizures. Concomitant administration of phenytoin and corticosteroids diminishes efficacy of both drugs. Valproic acid inhibits CYP enzymes and increases the toxicity of nitrosoureas, cisplatin, and etoposide. Thus, the newer AEDs (levetiracetam, pregabalin, lamotrigine, lacosamide, topiramate) are generally preferred over carbamazepine, phenytoin, phenobarbital, or valproic acid. Levetiracetam (Keppra) has gained wide acceptance as the optimum initial AED treatment in patients with brain tumors because of its efficacy, favorable toxicity profile, and absence of drug interactions.[56,57]

In addition to drug interactions, other adverse events from AEDs occur with increased frequency in patients with brain tumors compared with the general population. Approximately 20% of patients will require a change in initial AED because of adverse effects.[48] Drug rashes are common, occurring in 20% of patients with brain tumors compared with 5% to 10% of the general population taking AEDs.[58] Importantly, the risk of serious and rarely fatal cutaneous reactions, including erythema multiforme, Stevens-Johnson syndrome, and toxic epidermal necrolysis is increased with phenytoin, carbamazepine, and phenobarbital, especially during the first 8 weeks of AED therapy and during radiotherapy.[59–61] Cognitive impairment and neuropsychiatric effects from AEDs are often exaggerated in patients with brain tumors because of the underlying tumor and administration of concomitant neuropsychiatric medications. Similarly, the risk of bone marrow suppression and liver dysfunction may also be increased, likely due to additive or synergistic effects of multiple concomitant medications that are often prescribed in this patient population compared with the general population on AEDs.

Role of Antitumor Treatment

Although pharmacologic therapy is the cornerstone of seizure management in patients with brain tumors, surgery, radiotherapy, and chemotherapy may have a positive impact. Epilepsy surgery with maximal resection is an established modality for refractory seizures in patients with low-grade temporal lobe neuroepithelial tumors,[62,63] whereas resection of high-grade or nontemporal lobe tumors is less effective. Although the impact of cranial irradiation or chemotherapy on seizure control has not been well studied, retrospective series and clinical experience support a positive effect of these modalities in patients with AED-resistant tumor-associated epilepsy.[64–67] In one retrospective cohort study, the use of temozolomide in patients with low-grade gliomas was associated with a significant decrease in seizure frequency.[67] However, the use of radiotherapy or chemotherapy to control seizures, in the absence of other indications, should be avoided, and if deemed necessary, the acute and chronic risks of treatment must be carefully balanced against the morbidity of uncontrolled seizures.

Seizure Prophylaxis

Given the frequency of seizures in patients with brain tumors, the role of prophylactic AEDs in patients who never experienced a seizure has been evaluated in retrospective and prospective studies and in 3 meta-analyses.[48,68,69] These studies in the aggregate failed to demonstrate efficacy of prophylactic AEDs in preventing seizures, although confirming a significant incidence of adverse events. Thus, consensus guidelines from the American Academy of Neurology recommend that prophylactic AEDs not be routinely administered to patients with primary or metastatic brain tumors who have never had a seizure.[48] In patients undergoing craniotomy, prophylactic AEDs are often prescribed because of the potential for devastating sequelae of seizures in this setting. However, in the absence of a seizure history, AEDs administered perioperatively should be tapered and discontinued, given lack of proven benefit of extended AED prophylaxis following craniotomy.[48,68] Unresolved questions regarding the use of prophylactic AEDs is whether the newer AEDs may be more effective in seizure prevention and whether specific subsets of patients at highest risk of seizures benefit from prophylaxis.

RADIATION-RELATED COMPLICATIONS

Radiation therapy is a commonly used, noninvasive modality for the treatment of primary and metastatic brain tumors. As radiation technology has improved, the radiation oncologist is increasingly able to target the tumor while reducing the dose of radiation delivered to normal brain. Unfortunately, photon radiotherapy (also known as x-ray and gamma ray irradiation) deposits radiation dose along the entry path and exit path through the brain, causing acute and chronic radiation injury to normal brain tissue surrounding the tumor itself. An understanding of the spectrum of radiation-related CNS complications is important in their diagnosis, optimum management, and appropriate counseling before treatment. Importantly, when reporting radiation-induced toxicities, a standard scoring system, either the National Cancer Institute Common Terminology Criteria for Adverse Events or the Radiation Therapy Oncology Group CNS toxicity grading, should be used for comparability with current and future studies (**Box 1**).

Many issues regarding radiotherapy of brain tumors in children are distinct from that of adults. Children experience more neurocognitive sequelae as well as side effects because of the restriction of skull growth. Irradiation of children has specific and complex age and dose-volume effects that are beyond the scope of this article.[70,71]

Radiation-related CNS toxicities encompass diverse pathogenetic mechanisms and are temporally classified as follows: (1) *acute effects* that occur during or shortly after radiation, (2) *early delayed effects* that occur weeks to 4 months after treatment, and (3) *late effects* that appear more than 6 months after radiation. This article provides an overview of these toxicities, as well as strategies to treat and mitigate radiation-related CNS injury.

Acute Radiation-Related Complications

Acute radiation-induced effects typically are those that are associated with inflammation and edema caused in part by disruption of the BBB.[72] In addition, within a few weeks of radiotherapy, early demyelination occurs, with breakdown of neural tissue and degeneration of glial cells.[73]

The clinical effects associated with acute inflammation and edema typically include headache, worsening focal neurologic deficits, subtle changes in neurocognition, and seizures. These symptoms can be mitigated by a course of corticosteroids. The release of radiation-induced cytokines can also induce global side effects, such as somnolence that may begin during radiotherapy and last for several months after the completion of radiotherapy.[74] Because of the possibility of transient radiation-induced edema and swelling, special care should be taken in irradiating tumors causing mass effect or threatening cerebral spinal flow through the brain, including the initiation of corticosteroids before radiation.

Other acute reactions occur infrequently and relate to the dose and target volume. These reactions include a metallic taste or loss of taste, anorexia, nausea and vomiting, serous otitis media, parotitis, and mucositis. Myelosuppression is uncommon in the absence of concurrent chemotherapy or craniospinal irradiation.

Early Delayed Radiation-Related Complications (Pseudoprogression)

Early delayed reactions occur within weeks and up to 4 months after radiation. Their pathogenesis is likely multifactorial, including radiation-induced demyelination,

---

Box 1
Radiation-induced CNS toxicity grading criteria

RTOG Common Toxicity Criteria (CTC v2.0) Grading System

Neurologic/Cortical

Grade 1: Mild somnolence or agitation

Grade 2: Moderate somnolence or agitation

Grade 3: Severe somnolence, agitation, confusion, disorientation, hallucinations

Grade 4: Coma, seizures, toxic paralysis

Grade 5: Death

Neurologic/Headache

Grade 1: Mild headache

Grade 2: Moderate or severe but transient headache

Grade 3: Unrelenting and severe headache

Grade 4: —

Grade 5: Death

National Cancer Institute Common Terminology Criteria for Adverse Events (CTCAE) v4.0

Memory Impairment

Grade 1: Mild memory impairment

Grade 2: Moderate memory impairment; limiting instrumental activities of daily living (ADL)

Grade 3: Severe memory impairment; limiting self-care ADL

Grade 4/5: —

CNS Necrosis

Grade 1: Asymptomatic; clinical or diagnostic observations only; intervention not indicated

Grade 2: Moderate symptoms; corticosteroids indicated

Grade 3: Severe symptoms; medical intervention indicated

Grade 4: Life-threatening consequences; urgent intervention indicated

Grade 5: Death

Data from Cooperative Group Common Toxicity Criteria. 2011. Available at: http://www.rtog. org/ResearchAssociates/AdverseEventReporting/CooperativeGroupCommonToxicityCriteria. aspx. Accessed November 16, 2011; and Common terminology criteria for adverse events (CTCAE) Version 4.0. Published: May 28, 2009 (v.4.0.3: June 14, 2010). 2011. Available at: http://ctep.cancer.gov/protocolDevelopment/electronic_applications/ctc.htm#ctc_40. Accessed November 16, 2011.

---

altered capillary permeability, inflammation, and radionecrosis. Clinical manifestations include somnolence or exacerbation of tumor-associated symptoms. Radiographically, there may be changes on MRI that are indistinguishable from tumor progression (increasing enhancement, vasogenic edema, mass effect), a phenomenon referred to as "pseudoprogression."[75,76] Pseudoprogression occurs in approximately 20% of patients who receive temozolomide chemoradiotherapy for high-grade gliomas, and approximately half of the cases of radiographic progression seen on early imaging after chemoradiotherapy represent pseudoprogression rather than tumor growth.[77]

Failure to appreciate early delayed radiation reactions may lead to premature discontinuation of effective therapy or, in some cases, unnecessary surgical intervention. Criteria for the diagnosis of pseudoprogression have been defined for high-grade gliomas,[78] and recently, pseudoprogression has also been characterized for the treatment of brain metastases after radiosurgery.[79] Patients with pseudoprogression may have an improved prognosis compared with those who do not, perhaps indicating a robust treatment response.[79,80] Thus, patients with malignant gliomas who develop radiographic findings consistent with pseudoprogression within 3 months of radiation should continue on adjuvant temozolomide until there is unequivocal evidence of tumor progression on serial MRIs or unless there is biopsy confirmation of progressing tumor.[76]

Late Radiation-Related Complications

Late radiation-related complications are those typically occurring more than 6 months after the completion of radiotherapy. The spectrum of late complications includes radionecrosis, diffuse white matter injury, and neurocognitive decline. Additional late complications include cerebrovascular events, optic toxicities, and endocrinopathies.

The proper diagnosis of late radiation effects and subsequent management depend on identifying whether radiation is responsible for the clinical symptoms or whether disease progression or other systemic disease is responsible. One such paradigm to guide the approach to the diagnosis and management of late radiation complications is known as the LENT-SOMA scale (Late Effects of Normal Tissue – Subjective, Objective, Management, Analytic scale).[81] The recognition of radiation-induced toxicity is based on whether the clinical symptoms, time course, radiation dose delivered, laboratory tests, and imaging are consistent with radiation-induced toxicity. If side effects occur before 5 years have elapsed, cancer recurrence and metastatic disease must be considered. If side effects occur more than 5 years after radiotherapy, radiation-induced second malignancies must also be considered.

Late radiation-related reactions that involve brain necrosis and gliosis as a response to radiotherapy typically take at least 6 months to develop. The loss of capillary endothelial cells and microvascular degeneration eventually leads to cortical atrophy, and in its extreme, necrosis of nervous tissue.[73] Although difficult to predict, doses of at least 72 gray (Gy) (in 2 Gy/d fractions) are needed to place a patient at a 5% risk of symptomatic radiation necrosis. The brain is particularly sensitive to larger fraction sizes and accelerated (twice daily) treatment.[82] When imaged, late radiation treatment effects include white matter demyelination and leukoencephalopathy, with resultant ventricular dilatation and cortical atrophy.[83,84] Interestingly, these changes are also found in patients who do not undergo radiotherapy.[85] Radionecrosis may appear as a contrast-enhancing mass with surrounding white matter changes and edema, which is difficult to differentiate from recurrent tumor in the absence of a biopsy or resection.

In addition to neurologic effects, secondary malignancies can occur as a result of radiotherapy, including meningiomas, gliomas, and nerve sheath tumors. The absolute risk of a second malignancy attributable to radiotherapy is unknown, given the additional factors that may contribute, including exposure to chemotherapy and late recurrences of the original cancer. One large analysis of the National Cancer Institute's Surveillance, Epidemiology, and End Results (SEER) database found that patients who had radiotherapy as initial treatment for their CNS tumor were not significantly more likely than those who did not have radiotherapy to develop a second malignancy.[86] Specifically, 9% [95% confidence interval (CI), 3%–21%] of all subsequent solid tumors in patients treated with cranial radiotherapy were attributable to the radiotherapy, with the 95% CI crossing 0. These findings indicate that although cranial radiotherapy does indeed increase the risk of a second malignancy in long-surviving patients, the risk is modest and is highest in young children.

The total radiation dose, fractionation schedule, and volume and location of treatment are all critical variables in the development of radiation damage. Studies have shown that partial brain radiotherapy with doses of 50 to 60 Gy is associated with a low incidence of late neurocognitive decline in the absence of tumor progression,[87,88] although caution should be used when extrapolating these results to patients treated with fraction sizes greater than 2 Gy/d.[89] Structures without redundancy, particularly those with functional units in series (analogous to the serial electrical circuit) require extra care in avoidance of overdose. These structures include the optic nerves and chiasm, spinal cord and brainstem, and when radiosurgery is used, the pituitary stalk.

Avoidance and Treatment of Radiation Treatment Toxicity

The differential response and importance of different regions of the cerebrum to radiation damage is an area of continued study. The hippocampus has been highlighted as a region associated with memory function. As such, hippocampal-sparing radiotherapy has been suggested as a method to optimize currently available radiation dose–shaping techniques in the interest of neuropreservation.[90] Attempts to avoid extensive irradiation of surrounding normal brain must be balanced against the need to adequately treat the tumor and areas at risk for microscopic tumor extension, particularly because tumor control is the most critical factor predicting neurologic preservation.[91]

Treatment of Late Radiation Effects

The palliative treatment of late radiation effects involves the use of analgesics, antiseizure medications, and corticosteroids. Methylphenidate and donepezil have been reported to improve neurocognitive function. Surgical resection can relieve mass effect and is the only definitive means to confirm radiation necrosis, although positron emission tomography and MRI single-photon emission computed tomography, along with other advanced imaging techniques,[92] can be helpful in differentiating recurrent tumor from radiation necrosis. Bevacizumab has been reported to provide clinical benefit and radiographic response in patients with biopsy-proven radiation necrosis.[93] Hyperbaric oxygen has also been used for this difficult clinical situation.[94]

SUMMARY

The extent and attribution of radiation-induced side effects is an area of continued study. Although radiation-induced neurotoxicity is a widely accepted concept, high-quality prospective studies quantifying the actual progression of neurocognitive decline and injury in patients receiving radiotherapy compared with those who have not are limited. As the antitumor effects of radiotherapy can actually improve cognition,[91,95] fear of radiation side effects relative to their benefits should not cause hesitation in the appropriate use of cranial irradiation, particularly when its use has been proved to improve survival and progression-free survival in randomized trials. In patients who are expected to have long survival, fraction sizes of 2 Gy/dy or less should be used to mitigate the risk of late neurotoxicity.[82,89]

REFERENCES

1. Bertossi M, Virgintino D, Maiorano E, et al. Ultrastructural and morphometric investigation of human brain capillaries in normal and peritumoral tissues. Ultrastruct Pathol 1997;21:41–9.

2. Boucher Y, Salehi H, Witwer B, et al. Interstitial fluid pressure in intracranial tumours in patients and in rodents. Br J Cancer 1997;75:829–36.

3. Strugar JG, Criscuolo GR, Rothbart D, et al. Vascular endothelial growth/permeability factor expression in human glioma specimens: correlation with vasogenic brain edema and tumor-associated cysts. J Neurosurg 1995;83:682–9.

4. Dobrogowska DH, Lossinsky AS, Tarnawski M, et al. Increased blood-brain barrier permeability and endothelial abnormalities induced by vascular endothelial growth factor. J Neurocytol 1998;27:163–73.

5. Machein MR, Kullmer J, Fiebich BL, et al. Vascular endothelial growth factor expression, vascular volume, and, capillary permeability in human brain tumors. Neurosurgery 1999;44:732–40.

6. Carlson MR, Pope WB, Horvath S, et al. Relationship between survival and edema in malignant gliomas: role of vascular endothelial growth factor and neuronal pentraxin 2. Clin Cancer Res 2007;13:2592–8.

7. Gerstner ER, Duda DG, di Tomaso E, et al. VEGF inhibitors in the treatment of cerebral edema in patients with brain cancer. Nat Rev Clin Oncol 2009;6:229–36.

8. Chan AS, Leung SY, Wong MP, et al. Expression of vascular endothelial growth factor and its receptors in the anaplastic progression of astrocytoma, oligodendroglioma, and ependymoma. Am J Surg Pathol 1998;22:816–26.

9. Jarden JO, Dhawan V, Moeller JR, et al. The time course of steroid action on blood-to-brain and blood-to-tumor transport of 82Rb: a positron emission tomographic study. Ann Neurol 1989;25:239–45.

10. Sinha S, Bastin ME, Wardlaw JM, et al. Effects of dexamethasone on peritumoural oedematous brain: a DT-MRI study. J Neurol Neurosurg Psychiatry 2004;75:1632–5.

11. Kim H, Lee JM, Park JS, et al. Dexamethasone coordinately regulates angiopoietin-1 and VEGF: a mechanism of glucocorticoid-induced stabilization of blood-brain barrier. Biochem Biophys Res Commun 2008;372:243–8.

12. Heiss JD, Papavassiliou E, Merrill MJ, et al. Mechanism of dexamethasone suppression of brain tumor-associated vascular permeability in rats. Involvement of the glucocorticoid receptor and vascular permeability factor. J Clin Invest 1996;98:1400–8.

13. Ryken TC, McDermott M, Robinson PD, et al. The role of steroids in the management of brain metastases: a systematic review and evidence-based clinical practice guideline. J Neurooncol 2010;96:103–14.

14. Vecht CJ, Hovestadt A, Verbiest HB, et al. Dose-effect relationship of dexamethasone on Karnofsky performance in metastatic brain tumors: a randomized study of doses of 4, 8, and 16 mg per day. Neurology 1994;44:675–80.

15. Hempen C, Weiss E, Hess CF. Dexamethasone treatment in patients with brain metastases and primary brain tumors: do the benefits outweigh the side-effects? Support Care Cancer 2002;10:322–8.

16. Sturdza A, Millar BA, Bana N, et al. The use and toxicity of steroids in the management of patients with brain metastases. Support Care Cancer 2008;16:1041–8.

17. Dropcho EJ, Soong SJ. Steroid-induced weakness in patients with primary brain tumors. Neurology 1991;41:1235–9.

18. Henson JW, Jalaj JK, Walker RW, et al. Pneumocystis carinii pneumonia in patients with primary brain tumors. Arch Neurol 1991;48:406–9.

19. Schiff D. Pneumocystis pneumonia in brain tumor patients: risk factors and clinical features. J Neurooncol 1996;27:235.

20. Stupp R, Dietrich PY, Ostermann Kraljevic S, et al. Promising survival for patients with newly diagnosed glioblastoma multiforme treated with concomitant radiation

plus temozolomide followed by adjuvant temozolomide. J Clin Oncol 2002;20: 1375–82.

21. Piper JM, Ray WA, Daugherty JR, et al. Corticosteroid use and peptic ulcer disease: role of nonsteroidal anti-inflammatory drugs. Ann Intern Med 1991;114:735–40.

22. Weiner HL, Rezai AR, Cooper PR. Sigmoid diverticular perforation in neurosurgical patients receiving high-dose corticosteroids. Neurosurgery 1993;33:40–3.

23. ReMine SG, McIlrath DC. Bowel perforation in steroid-treated patients. Ann Surg 1980;192:581–6.

24. Kamoun WS, Ley CD, Farrar CT, et al. Edema control by cediranib, a vascular endothelial growth factor receptor-targeted kinase inhibitor, prolongs survival despite persistent brain tumor growth in mice. J Clin Oncol 2009;27:2542–52.

25. Vredenburgh JJ, Desjardins A, Herndon JE 2nd, et al. Bevacizumab plus irinotecan in recurrent glioblastoma multiforme. J Clin Oncol 2007;25:4722–9.

26. Norden AD, Young GS, Setayesh K, et al. Bevacizumab for recurrent malignant gliomas: efficacy, toxicity, and patterns of recurrence. Neurology 2008;70:779–87.

27. Friedman HS, Prados MD, Wen PY, et al. Bevacizumab alone and in combination with irinotecan in recurrent glioblastoma. J Clin Oncol 2009;27:4733–40.

28. Batchelor TT, Duda DG, di Tomaso E, et al. Phase II study of cediranib, an oral pan-vascular endothelial growth factor receptor tyrosine kinase inhibitor, in patients with recurrent glioblastoma. J Clin Oncol 2010;28:2817–23.

29. Nowosielski M, Recheis W, Goebel G, et al. ADC histograms predict response to anti-angiogenic therapy in patients with recurrent high-grade glioma. Neuroradiology 2011;53:291–302.

30. Prandoni P, Falanga A, Piccioli A. Cancer and venous thromboembolism. Lancet Oncol 2005;6:401–10.

31. Jenkins EO, Schiff D, Mackman N, et al. Venous thromboembolism in malignant gliomas. J Thromb Haemost 2010;8:221–7.

32. Gerber DE, Grossman SA, Streiff MB. Management of venous thromboembolism in patients with primary and metastatic brain tumors. J Clin Oncol 2006;24:1310–8.

33. Marras LC, Geerts WH, Perry JR. The risk of venous thromboembolism is increased throughout the course of malignant glioma: an evidence-based review. Cancer 2000;89:640–6.

34. Simanek R, Vormittag R, Hassler M, et al. Venous thromboembolism and survival in patients with high-grade glioma. Neuro Oncol 2007;9:89–95.

35. Lazio BE, Simard JM. Anticoagulation in neurosurgical patients. Neurosurgery 1999;45:838–47.

36. Lyman GH, Khorana AA, Falanga A, et al. American Society of Clinical Oncology guideline: recommendations for venous thromboembolism prophylaxis and treatment in patients with cancer. J Clin Oncol 2007;25:5490–505.

37. Prandoni P. How I treat venous thromboembolism in patients with cancer. Blood 2005;106:4027–33.

38. Noble SI, Shelley MD, Coles B, et al. Management of venous thromboembolism in patients with advanced cancer: a systematic review and meta-analysis. Lancet Oncol 2008;9:577–84.

39. Kearon C, Kahn SR, Agnelli G, et al. Antithrombotic therapy for venous thromboembolic disease: American College of Chest Physicians Evidence-Based Clinical Practice Guidelines (8th Edition). Chest 2008;133(Suppl 6):454S–545S.

40. Ruff RL, Posner JB. Incidence and treatment of peripheral venous thrombosis in patients with glioma. Ann Neurol 1983;13:334–6.

41. Levin JM, Schiff D, Loeffler JS, et al. Complications of therapy for venous thromboembolic disease in patients with brain tumors. Neurology 1993;43:1111–4.

42. Monreal M, Zacharski L, Jiménez JA, et al. Fixed-dose low-molecular-weight heparin for secondary prevention of venous thromboembolism in patients with disseminated cancer: a prospective cohort study. J Thromb Haemost 2004;2:1311–5.

43. Lee AY, Levine MN, Baker RI, et al. Low-molecular-weight heparin versus a coumarin for the prevention of recurrent venous thromboembolism in patients with cancer. N Engl J Med 2003;349:146–53.

44. Akl EA, Labedi N, Barba M, et al. Anticoagulation for the long-term treatment of venous thromboembolism in patients with cancer. Cochrane Database Syst Rev 2011;6:CD006650.

45. Nghiemphu PL, Green RM, Pope WB, et al. Safety of anticoagulation use and bevacizumab in patients with glioma. Neuro Oncol 2008;10:355–60.

46. Perry JR, Julian JA, Laperriere NJ, et al. PRODIGE: a randomized placebo-controlled trial of dalteparin low-molecular-weight heparin thromboprophylaxis in patients with newly diagnosed malignant glioma. J Thromb Haemost 2010;8:1959–65.

47. van Breemen MS, Wilms EB, Vecht CJ. Epilepsy in patients with brain tumours: epidemiology, mechanisms, and management. Lancet Neurol 2007;6:421–30.

48. Glantz MJ, Cole BF, Forsyth PA, et al. Practice parameter: anticonvulsant prophylaxis in patients with newly diagnosed brain tumors. Report of the Quality Standards Subcommittee of the American Academy of Neurology. Neurology 2000; 54(10):1886–93.

49. Lote K, Stenwig AE, Skullerud K, et al. Prevalence and prognostic significance of epilepsy in patients with gliomas. Eur J Cancer 1998;34:98–102.

50. Pace A, Bove L, Innocenti P, et al. Epilepsy and gliomas: incidence and treatment in 119 patients. J Exp Clin Cancer Res 1998;17:479–82.

51. Oberndorfer S, Schmal T, Lahrmann H, et al. The frequency of seizures in patients with primary brain tumors or cerebral metastases. An evaluation from the Ludwig Boltzmann Institute of Neuro-Oncology and the Department of Neurology, Kaiser Franz Josef Hospital, Vienna. Wien Klin Wochenschr 2002;114(21–22):911–6 [in German].

52. Cascino GD. Epilepsy and brain tumors: implications for treatment. Epilepsia 1990;31(Suppl 3):S37–44.

53. Cavaliere R, Farace E, Schiff D. Clinical implications of status epilepticus in patients with neoplasms. Arch Neurol 2006;63:1746–9.

54. Karceski S, Morrell MJ, Carpenter D. Treatment of epilepsy in adults: expert opinion, 2005. Epilepsy Behav 2005;7(Suppl 1):S1–64.

55. Vecht CJ, Wagner GL, Wilms EB. Interactions between antiepileptic and chemotherapeutic drugs. Lancet Neurol 2003;2:404–9.

56. Rosati A, Buttolo L, Stefini R, et al. Efficacy and safety of levetiracetam in patients with glioma: a clinical prospective study. Arch Neurol 2010;67:343–6.

57. Usery JB, Michael LM 2nd, Sills AK, et al. A prospective evaluation and literature review of levetiracetam use in patients with brain tumors and seizures. J Neurooncol 2010;99:251–60.

58. Mamon HJ, Wen PY, Burns AC, et al. Allergic skin reactions to anticonvulsant medications in patients receiving cranial radiation therapy. Epilepsia 1999;40:341–4.

59. Rzany B, Correia O, Kelly JP, et al. Risk of Stevens-Johnson syndrome and toxic epidermal necrolysis during first weeks of antiepileptic therapy: a case-control study. Study Group of the International Case Control Study on Severe Cutaneous Adverse Reactions. Lancet 1999;353(9171):2190–4.

60. Delattre JY, Safai B, Posner JB. Erythema multiforme and Stevens-Johnson syndrome in patients receiving cranial irradiation and phenytoin. Neurology 1988;38:194–8.

61. Khafaga YM, Jamshed A, Allam AA, et al. Stevens-Johnson syndrome in patients on phenytoin and cranial radiotherapy. Acta Oncol 1999;38:111–6.
62. Phi JH, Kim SK, Cho BK, et al. Long-term surgical outcomes of temporal lobe epilepsy associated with low-grade brain tumors. Cancer 2009;115:5771–9.
63. Luyken C, Blümcke I, Fimmers R, et al. The spectrum of long-term epilepsy-associated tumors: long-term seizure and tumor outcome and neurosurgical aspects. Epilepsia 2003;44:822–30.
64. Chalifoux R, Elisevich K. Effect of ionizing radiation on partial seizures attributable to malignant cerebral tumors. Stereotact Funct Neurosurg 1996–1997;67(3–4): 169–82.
65. Rogers LR, Morris HH, Lupica K. Effect of cranial irradiation on seizure frequency in adults with low-grade astrocytoma and medically intractable epilepsy. Neurology 1993;43:1599–601.
66. Pace A, Vidiri A, Galiè E, et al. Temozolomide chemotherapy for progressive low-grade glioma: clinical benefits and radiological response. Ann Oncol 2003;14: 1722–6.
67. Sherman JH, Moldovan K, Yeoh HK, et al. Impact of temozolomide chemotherapy on seizure frequency in patients with low-grade gliomas. J Neurosurg 2011;114: 1617–21.
68. Sirven JI, Wingerchuk DM, Drazkowski JF, et al. Seizure prophylaxis in patients with brain tumors: a meta-analysis. Mayo Clin Proc 2004;79:1489–94.
69. Kuijlen JM, Teernstra OP, Kessels AG, et al. Effectiveness of antiepileptic prophylaxis used with supratentorial craniotomies: a meta-analysis. Seizure 1996;5: 291–8.
70. Merchant TE, Kiehna EN, Li C, et al. Modeling radiation dosimetry to predict cognitive outcomes in pediatric patients with CNS embryonal tumors including medulloblastoma. Int J Radiat Oncol Biol Phys 2006;65:210–21.
71. Silber JH, Radcliffe J, Peckham V, et al. Whole-brain irradiation and decline in intelligence: the influence of dose and age on IQ score. J Clin Oncol 1992;10:1390–6.
72. Wong CS, Van der Kogel AJ. Mechanisms of radiation injury to the central nervous system: implications for neuroprotection. Mol Interv 2004;4:273–84.
73. Coderre JA, Morris GM, Micca PL, et al. Late effects of radiation on the central nervous system: role of vascular endothelial damage and glial stem cell survival. Radiat Res 2006;166:495–503.
74. Hong JH, Chiang CS, Campbell IL, et al. Induction of acute phase gene expression by brain irradiation. Int J Radiat Oncol Biol Phys 1995;33:619–26.
75. Chamberlain MC, Glantz MJ, Chalmers L, et al. Early necrosis following concurrent Temodar and radiotherapy in patients with glioblastoma. J Neurooncol 2007; 82:81–3.
76. Brandsma D, Stalpers L, Taal W, et al. Clinical features, mechanisms, and management of pseudoprogression in malignant gliomas. Lancet Oncol 2008; 9:453–61.
77. Taal W, Brandsma D, de Bruin HG, et al. Incidence of early pseudo-progression in a cohort of malignant glioma patients treated with chemoirradiation with temozolomide. Cancer 2008;113:405–10.
78. Wen PY, Macdonald DR, Reardon DA, et al. Updated response assessment criteria for high-grade gliomas: response assessment in neuro-oncology working group. J Clin Oncol 2010;28:1963–72.
79. Patel TR, McHugh BJ, Bi WL, et al. A Comprehensive Review of MR Imaging Changes following Radiosurgery to 500 Brain Metastases. AJNR Am J Neuroradiol 2011;32:1885–92.

80. Brandes AA, Franceschi E, Tosoni A, et al. MGMT promoter methylation status can predict the incidence and outcome of pseudoprogression after concomitant radiochemotherapy in newly diagnosed glioblastoma patients. J Clin Oncol 2008; 26:2192–7.
81. LENT. SOMA scales for all anatomic sites. Int J Radiat Oncol Biol Phys 1995;31: 1049–91.
82. Lawrence YR, Li XA, el Naqa I, et al. Radiation dose-volume effects in the brain. Int J Radiat Oncol Biol Phys 2010;76:S20–7.
83. Wassenberg MW, Bromberg JE, Witkamp TD, et al. White matter lesions and encephalopathy in patients treated for primary central nervous system lymphoma. J Neurooncol 2001;52:73–80.
84. Shibamoto Y, Baba F, Oda K, et al. Incidence of brain atrophy and decline in mini-mental state examination score after whole-brain radiotherapy in patients with brain metastases: a prospective study. Int J Radiat Oncol Biol Phys 2008;72: 1168–73.
85. Armstrong CL, Hunter JV, Hackney D, et al. MRI changes due to early-delayed conformal radiotherapy and postsurgical effects in patients with brain tumors. Int J Radiat Oncol Biol Phys 2005;63:56–63.
86. Berrington de Gonzalez A, Curtis RE, Kry SF, et al. Proportion of second cancers attributable to radiotherapy treatment in adults: a cohort study in the US SEER cancer registries. Lancet Oncol 2011;12:353–60.
87. Armstrong CL, Hunter JV, Ledakis GE, et al. Late cognitive and radiographic changes related to radiotherapy: initial prospective findings. Neurology 2002;59:40–8.
88. Brown PD, Buckner JC, O'Fallon JR, et al. Effects of radiotherapy on cognitive function in patients with low-grade glioma measured by the folstein mini-mental state examination. J Clin Oncol 2003;21:2519–24.
89. Surma-aho O, Niemela M, Vilkki J, et al. Adverse long-term effects of brain radiotherapy in adult low-grade glioma patients. Neurology 2001;56:1285–90.
90. Gondi V, Tolakanahalli R, Mehta MP, et al. Hippocampal-sparing whole-brain radiotherapy: a "how-to" technique using helical tomotherapy and linear accelerator-based intensity-modulated radiotherapy. Int J Radiat Oncol Biol Phys 2010;78:1244–52.
91. Li J, Bentzen SM, Renschler M, et al. Regression after whole-brain radiation therapy for brain metastases correlates with survival and improved neurocognitive function. J Clin Oncol 2007;25:1260–6.
92. Gahramanov S, Raslan AM, Muldoon LL, et al. Potential for differentiation of pseudoprogression from true tumor progression with dynamic susceptibility-weighted contrast-enhanced magnetic resonance imaging using ferumoxytol vs. gadoteridol: a pilot study. Int J Radiat Oncol Biol Phys 2011;79:514–23.
93. Torcuator R, Zuniga R, Mohan YS, et al. Initial experience with bevacizumab treatment for biopsy confirmed cerebral radiation necrosis. J Neurooncol 2009;94: 63–8.
94. Chuba PJ, Aronin P, Bhambhani K, et al. Hyperbaric oxygen therapy for radiation-induced brain injury in children. Cancer 1997;80:2005–12.
95. Khuntia D, Brown P, Li J, et al. Whole-brain radiotherapy in the management of brain metastasis. J Clin Oncol 2006;24:1295–304.

Low-Grade Gliomas
When and How to Treat

Sacit Bulent Omay, MD[a], Joseph M. Piepmeier, MD[a],
Jonathan P.S. Knisely, MD[b],*

KEYWORDS

- Low-grade glioma • Glioma ontogeny • Glioma imaging • Glioma surgery
- Glioma radiotherapy • Glioma chemotherapy

KEY POINTS

- Low-grade gliomas are slow-growing primary brain tumors and are most commonly diagnosed in young adults after new-onset seizures.
- A complete resection of a low-grade glioma may confer a survival benefit; at least one phase III trial is under way to test this.
- Chromosomal codeletion of 1p19q (oligodendroglial histology), isocitrate dehydrogenase (IDH) mutations, and smaller tumor size all predict an improved survival.
- Phase III trials have showed no survival benefit for early postoperative irradiation or for radiotherapy doses exceeding approximately 45 to 50 Gy.
- Clinical trial-based data guiding decisions about the use of systemic chemotherapy are lacking.

INTRODUCTION

Low-grade gliomas (LGGs) are primary brain tumors that most commonly arise in the cerebral hemispheres. According to the World Health Organization (WHO), LGGs are classified as Grade I and II tumors. Grade I LGGs are well circumscribed and include pilocytic astrocytomas, subependymomas, and dysembryoplastic neuroepithelial tumors. Grade II LGGs are far more common and represent diffusely infiltrating glial neoplasms with atypical nuclei.

The most common WHO II LGGs are astrocytomas, oligodendrogliomas, and mixed oligoastrocytic tumors.[1] This article focuses on WHO Grade II gliomas located in the

Funding sources: None.
Conflict of interest: None.
[a] Department of Neurosurgery, Yale University School of Medicine, PO Box 208082, New Haven, CT 06520, USA; [b] Division of Radiosurgery and Stereotactic Program, Department of Radiation Medicine, Hofstra North Shore-LIJ School of Medicine, North Shore University Hospital, 300 Community Drive, Manhasset, NY 11030, USA
* Corresponding author.
E-mail address: jknisely@nshs.edu

Hematol Oncol Clin N Am 26 (2012) 797–809
doi:10.1016/j.hoc.2012.05.001
0889-8588/12/$ – see front matter © 2012 Elsevier Inc. All rights reserved.

supratentorial area in adults, because they are the most common form of this disease. These gliomas are slow-growing primary brain tumors that represent approximately 15% to 25% of gliomas.[2]

CLINICAL FINDINGS, EPIDEMIOLOGY, AND NATURAL HISTORY

The typical LGG patient is a young adult between age 20 and 40 years who reaches medical attention following the new onset of seizures.[2,3] In a study that compared the prevalence of seizures in glioma patients, LGGs were more likely to present with seizures (85% vs 69% and 49%, in patients with anaplastic glioma and glioblastoma, respectively).[4] These patients classically present with modest or only slight neurologic deficits. Some patients demonstrate changes in mental status (10%), headaches (40%), and nausea. Weakness, dysarthria, and personality changes can be detected with frontal lobe tumors; difficulty with speech, vision changes, and frequent seizures may be seen in temporal lobe lesions, and sensory deficits and visual symptoms are reported in patients with parietal lobe gliomas. Visual changes are seen with involvement of the occipital lobes, and cerebellar tumors can cause hydrocephalus.[3]

The natural history of a WHO Grade II LGG ultimately results in transformation into a high-grade tumor. This transition is the major factor in determining a patient's survival. Whereas the timing of change to a high-grade tumor may be unpredictable, the outcome once this has occurred is nearly universally fatal. Several factors have been useful in anticipating the biological behavior in LGG patients, and these are addressed in this article.

The prognosis for LGG patients is classically determined by age, tumor size, and preoperative neurologic functional impairment. Patients younger than of 40 years with complete resection and an oligodendroglioma generally have a more favorable prognosis. The cumulative 5-, 10-, 15-, and 20-year survival rates from the Surveillance, Epidemiology, and End Results (SEER) database among all individuals initially diagnosed with a supratentorial low-grade glioma at the end of the twentieth century were 59.9%, 42.6%, 31.9%, and 26.0%, respectively.[5] Patients diagnosed with histologically mixed tumors or oligodendrogliomas enjoy longer survival than patients diagnosed with astrocytomas. Histopathologic classification of LGGs is historically based on morphologic findings. This method has been inadequate to provide optimal guidance for prognosis, because of ambiguity in interpretation of biopsy findings.[6] Immunohistochemical markers and analyses of tumor genetic and epigenetic changes have proved to be of prognostic value and often help guide treatment strategies.

It is now well recognized that LGGs containing deletions of chromosomal arms 1p and 19q have a more favorable prognosis. Tumors that share these deletions have a more indolent clinical course regardless of treatment methods.[7,8] Codeletion of 1p/19q is highly correlated with oligodendroglioma histopathology and is observed in only 7% of fibrillary astrocytomas.[9] Isocitrate dehydrogenase active-site mutations have been recently demonstrated in a majority of WHO Grade II gliomas.[10] These mutations have been found to be an independent favorable prognostic factor.[11]

Immunohistochemical assessment of the proliferation index (PI) with Ki-67/MIB-1 markers also provides diagnostic and prognostic value. LGGs usually have a PI of less than 4%, and the prognosis is poorer for patients whose tumors have a high PI in comparison with those with a low PI.[12–14]

Alkylating agents (eg, temozolomide [TMZ] and the nitrosoureas carmustine [BCNU] and lomustine [CCNU]) inhibit growth primary through DNA alkylation. A method of intrinsic resistance of most gliomas is the expression of O^6-methylguanine DNA methyltransferase (MGMT), which is a DNA repair enzyme that cleaves alkyl groups. MGMT levels in tumors are now used as a marker of chemotherapeutic response to TMZ in LGG and have been shown to correlate with progression-free survival (PFS).[15,16]

MOLECULAR PATHOGENESIS OF LOW-GRADE GLIOMA

Until recently, it was commonly held that most LGGs harbored either a tp53 mutation (astrocytoma) or loss of chromosomal arms 1p and 19q (oligodendroglioma). The recent identification of isocitrate dehydrogenase (IDH) mutations early in LGG molecular pathogenesis has changed the general understanding; and indeed, IDH mutations appear to arise before subsequent genetic alterations, and are present in the vast majority of secondary glioblastomas.[10,17,18] Of interest is the nature of the mutations: they change the molecular substrate of the IDH enzyme. It normally catalyzes the conversion of isocitrate to α-ketoglutarate, but when mutated, catalyzes the conversion of α-ketoglutarate to 2-hydroxyglutarate (2HG). 2HG is an oncometabolite whose accumulation is now linked to the formation and malignant progression of gliomas. The mechanistic link between 2HG accumulation and the development of malignancy is still uncertain, but interference with the respiratory chain and the induction of redox stress via hypoxia-inducible factor 1α has been identified as a plausible mechanism.[19]

Recently, the possibility of oncogene addiction in gliomas has been broached.[20] If this is found to be true for subsets of LGGs, it would have significant implications for targeting the critical molecular pathways maintaining the aberrant phenotype.

IMAGING OF LOW-GRADE GLIOMA

LGGs may be difficult to delineate on computed tomography (CT) scan. Most LGGs do not enhance with contrast administration, and although there may be evidence of calcification in some tumors (oligodendrogliomas), most LGGs appear only as areas of low density with indistinct margins. For this reason, magnetic resonance imaging (MRI) has supplanted CT imaging for establishing the anatomic distribution of the tumor, as well as for surgical planning and monitoring.

Most LGGs have a classic appearance on MRI of the brain (**Fig. 1**). The typical findings are of an infiltrative, nonenhancing mass lesion that arises in white matter and often extends into the cortex. These tumors are hypointense on T1 spin-echo sequences, and hyperintense on T2 and proton-density sequences, with varying degrees of white matter infiltration and edema around the central part of the tumor. As already stated, unlike high-grade lesions LGGs generally do not enhance with contrast administration, although up to 25% of oligodendrogliomas may have partial contrast enhancement.[21]

It is generally found that the acquisition of contrast enhancement in a previously nonenhancing LGG is evidence for transition to a high-grade lesion, and even if a contrast-enhancing tumor is histopathologically low grade, the behavior has often become that of a more aggressive glioma.[22] Because of their relatively slow growth rate they are less likely higher-grade tumors to cause vasogenic edema. Fluid-attenuated inversion recovery (FLAIR) or T2-weighted MRI sequences are optimal for revealing the contours of these tumors, which typically appear on these pulse sequences as hyperintense lesions.

Some oligodendrogliomas are often associated with intratumoral calcifications that can be seen on MRI and CT scans. Loss of chromosomal arms 1p and 19q has been reported to be associated with an indistinct border on T1-weighted images and mixed-intensity signal on T1 and T2 imaging. Loss of 1p and 19q was also associated with a paramagnetic susceptibility effect and with calcification, which is, as noted earlier, a common histopathologic finding in oligodendrogliomas.[23]

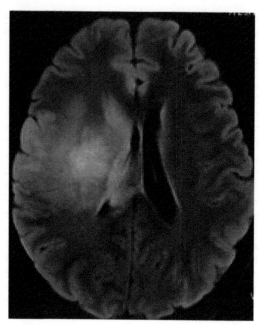

Fig. 1. Fluid-attenuated inversion recovery (FLAIR)-sequence MRI demonstrating a diffuse infiltrative LGG in the right hemisphere. The size and location of this tumor precludes surgical removal.

LGGs are typically hypometabolic on ^{18}F-fluorodeoxyglucose positron emission tomography (PET) scans. The use of radiolabeled amino acids and other tracers in the diagnosis and management of patients with low-grade gliomas is still largely investigational, with only small, single-institution series providing glimpses of how metabolic imaging may be of value in the future.[24,25] For example, the identification of radiolabeled fluoroethyltyrosine (^{18}F-FET) hot spots within an LGG may help to direct biopsy of a more aggressive subcomponent that will affect management decisions and alter prognosis.[26] PET imaging is still in the developmental phase for low-grade glioma assessment, but in additional attempts to go beyond checking integrity of the blood-brain barrier (ie, the absence or presence of contrast enhancement) in assessing low-grade glioma biological activity, other advanced imaging techniques are being used to evaluate tumors.[27]

Magnetic resonance spectroscopy (MRS) is a noninvasive MRI technology that assesses metabolite levels within lesions. LGGs demonstrate a decrease in N-acetylaspartate (NAA) and creatine levels and an increase in choline (Cho) levels, secondary to increased proliferation of cells within the tumor; this profile is increasingly prominent the higher the grade of the glioma. Responses to TMZ therapy in patients with LGGs have been reported to be detectable with MRS at 3 months. These early changes predicted responses at 14 months, and were more informative than tumor T2-weighted or FLAIR volume changes.[28] Perhaps MRS will prove valuable in determining which patients may require changes in therapy before conventional radiographic or clinical assessments can reliably determine whether a given therapy is efficacious.

Diffusion-weighted and perfusion-weighted MRI are techniques that, respectively, evaluate the mobility of water molecules within the tumor's interstitial space and evaluate tumor-induced neovascularization. Diffusion tensor imaging is especially important for patients with tumors near critical language, motor, and other eloquent areas, and when normal anatomic landmarks may be distorted by the presence of the tumor and associated edema.[29,30] An elevated baseline relative cerebral blood volume (rCBV) within a low-grade glioma has been shown to be predictive of a shorter PFS and overall survival.[31] Longitudinal assessment of rCBV in patients with LGGs has also been able to detect early progression to high-grade gliomas using conventional assessment techniques.[32]

Postoperative imaging of patients with LGGs can provide prognostic information as well. In a prospective multicenter phase II study, conducted by the Radiation Therapy Oncology Group, of patients younger than 40 years with a neurosurgeon-ascertained gross total resection who had preoperative and postoperative imaging, 59% of patients were found to have less than 1 cm of residual disease, whereas 32% had 1 to 2 cm of residual disease and 9% had more than 2 cm of residual disease. The recurrence rates for these subsets were 26%, 68%, and 89%, respectively. Two-year and 5-year survival rates of the 111 patients enrolled on this trial were 99% and 93%.[33]

SURGICAL MANAGEMENT

The optimal treatment for an LGG is a controversial topic, but there is growing evidence that aggressive surgical resection provides the best chances for minimizing the risk of radiographic or clinical progression and malignant transformation. There have been no randomized controlled trials evaluating whether aggressive surgery provides a better outcome than less aggressive surgery that establishes the diagnosis and avoids risking operative injury, and it is doubtful that any study will ever document that this is the case. The most recent evidence-based review of treatment options[34] suggests that if a patient is to receive treatment for a presumed LGG and surgical resection is not considered possible, a biopsy should still be obtained to confirm the tissue diagnosis (**Figs. 2** and **3**).

Biopsy of an LGG is commonly directed by stereotactic guidance. Because gliomas may contain regions of variable histopathologic findings, stereotactic biopsy of a diffusely infiltrating glioma carries a risk that any small sample may not contain the component with the greatest prognostic importance.[35] Although most of these tumors have a homogeneous appearance on MRI, specific imaging characteristics can help guide the surgeon to target the areas of highest risk for anaplasia. A region of contrast enhancement within an otherwise nonenhancing LGG is commonly

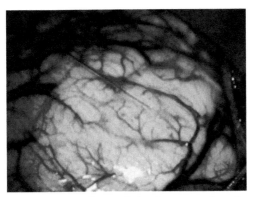

Fig. 2. Operative view of a WHO Grade II LGG that has grown into the subpial layer of the hemisphere. The tumor is identified as the white tissue surrounded by cortical veins.

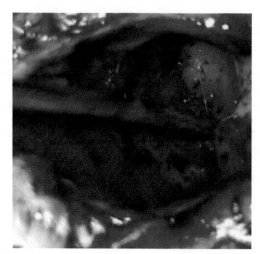

Fig. 3. Operative view of an LGG (gray tissue).

targeted, as it is suggestive of transformation to a more anaplastic tumor. Alternatively, when spectroscopic imaging is used to assist target selection, the region of the highest Cho/NAA ratio is considered to be the area of highest cellularity, and more likely to result in appropriate tumor grading from a small sample of a larger lesion.[36] As noted earlier, dynamic ^{18}F-FET PET has also been reported as useful in identifying biopsy targets in LGGs.[37]

There is abundant level-2 and level-3 evidence, but no data from randomized controlled trials, to indicate that extensive resection of an LGG is associated with improved survival when compared with subtotal resection or biopsy. In retrospective studies, extensive resection was found to have a positive impact on survival, and when preoperative and postoperative tumor volumes and extent of resection have been analyzed, patients who had 90% or more of their tumor resected were found to have a significant survival advantage.[38,39]

The survival benefit from aggressive resection of LGG has motivated surgeons to use stereotactic imaging, functional imaging, physiologic monitoring, and intraoperative imaging to maximize their ability to remove tumors safely while minimizing neurologic impairment. During surgical resection many LGGs are difficult to distinguish from normal white matter. The difficulty in detecting tumor margins can result in problems in deciding how much tissue to remove. Stereotactic localization (frameless or frame-based) can provide guidance to the lesion and its margins based on preoperative imaging data. These techniques have become the standard of care for resection of large tumors and lesions that reside below the cortex. When tumors arise near critical cortical and subcortical regions that serve motor, language, and vision, diffusion tensor imaging and functional MRI (**Fig. 4**) are often obtained before surgery to illustrate the topographic relationship between these areas and the tumor.

When a high risk of impairment is anticipated, direct cortical and subcortical mapping during surgery is performed to minimize the risk. Cortical and subcortical mapping is commonly performed with bipolar electrode stimulation to the brain, to detect language and motor regions with precision. These techniques are particularly useful when the tumor mass has displaced or distorted normal anatomy. It is commonly observed that resection of mass lesions in the brain will create changes in anatomic relationships. This alteration (brain shift) diminishes the reliability of

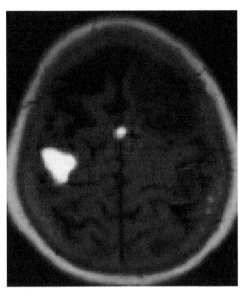

Fig. 4. Functional MRI of primary motor regions for the hand in a patient with an LGG in the left frontal lobe.

preoperative imaging to guide tumor resection. Intraoperative imaging with MRI has been developed to provide the surgeon with accurate and immediate imaging during surgery to provide critical guidance.[40]

Investigational efforts to improve the intraoperative ability to discern the boundary between tumor and normal brain have also used techniques such as the administration of 5-aminolevulinic acid (5-ALA), which fluoresces under appropriate blue light and can help with a macroscopic resection of malignant gliomas. Although macroscopic fluorescence is not manifested by LGGs after the administration of 5-ALA, the use of confocal microscopy can detect fluorescence at a cellular level.[41] It remains to be seen whether the extent of resection will be improved with this approach, and whether local control and survival will be favorably affected.[42] Fluorescent quantum dots linked to moieties that will bind to endothelial growth factor receptors are another approach that may eventually prove useful in assisting surgeons to obtain complete resections of LGGs.[43]

RADIOTHERAPY

Several randomized controlled trials have been performed to evaluate the role of radiation therapy in the management of LGGs. Studies have been conducted to assess the value of various radiotherapy doses and of the timing of delivery of radiation therapy. Data have been collected on neurocognitive outcomes and quality of life, and the data from these trials inform recommendations on present-day management of patients with LGGs.

Before the use of MRI technology, LGGs were often not identified early in their natural history. Patients harboring LGGs often have only very subtle neurologic findings at the time of their initial presentation (often new-onset seizure). Even if an LGG was suspected, diagnostic imaging before the MRI era often was barely able to detect the presence of a nonenhancing mass lesion nearly isodense with normal brain on CT. However, T2 and FLAIR pulse sequences show an LGG even in the absence of any blood-brain barrier breakdown by neovascularization; the slight amount of edema within the LGG causes it to stand out brightly.

As already noted, once a patient is identified to have a clinical and radiographic picture consistent with an LGG, to guide treatment decisions a biopsy is recommended. There were sharp disagreements about the appropriateness of proceeding with radiation therapy for a patient with an LGG immediately after a tissue diagnosis was made.[44,45] Arguments were put forth that maximal surgical debulking of the tumor should be followed by radiotherapy to address what was arguably the lowest residual disease burden that could be achieved. Countervailing arguments were mounted to support delaying radiotherapy in diffuse LGGs because the treatment was not curative and had recognized side effects. Randomized trials on the timing of radiation therapy after initial surgical management could not be completed in the United States, but European investigators were able to mount and complete such a study.[46]

European and North American investigators both were able to mount studies to evaluate various doses of radiation therapy for LGGs.[47,48] It was hoped that maximal safe surgical debulking followed by radiation therapy to higher doses would improve disease-free and overall survival by more completely eradicating any remaining tumor clonogens that would not have been sterilized by lower doses of radiation therapy. However, this was not the case. These studies showed no survival advantage or local control advantage for dose escalation of radiation therapy beyond localized treatment to 45 to 50 Gy delivered in 25 to 28 fractions. Median PFS for both studies were statistically equivalent at 52 to 55 months. Five-year overall survival was 65% to 72% in the North American trial, and 5-year PFS in the European trial was 47% to 50% with a 5-year overall survival rate of 58% to 59%. Perhaps not surprisingly, higher doses of radiation were correlated with higher rates of radiation injury in both trials, and a lower quality of life for patients randomized to the higher dose of radiation was observed in an ancillary study performed as part of the European trial.[49]

Other investigators have also prospectively evaluated neurocognitive outcomes in prospective trials for LGG patients, and have had diverging opinions about whether radiation therapy is associated with adverse sequelae.[50,51] Attention to certain technical aspects of radiotherapy planning and delivery may help minimize the risk of side effects of radiotherapy for LGGs.

Only with the advent of cross-sectional imaging, and in particular, MRI, could partial brain radiotherapy portals be rationally designed for LGGs. Precise localization of a radiographically indistinct tumor was challenging, and it was common to use whole-brain radiation therapy or radiotherapy schemes that were simple to plan and deliver, perhaps just centering on the craniotomy site, but which unwittingly gave the same dose of radiation to the tumor and also to significant volumes of normal brain. It can be readily discerned that lowering the volume of normal brain that receives high-dose irradiation through the use of modern 3-dimensional radiotherapy planning tools should improve the risk-benefit ratio for LGG radiotherapy.

It is prudent for physicians to bear in mind the potential for delayed neurocognitive morbidity when considering radiation as part of the management of an LGG; the side effects of radiation may remit in the short term, but can be progressive in the long term.[48,49,51,52] Approaches such as avoiding incidental irradiation of eloquent cortical areas and stem-cell niches in the hippocampi may help minimize the risk of side effects of radiotherapy for LGGs, but these theoretically appealing approaches have not been tested and found to be superior.

At present, it is recognized that for certain patients with LGGs, irradiation may be reasonably deferred after initial surgical management. An analysis of the European Organization for Research and Treatment of Cancer (EORTC) data on the aforementioned LGG trials evaluating radiation dose and radiation timing identified adverse prognostic factors that were associated with early progression.[53] These factors included astrocytoma histology, age of 40 years and older, maximal tumor dimension of 6 cm or greater, extension across the midline, and the presence of a neurologic deficit preoperatively. The extent of resection was not prognostically significant, but this was assessed only by the neurosurgeon and was not confirmed with postoperative imaging. The analysis showed that for a given patient, having none to 2 of these adverse factors was associated with a median survival of longer than 7.5 years, but the presence of 3 or more of these factors was associated with a median survival approximately half that of the low-risk group.

These prognostic factors were assessed using data from a North American phase III trial comparing low-dose and high-dose radiotherapy for LGG.[7] The investigators also analyzed the extent of resection, Mini-Mental Status Examination (MMSE) score, and the influence of loss of chromosomal arms 1p and 19q. Multivariate analysis showed that tumor size and an MMSE score of 27 to 30 were significant predictors of overall survival whereas tumor size, astrocytoma histology, and MMSE score were significant predictors of PFS. When the EORTC risk criteria were used to stratify patients into high-risk and low-risk groups, the median PFS was 1.9 versus 6.2 years and median overall survival was 7.2 versus 12.6 years. Their evaluation identified that the high-risk group's poorer outcome was predominantly attributable to the influence of histology and tumor size. Codeletion of 1p and 19q was statistically significantly associated with an improved survival relative to single deletion or no deletion (12.6 vs 7.2 years; $P = .03$).

Several attempts have been made to test the validity of the EORTC criteria using the SEER database.[54–56] Using these criteria in patients in the SEER database who had not received radiation therapy resulted in a high-risk group with a median survival of 4.8 years, whereas the low-risk group's median survival had not yet been reached.[54] Another group's analysis looked at the early use of radiation therapy and found that additional poor prognostic factors included male gender and nonfrontal lobe location. Radiotherapy delivery within 4 months of surgery was found to be associated with a poorer overall and cause-specific survival, but it is unclear which confounding variables not captured in the SEER database might have contributed to the early use of radiotherapy in at least some patients who received this treatment. One additional assessment of the SEER database of patients with LGGs found that radiotherapy was associated with a decreased survival for all histologies. The overall hazard ratio for survival associated with the use of radiotherapy was 1.5; the investigators considered that it was difficult to discern a clear benefit from the use of radiotherapy in the initial management of patients with LGGs.[56]

It is very reasonable to use predictive data that has been validated in numerous databases to make clinical decisions about which patients should be given early radiation therapy, but as yet there have been no studies done that document whether early radiotherapy provides a better outcome in this poor-prognosis subset. It may be possible that early radiotherapy in this cohort will delay progression and tumor-related morbidity. The relative importance and success at achieving these end points will need to be assessed relative to the side effects associated with partial brain radiotherapy to doses of approximately 45 to 50 Gy, and it is entirely possible that more conformal treatments that avoid incidental irradiation of eloquent cortex and areas known to contain important stem-cell populations for the brain will prove effective at achieving uncomplicated and protracted disease control. Perhaps additional advantage in identification of patients who will benefit from early, aggressive postoperative therapy will come through more exhaustive analysis of tumor molecular signatures and recognition of poor-prognosis characteristics from advanced MRI techniques.

CHEMOTHERAPY

Chemotherapy has historically not routinely been used for LGG patients. In patients who have failed radiation therapy, chemotherapy has been moderately effective in prolonging survival. Previous experience with a combination of agents (procarbazine, CCNU, and vincristine) has demonstrated activity, particularly against oligodendrogliomas that have transformed into anaplastic tumors.[57] More recently, a single agent, TMZ, has been used as the drug of choice. Several clinical studies have shown some activity of this drug against LGGs,[58–60] this being particularly true for oligodendrogliomas with 1p/19q deletions and for patients with MGMT promoter methylation.

Roughly 50% of patients will demonstrate a reduction in tumor size with chemotherapy, and the prediction of a response may be identified on magnetic resonance spectroscopy.[28] This response may take several months and is most often seen in tumors that are actively growing or are more biologically aggressive. TMZ is commonly delivered in cycles with repeat imaging after every second cycle to evaluate response. Perhaps through direct cytoreduction, TMZ has been shown to improve seizure control in patients with tumor-related refractory epilepsy.[61] It is conceivable that in the near future, therapy directed against tumor glutamate release, using drugs such as sulfasalazine, will be used to help control tumor-associated epilepsy.[62]

SUMMARY

The optimal treatment for a patient with an LGG remains to be determined. As treatment can rarely be considered curative, and as many innovative imaging, histopathologic, and operative techniques are still not routinely available, it may benefit patients with LGG to be managed at experienced medical centers for all or part of their care to ensure that appropriate recommendations are made using evidence-based medicine where available, and the expertise of seasoned clinicians where evidence-based medicine is still lacking.

REFERENCES

1. Louis DN, Ohgaki H, Wiestler OD, et al, editors. WHO classification of tumours. Lyon (France): International Agency for Research on Cancer Press; 2007.
2. Walker DG, Kaye AH. Low grade glial neoplasms. J Clin Neurosci 2003;10:1–13.
3. DeAngelis LM. Brain tumors. N Engl J Med 2001;344:114–23.
4. Lote K, Stenwig AE, Skullerud K, et al. Prevalence and prognostic significance of epilepsy in patients with gliomas. Eur J Cancer 1998;34:98–102.
5. Claus EB, Black PM. Survival rates and patterns of care for patients diagnosed with supratentorial low grade gliomas: data from the SEER program, 1973-2001. Cancer 2006;106:1358–63.
6. Trembath D, Miller CR, Perry A. Gray zones in brain tumor classification: evolving concepts. Adv Anat Pathol 2008;15:287–97.
7. Daniels TB, Brown PD, Felten SJ, et al. Validation of EORTC prognostic factors for adults with low-grade glioma: a report using intergroup 86-72-51. Int J Radiat Oncol Biol Phys 2011;81:218–24.
8. Jenkins RB, Blair H, Ballman KV, et al. A t(1;19)(q10;p10) mediates the combined deletions of 1p and 19q and predicts a better prognosis of patients with oligodendroglioma. Cancer Res 2006;66:9852–61.
9. Kujas M, Lejeune J, Benouaich-Amiel A, et al. Chromosome1p loss: a favorable prognostic factor in low-grade gliomas. Ann Neurol 2005;58:322–6.

10. Balss J, Meyer J, Mueller W, et al. Analysis of the IDH1 codon 132 mutation in brain tumors. Acta Neuropathol 2008;116:597–602.
11. Sanson M, Marie Y, Paris S, et al. Isocitrate dehydrogenase 1 codon 132 mutation is an important prognostic biomarker in gliomas. J Clin Oncol 2009;27:4150–4.
12. Ohgaki H. Genetic pathways to glioblastomas. Neuropathology 2005;25:1–7.
13. Schiff D, Brown PD, Giannini C. Outcome in adult low-grade glioma: the impact of prognostic factors and treatment. Neurology 2007;69:1366–73.
14. Kros JM, Hop WC, Godschalk JJ, et al. Prognostic value of the proliferation-related antigen Ki-67 in oligodendrogliomas. Cancer 1996;78:1107–13.
15. Everhard S, Kaloshi G, Criniere E, et al. MGMT methylation: a marker of response to temozolomide in low-grade gliomas. Ann Neurol 2006;60:740–3.
16. Yokoyama T, Fukushima T. Promoter hypermethylation of the DNA repair gene O6-methylguanine-DNA methyltransferase is an independent predictor of shortened progression free survival in patients with low-grade diffuse astrocytomas. Brain Pathol 2003;13:176–84.
17. Yan H, Parsons DW, Jin G, et al. IDH1 and IDH2 mutations in gliomas. N Engl J Med 2009;360:765–73.
18. Dang L, White DW, Gross S, et al. Cancer-associated IDH1 mutations produce 2-hydroxyglutarate. Nature 2009;462:739–44.
19. Zhao S, Lin Y, Xu W, et al. Glioma-derived mutations in IDH1 dominantly inhibit IDH1 catalytic activity and induce HIF-1alpha. Science 2009;324:261–5.
20. Yan W, Zhang W, Jiang T. Oncogene addiction in gliomas: implications for molecular targeted therapy. J Exp Clin Cancer Res 2011;30:58.
21. Ricci PE, Dungan DH. Imaging of low- and intermediate-grade gliomas. Semin Radiat Oncol 2001;11:103–12.
22. Piepmeier JM. Observations on the current treatment of low-grade astrocytic tumors of the cerebral hemispheres. J Neurosurg 1987;67:177–81.
23. Megyesi JF, Kachur E, Lee DH, et al. Imaging correlates of molecular signatures in oligodendrogliomas. Clin Cancer Res 2004;10:4303–6.
24. Waldman AD, Jackson A, Price SJ, et al. Quantitative imaging biomarkers in neuro-oncology. Nat Rev Clin Oncol 2009;6:445–54.
25. laFougère C, Suchorska B, Bartenstein P, et al. Molecular imaging of gliomas with PET: opportunities and limitations. Neuro Oncol 2011;13:806–19.
26. Kunz M, Thon N, Eigenbrod S, et al. Hot spots in dynamic (18)FET-PET delineate malignant tumor parts within suspected WHO grade II gliomas. Neuro Oncol 2011;13:307–16.
27. Dhermain FG, Hau P, Lanfermann H, et al. Advanced MRI and PET imaging for assessment of treatment response in patients with gliomas. Lancet Neurol 2010;9:906–20.
28. Guillevin R, Menuel C, Taillibert S, et al. Predicting the outcome of grade II glioma treated with temozolomide using proton magnetic resonance spectroscopy. Br J Cancer 2011;104:1854–61.
29. Bode MK, Ruohonen J, Nieminen MT, et al. Potential of diffusion imaging in brain tumors: a review. Acta Radiol 2006;47:585–94.
30. Gupta A, Shah A, Young RJ, et al. Imaging of brain tumors: functional magnetic resonance imaging and diffusion tensor imaging. Neuroimaging Clin N Am 2010;20:379–400.
31. Caseiras GB, Chheang S, Babb J, et al. Relative cerebral blood volume measurements of low-grade gliomas predict patient outcome in a multi-institution setting. Eur J Radiol 2010;73:215–20.

32. Danchaivijitr N, Waldman AD, Tozer DJ, et al. Low-grade gliomas: do changes in rCBV measurements at longitudinal perfusion-weighted MR imaging predict malignant transformation? Radiology 2008;247:170–8.

33. Shaw EG, Berkey B, Coons SW, et al. Recurrence following neurosurgeon-determined gross-total resection of adult supratentorial low-grade glioma: results of a prospective clinical trial. J Neurosurg 2008;109:835–41.

34. Soffietti R, Baumert BG, Bello L, et al. Guidelines on management of low-grade gliomas: report of an EFNS-EANO Task Force. Eur J Neurol 2010;17:1124–33.

35. Muragaki Y, Chernov M, Maruyama T, et al. Low-grade glioma on stereotactic biopsy: how often is the diagnosis accurate? Minim Invasive Neurosurg 2008; 51:275–9.

36. Pirotte B, Goldman S, Massager N, et al. Comparison of ^{18}F-FDGand ^{11}C-methionine for PET-guided stereotactic brain biopsy of gliomas. J Nucl Med 2004;45: 1293–8.

37. McKnight TR, Lamborn KR, Love TD, et al. Correlation of magnetic resonance spectroscopic and growth characteristics within Grades II and III gliomas. J Neurosurg 2007;106:660–6.

38. Sanai N, Berger MS. Glioma extent of resection and its impact on patient outcome. Neurosurgery 2008;62:753–64.

39. Smith JS, Chang EF, Lamborn KR, et al. Role of extent of resection in the long term outcome of low-grade hemispheric gliomas. J Clin Oncol 2008;26:1338–45.

40. Claus EB, Horlacher A, Hsu L, et al. Survival rates in patients with low-grade glioma after intraoperative magnetic resonance image guidance. Cancer 2005; 103(6):1227–33.

41. Sanai N, Snyder LA, Honea NJ, et al. Intraoperative confocal microscopy in the visualization of 5-aminolevulinic acid fluorescence in low-grade gliomas. J Neurosurg 2011;115:740–8.

42. Available at: http://clinicaltrials.gov/ct2/show/NCT01502280. Accessed May 27, 2012.

43. Kantelhardt SR, Caarls W, de Vries AH, et al. Specific visualization of glioma cells in living low-grade tumor tissue. PLoS One 2010;5(6):e11323.

44. Cairncross JG, Laperriere NJ. Low-grade glioma. To treat or not to treat? Arch Neurol 1989;46:1238–9.

45. Shaw EG. Low-grade gliomas: to treat or not to treat? A radiation oncologist's viewpoint. Arch Neurol 1990;47:1138–9.

46. van den Bent MJ, Afra D, de Witte O, et al. Long-term efficacy of early versus delayed radiotherapy for low-grade astrocytoma and oligodendroglioma in adults: the EORTC 22845 randomised trial [Erratum in: Lancet 2006;367:1818]. Lancet 2005;366:985–90.

47. Karim AB, Maat B, Hatlevoll R. A randomized trial on dose-response in radiation therapy of low-grade cerebral glioma: European Organization for Research and Treatment of Cancer (EORTC) Study 22844. Int J Radiat Oncol Biol Phys 1996; 36:549–56.

48. Shaw E, Arusell R, Scheithauer B, et al. Prospective randomized trial of low-versus high-dose radiation therapy in adults with supratentorial low-grade glioma: initial report of a North Central Cancer Treatment Group/Radiation Therapy Oncology Group/Eastern Cooperative Oncology Group study. J Clin Oncol 2002;20:2267–76.

49. Kiebert GM, Curran D, Aaronson NK, et al. Quality of life after radiation therapy of cerebral low-grade gliomas of the adult: results of a randomised phase III trial on dose response (EORTC trial 22844). Eur J Cancer 1998;34:1902–9.

50. Laack NN, Brown PD, Ivnik RJ, et al. Cognitive function after radiotherapy for supratentorial low-grade glioma: a North Central Cancer Treatment Group prospective study. Int J Radiat Oncol Biol Phys 2005;63:1175–83.
51. Douw L, Klein M, Fagel SS, et al. Cognitive and radiological effects of radio-therapy in patients with low-grade glioma: long-term follow-up. Lancet Neurol 2009;8:810–8.
52. Armstrong CL, Ruffer JE, Corn B, et al. Biphasic patterns of memory deficits following moderate dose/partial brain irradiation: neuropsychologic outcome and proposed mechanisms. J Clin Oncol 1995;13:2263–71.
53. Pignatti F, van den Bent M, Curran D, et al. Prognostic factors for survival in adult patients with cerebral low-grade glioma. J Clin Oncol 2002;20:2076–84.
54. Knisely JP, Lally BE, Zelterman D. Validation of the European Organization for Research and Treatment of Cancer (EORTC) prognostic factors for low grade gliomas utilizing the surveillance, epidemiology, and end results (SEER) data-base. Int J Radiat Oncol Biol Phys 2005;63(Suppl 1):S262–3.
55. Gondi V, Eickhoff J, Tome WA, et al. SEER database analysis of survival impact of early adjuvant radiotherapy (EART) for resected supratentorial low-grade glioma (SLGG) in adults. Int J Radiat Oncol Biol Phys 2011;81(Suppl 2):S270.
56. Lally B, Baehring J, Zelterman D, et al. Observations on the relationship between radiotherapy and survival in patients with low-grade gliomas from the Surveil-lance, Epidemiology, and End Results (SEER) program. Neuro-Oncol 2005; 7(3):389.
57. Buckner JC, Gesme D Jr, O'Fallon JR, et al. Phase II trial of procarbazine, lomus-tine, and vincristine as initial therapy for patients with low-grade oligodendro-glioma or oligoastrocytoma: efficacy and associations with chromosomal abnormalities. J Clin Oncol 2003;21:251–5.
58. Kaloshi G, Benouaich-Amiel A, Diakite F, et al. Temozolomide for low-grade gliomas: predictive impact of 1p/19q loss on response and outcome. Neurology 2007;68:1831–6.
59. Huang L, Jiang T, Yuan F, et al. Correlation of chromosomes 1p and 19q status and expressions of O6-methylguanine DNA methyltransferase (MGMT), p53 and Ki-67 in diffuse gliomas of World Health Organization (WHO) grades II and III: a clinicopathological study. Neuropathol Appl Neurobiol 2009;35:367–79.
60. Ochsenbein AF, Schubert AD, Vassella E, et al. Quantitative analysis of O6-methylguanine DNA methyltransferase (MGMT) promoter methylation in patients with low-grade gliomas. J Neurooncol 2011;103:343–51.
61. Sherman JH, Moldovan K, Yeoh HK, et al. Impact of temozolomide chemotherapy on seizure frequency in patients with low-grade gliomas. J Neurosurg 2011;114: 1617–21.
62. Buckingham SC, Campbell SL, Haas BR, et al. Glutamate release by primary brain tumors induces epileptic activity. Nat Med 2011;17:1269–74.

Anaplastic Gliomas
Radiation, Chemotherapy, or Both?

Nicholas A. Blondin, MD*, Kevin P. Becker, MD, PhD

KEYWORDS

- Anaplastic glioma • Anaplastic astrocytoma • Anaplastic oligodendroglioma
- Anaplastic oligoastrocytoma • Treatment

KEY POINTS

- Anaplastic gliomas have a unique natural history compared with glioblastomas and low-grade gliomas, but have historically been grouped together with either of these tumor types in treatment studies.
- Survival differences exist between anaplastic astrocytomas and anaplastic oligodendrogliomas, which are caused by the differing molecular features of these tumors.
- Current evidence indicates that there is no benefit to radiotherapy with concurrent or adjuvant chemotherapy in patients with anaplastic gliomas.
- Initial treatment with chemotherapy or radiation alone is an appropriate treatment strategy, and temozolomide is the first-line chemotherapy agent. The other treatment modality should be used when relapse occurs.

INTRODUCTION
Background

Anaplastic gliomas comprise World Health Organization (WHO) grade III astrocytomas, oligodendrogliomas, and oligoastrocytomas (referred to as mixed gliomas). Typical microscopic features of anaplastic gliomas include moderate hypercellularity, moderate cellular and nuclear pleomorphism, increased mitotic activity, and microvascular proliferation without necrosis.[1] These features are in contrast with WHO grade II gliomas, which are low in mitotic activity, and WHO grade IV gliomas, referred to as glioblastomas, which show vascular proliferation and necrosis.

In most studies conducted before the year 2000, anaplastic gliomas were grouped with glioblastomas as high-grade gliomas or malignant gliomas. Patients with glioblastoma typically comprise most of the patients in these studies, causing difficulty in the interpretation of treatment results. Some studies have also grouped anaplastic

Department of Neurology, Yale University School of Medicine, PO Box 208018, 15 York Street, LCI-9, New Haven, CT 06520, USA
* Corresponding author.
E-mail address: nicholas.blondin@yale.edu

Hematol Oncol Clin N Am 26 (2012) 811–823
doi:10.1016/j.hoc.2012.04.003
0889-8588/12/$ – see front matter © 2012 Elsevier Inc. All rights reserved.

hemonc.theclinics.com

gliomas as a single entity. However, it is now evident that anaplastic astrocytomas have a distinct prognosis compared with anaplastic oligodendrogliomas and mixed gliomas, which are more susceptible to chemotherapy and radiotherapy. In addition to tumor grade and histologic type of anaplastic glioma, other prognostic indicators of survival include patient age at diagnosis and the Karnofsky Performance Score (KPS) of the patient.[2]

Although a widely accepted standard of care currently exists for the initial treatment of glioblastomas,[3] the optimal treatment of anaplastic gliomas remains controversial. Options for treatment include radiotherapy, which is currently used in most patients diagnosed with an anaplastic glioma, as well as chemotherapy or a combination of modalities (**Table 1**). This article describes how treatment algorithms for anaplastic gliomas have evolved and reviews the recent studies that have established the current standard of care.

Molecular Features

Important molecular differences exist between anaplastic astrocytomas and anaplastic oligodendrogliomas. Mixed gliomas typically share features of anaplastic oligodendrogliomas, as well as having a better prognosis compared with anaplastic astrocytomas. Important molecular features include 1p/19q codeletion, isocitrate dehydrogenase mutations (IDH1/IDH2), and O^6-methylguanine-DNA-methyltransferase (MGMT) promoter methylation.

Loss of the short arm of chromosome 1 and long arm of chromosome 19, referred to as 1p/19q codeletion, is caused by an unbalanced chromosomal translocation resulting in a loss of genetic material.[4] 1p/19q Codeletion is commonly found in anaplastic oligodendrogliomas and mixed gliomas and is associated with increased chemosensitivity and radiosensitivity of the tumor.[5,6] The presence of 1p/19q codeletion has been found to be the most important prognostic factor associated with improved survival in patients with anaplastic oligodendrogliomas.[7]

Mutation in the IDH1 and IDH2 genes currently has an unknown mechanism affecting tumor biology, and the presence of mutation is associated with a better prognosis.[8] MGMT promoter methylation results in MGMT gene silencing and is commonly found in anaplastic gliomas.[9] It is presumed to increase tumor susceptibility to alkylating chemotherapy agents, and is associated with a better prognosis.[3]

Surgery

The diagnosis of an anaplastic glioma is made histologically. Although biopsy may suffice for diagnosis, maximal safe resection significantly improves both progression-free survival and overall survival.[10] Quality of life is also improved in patients treated with maximal surgical resection.[11] The use of agents to improve visualization of tumor, such as 5-aminolevulinic acid (which causes tumor fluorescence), can lead to an improvement in achieving gross total resection and improves progression-free survival.[12] However, because of the infiltrative nature of anaplastic gliomas, surgical resection is not curative, and treatment with radiotherapy, chemotherapy, or both modalities is required for further treatment of the tumor.

EVOLUTION OF TREATMENT STRATEGIES FOR ANAPLASTIC GLIOMAS
Radiation

Radiotherapy volume (whole brain radiotherapy vs external beam radiotherapy)
Whole brain radiotherapy (WBRT) following surgery for anaplastic gliomas was developed in the early 1970s and used through the early 1980s. Studies evaluating WBRT for malignant gliomas consistently showed a survival benefit, albeit modest.[13–15]

Table 1
Large studies of postoperative treatment of anaplastic gliomas

Author	Study Year	Tumor Type	Number of Patients	Initial Therapy	OS	P Value
Walker et al[14]	1980	AG	94	RT	9	—
			92	RT + BCNU	12.75	P = .108, vs RT alone
			91	RT + MeCCNU	10.5	P = .668, vs RT alone
Cairncross et al[56] RTOG 9402	2006	AO	142	RT	56.4	—
			147	RT + PCV	58.8	P = .26
van den Bent et al[57] EORTC 26951	2006	AO	183	RT	30.6	—
			185	RT + PCV	40.3	P = .23
Wick et al[61] NOA-04	2009	AG	139	RT	72.1	—
			135	PCV or TMZ	82.6	P = NS
Lassman et al[65]	2011	AG	200	RT	52.8	—
			528	RT + PCV or TMZ	85.2	P<.0001, vs RT alone
			201	PCV or TMZ	84	P = .0008, vs RT alone

Abbreviations: AG, anaplastic glioma; AO, anaplastic oligodendroglioma and mixed glioma; BCNU, N,N'-bis(2-chloroethyl)-N-nitrosourea; EORTC, European Organisation for Research and Treatment of Cancer; MeCCNU, 1-(2-chloroethyl)-3-(4-methylcyclohexyl)-1-nitrosoureanvbn; NOA, Neurooncology Working Group of the German Cancer Society; NS, nonsignificant; OS, overall survival in months; PCV, combination procarbazine, lomustine, and vincristine; RT, radiotherapy; RTOG, Radiation Therapy Oncology Group; TMZ, temozolomide.

However, radiotherapy can have serious long-term neurotoxic effects, particularly in large treatment fields such as WBRT. These effects can include a progressive neuro-degenerative process characterized by neuronal loss and demyelination, as well as both small and large vessel disease.[16] In patients with expected long-term survival, such as those with anaplastic gliomas, and particularly those with anaplastic oligoden-drogliomas, radiotherapy-induced neurotoxicity must be considered when making treatment decisions.

In patients treated with WBRT, tumor recurrence was recognized to commonly develop within 2 cm of the original tumor site.[17] Because of this observation, as well as the significant risk of neurotoxicity with WBRT, external beam radiotherapy (EBRT) was developed to maximize treatment to the tumor and minimize radiation to sur-rounding brain tissue.[18] A study of 50 patients with malignant glioma randomized to receive either EBRT 50 Gy followed by a boost of 10 Gy, or WBRT 40 Gy followed by a boost of 20 Gy, found no 6-month overall survival benefit in the EBRT group (66.7% vs 50.7%, $P>.1$), but there was a significant improvement in the KPS of patients treated with EBRT (80% vs 56% improved, $P<.01$).[19]

The development of neuroimaging techniques, such as computed tomography (CT) and magnetic resonance imaging (MRI) has led to further refinement in the accuracy of EBRT.[20] Using CT planning, three-dimensional (3D) conformal radiotherapy is now used to maximize radiotherapy to the tumor.[21] Intensity-modulated radiotherapy (IMRT), in which radiation intensity is varied across the treatment field to further reduce the risk of radiation injury to critical adjacent brain structures, is also commonly used in many centers.[22]

Radiotherapy dosing

The initial radiotherapy studies using WBRT typically used a treatment dosing of 50 to 60 Gy. Larger doses of radiotherapy were found to have higher toxicity rates with no improvement in survival.[23,24] After EBRT became the accepted standard of care, a large trial of patients with malignant gliomas was conducted to establish the optimal radiotherapy dosing. In this study, 474 patients were randomized to receive either a low dose of 45 Gy in 20 fractions over 4 weeks or a high dose of 60 Gy in 30 fractions over 6 weeks.[25] There was a significant increase in median survival in the high-dose group (12 vs 9 months, $P = .007$), establishing 60 Gy as the optimal target dose. The increase in survival was still evident in a subgroup analysis of patients with poor prognosis. More recent studies have confirmed that radiotherapy doses of more than 60 Gy do not confer a significant survival benefit for patients with anaplastic gliomas. A trial using a 3D conformal IMRT technique found no survival benefit in patients with malignant gliomas treated with 70, 80, or 90 Gy.[26]

Fractionation schemes

Conventional fractionation refers to the once daily delivery of radiotherapy, typically with a dose of 1.8 to 2.0 Gy per day, for a total up to 60 Gy. Hyperfractionation refers to the delivery of 2 smaller doses of radiation per day, which can allow for an increase in the maximal dose of radiation that can be safely delivered. In a study of several hyperfractionation schemes with adjuvant carmustine, there was no survival benefit to patients with malignant gliomas treated to 72 Gy (with hyperfractionation of 1.2 Gy twice-daily dosing) compared with conventional radiotherapy at 60 Gy.[27]

Additional smaller studies have also found no clear benefit to hyperfractionation versus conventional fractionation schemes.[28,29] A review of fractionation schemes found that, although hyperfractionation can shorten the treatment time of radiotherapy for patients with malignant gliomas, it does not result in an improvement in overall survival.[30]

Radiosensitizers
Radiosensitizers are compounds given concurrently with radiotherapy to increase the therapeutic effect of radiation. In the past 2 decades, several compounds have been investigated. However, none showed a clear benefit in survival.

In a small study of patients with recurrent malignant gliomas, α-difluoromethylornithine (DFMO), in combination with carmustine, was associated with a survival benefit.[31] However, myelosuppression and hearing loss were dose-limiting toxicities. A larger study of 249 patients with anaplastic glioma randomized to receive either PCV (procarbazine, lomustine (1-(2-chloro-ethyl)-3-cyclohexyl-1-nitrosourea [CCNU]), and vincristine) chemotherapy or DFMO-PCV after surgery and radiotherapy found no difference in overall survival between the 2 groups, and a significant increase in gastrointestinal and hematologic toxicities in the DFMO-PCV group.[32]

Other radiosensitizers include 5-bromo-2'-deoxyuridine (BrdU, bromodeoxyuridine) and misonidazole. BrdU was found to have no survival benefit, and likely worsened toxicity of radiation.[33,34] Misonidazole was also found to trend toward worsened survival.[35] At this time, radiosensitizers are not used in conventional therapy.

Current standard of care for radiation
Despite many years of research related to radiotherapy dosing and fractionation, there does not seem to be a significant benefit to any scheme other than EBRT given in conventional fractionation to a maximum dose of 60 Gy to a focal radiation field using 3D conformal planning techniques. Radiotherapy remains a frequent choice of the initial therapy for anaplastic gliomas, and this is discussed further later.

For slow-growing tumors such as anaplastic oligodendrogliomas, reirradiation may be considered for patients with an interval of at least several years since the prior radiotherapy. In a study of patients with recurrent glioma after cranial radiation treated with repeat radiotherapy at a median of 9 years, there was modestly improved overall survival, although most patients died of tumor progression before the onset of late effects from the reirradiation.[36]

Chemotherapy

Carmustine
The earliest chemotherapy to show a survival benefit in anaplastic gliomas (included in trials of malignant gliomas) was carmustine (N,N'-bis(2-chloroethyl)-N-nitrosourea [BCNU]). From 1970 to 1990, no single chemotherapy agent or combination was found to confer a survival benefit that was superior to BCNU alone. However, BCNU has only a modest survival benefit, and a substantial risk of toxicity. In the German-Austrian Glioma (GAG) trial, patients with malignant glioma treated with surgery and WBRT were randomized to combination chemotherapy with BCNU plus teniposide or BCNU alone. There was no difference in overall survival and 36% of patients treated with BCNU experienced symptoms of pulmonary fibrosis within 12 months, in some cases after a single dose. The trial results are available, but are not published in peer-reviewed literature.

The high rate of pulmonary toxicity of BCNU in the GAG trial, as well as its modest efficacy, led to the study of alternative nitrosoureas. In the NOA-01 trial, patients with malignant glioma treated with surgery and EBRT were randomized to receive nimustine ((1-4-amino-2-methyl-5-pyrimidinyl)-methyl-3-(2-chloroethyl)-3-nitrosourea [ACNU]) plus teniposide or ACNU plus cytarabine.[37] There was a modest overall survival advantage in both groups compared with historical controls in this trial, but, as with BCNU, ACNU has substantial toxicity and is not currently in clinical use in the United States.[38] Lomustine (CCNU) also had modest efficacy and is currently the most commonly used nitrosourea, as a component of the PCV chemotherapy regimen.

PCV regimen

The PCV regimen consists of procarbazine, CCNU, and vincristine. In 1990, a trial of PCV versus single-agent BCNU in patients with malignant gliomas found a significantly improved overall survival in patients with anaplastic gliomas treated with PCV compared with BCNU (157 vs 82 weeks, $P = .021$).[39] The study was small (only 36 and 37 patients in the PCV and BCNU arms, respectively) and it was not performed as an intention-to-treat analysis. Despite these limitations, this trial led to PCV replacing BCNU as the standard of care for chemotherapy, before the development of temozolomide.

As with radiotherapy, anaplastic oligodendrogliomas and mixed gliomas have a more favorable response to PCV compared with anaplastic astrocytomas in both progression-free and overall survival.[40–43] However, PCV also has a substantial risk of toxicity. In a regimen using a dose-intense scheme of PCV, central neurotoxic side effects in combination with severe hematologic and hepatic toxicity were frequently observed.[44] Many patients are thus unable to complete a full course of therapy.

Temozolomide

Temozolomide is an alkylating chemotherapy agent that has more recently been found to be effective in patients with anaplastic gliomas. In a retrospective analysis of 109 patients with anaplastic astrocytomas derived from 2 trials, adjuvant temozolomide was as effective as, and less toxic than, PCV.[10] There was no significant difference in 2-year progression-free survival or median progression-free survival. However, temozolomide was discontinued less often than PCV because of toxicity (0% vs 37%).

Varying dose schedules of temozolomide have been evaluated in malignant gliomas. In one study, temozolomide was given daily for either 5 days (200 mg/m^2/d) or 21 days (100 mg/m^2/d), in 28-day cycles, up to 9 months.[45] The 5-day-per-cycle dosing schedule had improved progression-free survival compared with the 21-day-per-cycle dosing (5.0 vs 4.2 months, $P = .023$), improved global quality of life (49% vs 19% improved, $P = .005$), and a trend toward improved overall survival (8.5 vs 6.6 months, $P = .056$). Temozolomide 5-day-per-cycle dosing also had improved progression-free survival compared with a standard PCV dosing regimen (5.0 vs 3.6 months, $P = .038$).

High-dose temozolomide (550 mg/m^2) in combination with BCNU (150 mg/m^2) given once in 42-day cycles was evaluated in a small study of patients with anaplastic gliomas.[46] Nearly half of patients experienced grade 3 or 4 (according to National Cancer Institute Common Toxicity Criteria) hematologic toxicities. The complete and partial response rates were 2% and 27% respectively, and an additional 54% of patients had stable disease. This regimen was thought to be excessively toxic, without a strong survival benefit. Thus, temozolomide 5-day-per-cycle dosing is currently the standard dosing schedule.

In addition to efficacy as an initial treatment, temozolomide has been shown to have efficacy after recurrence of tumor. In one study, 38 patients with anaplastic oligodendrogliomas or mixed gliomas who were chemotherapy naïve, previously treated with surgery and radiation, were treated with temozolomide after tumor recurrence.[47] More than half of patients had a complete (26.3%) or partial response to temozolomide. In another study, 67 patients with anaplastic oligodendrogliomas or mixed gliomas were treated with temozolomide after tumor recurrence.[48] The overall response rate was 46.3%, with a higher response rate seen in patients with anaplastic oligodendrogliomas and tumors with 1p/19q codeletion.

In certain patient populations, for example extensively infiltrative gliomas affecting the dominant or both hemispheres, radiotherapy can be associated with significant morbidity, and monotherapy with temozolomide may be considered. Patients with 1p/19q codeletion have a longer progression-free survival, making temozolomide monotherapy an attractive option to avoid radiation-induced neurotoxicity.[6,49] Temozolomide monotherapy may also be considered for elderly patients, because a significant number of patients can achieve a prolonged survival.[50]

Salvage agents

Studies of patients with anaplastic oligodendroglioma have evaluated salvage chemotherapy with temozolomide and PCV. In one study, 48 patients with anaplastic oligodendrogliomas or mixed gliomas who had received previous radiation and PCV chemotherapy were treated with temozolomide, with an objective response rate of 43.8%, a median progression-free survival of 6.7 months, and a median overall survival of 10 months.[51] PCV may also be used in recurrent anaplastic oligodendroglioma after radiation and temozolomide treatment.[52]

Patients who have progressed on both PCV and temozolomide should be considered for a clinical trial. Newer agents, such as bevacizumab (a monoclonal antibody against vascular endothelial growth factor [VEGF]) are being evaluated for efficacy in anaplastic gliomas. A recent retrospective evaluation of single-agent bevacizumab was performed in 22 adults with recurrent 1p/19q codeleted anaplastic oligodendroglioma.[53] Fifteen patients (68%) showed a partial radiographic response, with median time to progression of 6.75 months and median survival of 8.5 months. Other standard chemotherapy agents including irinotecan, carboplatin, paclitaxel, and etoposide plus cisplatin have failed to show survival benefit in patients with relapsed anaplastic gliomas.

Current standard of care for chemotherapy

For patients with anaplastic gliomas, temozolomide has been found to be at least as effective as the PCV regimen, with significantly less toxicity, improved ease of administration, and better tolerability.[10] Because of this, temozolomide is now considered to be the first-line chemotherapy agent for anaplastic gliomas. The conventional dosing for temozolomide is 200 mg/m^2/d once daily for 5 days in 28-day cycles, up to 9 months. If a patient has treatment failure with temozolomide, PCV or bevacizumab can be considered as salvage agents.

CONTROVERSIES IN INITIAL TREATMENT OF ANAPLASTIC GLIOMAS
Radiation, Chemotherapy, or Both?

Concurrent or adjuvant radiation and chemotherapy

Most trials evaluating treatment strategies for anaplastic gliomas have compared radiotherapy and concurrent or adjuvant chemotherapy versus radiotherapy alone. These studies have consistently shown no difference in overall survival between groups, even when adjusted for tumor histologic subgroup, patient age, or KPS.[54,55] Two large prospective trials of patients with anaplastic oligodendrogliomas and mixed gliomas have provided the strongest evidence against concurrent or adjuvant radiation and chemotherapy: the RTOG 9402 trial and the EORTC 26951 trial.

In the RTOG 9402 trial, 289 patients were randomized to radiotherapy (RT) versus PCV chemotherapy followed by radiotherapy.[56] Only 48% of patients assigned to the PCV/RT arm were able to complete 4 cycles of chemotherapy, because of substantial PCV toxicity. Patients in the PCV/RT arm were found to have a longer progression-free survival (2.6 vs 1.7 years, $P = .004$), but there was no difference in overall survival (4.9 vs 4.7 years, $P = .26$). Patients with 1p/19q codeletion had a significantly longer survival in both treatment arms (>7 vs 2.8 years, $P \leq .001$).

In the EORTC 26951 trial, 368 patients were randomized to radiotherapy versus radiotherapy and concurrent PCV.[57] As in the RTOG 9402 trial, RT/PCV increased progression-free survival time (23 vs 13.2 months, $P = .0018$) but did not significantly improve overall survival (40.3 vs 30.6 months, $P = .23$). In 38% of the patients in the RT/PCV arm, adjuvant PCV was discontinued because of toxicity. Patients with combined 1p/19q loss had longer survival, with no difference between the 2 treatment arms. A subset analysis also found that MGMT promoter hypermethylation was a prognostic factor associated with an improved outcome for both treatment arms.[58]

In both the RTOG 9402 and EORTC 26951 trials, there was no increase in overall survival in patients initially treated with concurrent radiation and PCV chemotherapy versus radiation alone. However, most patients assigned to the radiation-only arms in each trial (80% in RTOG 9402 and 82% in EORTC 26951) received PCV on disease progression. Thus, these 2 trials showed that a treatment strategy of radiation therapy followed by chemotherapy at relapse may be appropriate, rather than concurrent or adjuvant chemotherapy with radiation.

Sequential radiation or chemotherapy

Initial treatment with chemoradiation or radiation therapy, followed by the use of the other modality at relapse, can be referred to as sequential therapy. Although radiotherapy has historically been viewed as the first-line treatment of anaplastic gliomas, a treatment strategy of chemotherapy as the initial modality has also been studied.[59] In a small study, 20 patients with anaplastic oligodendrogliomas received temozolomide as their first modality of therapy, with radiation held until there was progression of disease.[60] Treatment was given for 5 days in 28-day cycles at a starting dose of 200 mg/m²/d, with an objective response rate of 75% and median time to progression of 24 months. Temozolomide was well tolerated, with only 2 events of grade 3/4 hematologic toxicity.

Initial treatment with chemotherapy, followed by radiation at tumor recurrence, was evaluated in the recent NOA-4 trial.[61] In this large prospective study, 318 patients with anaplastic gliomas were randomized to receive conventional radiotherapy or chemotherapy, either PCV or temozolomide, at initial diagnosis. At the occurrence of disease progression, or unacceptable toxicity, patients were switched from radiotherapy to chemotherapy or from chemotherapy to radiotherapy, with some exceptions in a small group of patients. The primary end point was the time to treatment failure, which was defined as progression of disease after radiotherapy and 1 chemotherapy regimen.

Between the radiotherapy and chemotherapy groups there was no significant difference between the median time to treatment failure (42.7 vs 43.8 months, $P = .28$), progression-free survival (30.6 vs 31.9 months, $P = .87$), and overall survival (72.1 vs 82.6 months, P reported as nonsignificant). Older age and incomplete surgical resection of tumor were associated with a shorter time to treatment failure. As expected, anaplastic oligodendrogliomas and mixed gliomas were found to have a significantly better prognosis than anaplastic astrocytomas. MGMT promoter hypermethylation, IDH1 gene mutation, and 1p/19q codeletion also reduced the risk of disease progression independently of treatment strategy. The study showed that chemotherapy alone is an acceptable initial treatment strategy for patients with anaplastic gliomas, with radiation therapy on progression of disease.

SUMMARY

In patients with WHO grade II gliomas, adjuvant chemotherapy or radiation therapy can be safely held until radiographic progression occurs or a tumor-related neurologic symptom occurs, which has been termed the wait-and-see approach.[62] However, in patients with anaplastic gliomas, delaying initial treatment significantly reduces survival.[63,64]

Based on the results of the RTOG 9402, EORTC 26951, and NOA-04 trials, there does not seem to be any benefit to radiotherapy and concurrent or adjuvant chemotherapy in patients with anaplastic gliomas. In these patients, initial treatment with chemotherapy or radiation alone is the preferred treatment modality. A limitation of the RTOG 9402 and EORTC 26951 trials is the choice of PCV chemotherapy, known to have significant toxicity limiting the effective dose that can be given. Temozolomide is now the preferred chemotherapy agent for the treatment of anaplastic gliomas, and must be evaluated in future studies.

Although the recent prospective clinical trial data have shown no benefit to concurrent or adjuvant chemotherapy with radiotherapy, a recent large retrospective study has suggested that there may be a survival advantage in certain histologic subgroups of anaplastic gliomas.[65] In this study, there was no difference in overall survival in patients with 1p/19q codeleted anaplastic oligodendrogliomas who received chemotherapy, radiation, or combination chemotherapy-radiation as their initial treatment modality, likely because patients received additional therapy on tumor recurrence. However, in patients without 1p/19q codeletion, overall survival was longer in patients who had been treated initially with concurrent chemotherapy and radiotherapy (median 5.0 years) versus chemotherapy (2.2 years, $P = .02$) or radiotherapy (1.9 years, $P<.0001$) alone. Two large prospective trials are currently underway to evaluate whether radiotherapy and concurrent temozolomide offers a survival advantage.

The CODEL (1p/19q codeleted tumors) trial is a phase III trial investigating patients diagnosed with anaplastic gliomas found to have 1p/19q codeletion, which will compare radiotherapy alone versus temozolomide alone versus radiotherapy with concurrent temozolomide.[66] The trial is estimating enrollment of 488 patients and has an estimated completion date of February 2014. The CATNON (concurrent adjuvant temozolomide chemotherapy for patients with NON-1p/19q deleted anaplastic glioma) trial is a phase III trial investigating patients with anaplastic gliomas without 1p/19q codeletion, and will compare radiotherapy alone versus concurrent or adjuvant temozolomide chemotherapy with radiotherapy.[67] The trial is estimating enrollment of 1360 patients and has an estimated completion date of June 2015.

At this time, the available prospective evidence indicates that patients with a newly diagnosed anaplastic glioma should undergo initial treatment with chemotherapy or radiotherapy, with the other modality used at relapse. For selected patient populations, such as patients with extensively infiltrative neoplasms of the dominant or both hemispheres, initial chemotherapy may be superior because it avoids the risk of radiation neurotoxicity, at least at the time of initial diagnosis. However, specific treatment algorithms for subpopulations await prospective evaluation. Refinement of the current treatment algorithm may occur when the results of the CODEL and CATNON trials are reported within the next few years.

REFERENCES

1. Louis DN, Ohgaki H, Wiestler OD, et al. The 2007 WHO classification of tumours of the central nervous system. Acta Neuropathol 2007;114(2):97–109.

2. Buckner JC. Factors influencing survival in high-grade gliomas. Semin Oncol 2003;30(6 Suppl 19):10–4.

3. Stupp R, Hegi ME, Mason WP, et al. Effects of radiotherapy with concomitant and adjuvant temozolomide versus radiotherapy alone on survival in glioblastoma in a randomised phase III study: 5-year analysis of the EORTC-NCIC trial. Lancet Oncol 2009;10(5):459–66.

4. Jenkins RB, Blair H, Ballman KV, et al. A t(1;19)(q10;p10) mediates the combined deletions of 1p and 19q and predicts a better prognosis of patients with oligodendroglioma. Cancer Res 2006;66(20):9852–61.

5. Cairncross G, Macdonald D, Ludwin S, et al. Chemotherapy for anaplastic oligodendroglioma. National Cancer Institute of Canada Clinical Trials Group. J Clin Oncol 1994;12(10):2013–21.

6. Cairncross JG, Ueki K, Zlatescu MC, et al. Specific genetic predictors of chemotherapeutic response and survival in patients with anaplastic oligodendrogliomas. J Natl Cancer Inst 1998;90(19):1473–9.

7. Smith JS, Perry A, Borell TJ, et al. Alterations of chromosome arms 1p and 19q as predictors of survival in oligodendrogliomas, astrocytomas, and mixed oligoastrocytomas. J Clin Oncol 2000;18(3):636–45.

8. Sanson M, Marie Y, Paris S, et al. Isocitrate dehydrogenase 1 codon 132 mutation is an important prognostic biomarker in gliomas. J Clin Oncol 2009;27(25): 4150–4.

9. Suri V, Jha P, Sharma MC, et al. O6-Methylguanine DNA methyltransferase gene promoter methylation in high-grade gliomas: a review of current status. Neurol India 2011;59(2):229–35.

10. Brandes AA, Nicolardi L, Tosoni A, et al. Survival following adjuvant PCV or temozolomide for anaplastic astrocytoma. Neuro Oncol 2006;8(3):253–60.

11. Tsitlakidis A, Foroglou N, Venetis CA, et al. Biopsy versus resection in the management of malignant gliomas: a systematic review and meta-analysis. J Neurosurg 2010;112(5):1020–32.

12. Stummer W, Pichlmeier U, Meinel T, et al. Fluorescence-guided surgery with 5-aminolevulinic acid for resection of malignant glioma: a randomised controlled multicentre phase III trial. Lancet Oncol 2006;7(5):392–401.

13. Walker MD, Alexander E Jr, Hunt WE, et al. Evaluation of BCNU and/or radiotherapy in the treatment of anaplastic gliomas. A cooperative clinical trial. J Neurosurg 1978;49(3):333–43.

14. Walker MD, Green SB, Byar DP, et al. Randomized comparisons of radiotherapy and nitrosoureas for the treatment of malignant glioma after surgery. N Engl J Med 1980;303(23):1323–9.

15. Sandberg-Wollheim M, Malmstrom P, Stromblad LG, et al. A randomized study of chemotherapy with procarbazine, vincristine, and lomustine with and without radiation therapy for astrocytoma grades 3 and/or 4. Cancer 1991;68(1):22–9.

16. Shapiro WR. Therapy of adult malignant brain tumors: what have the clinical trials taught us? Semin Oncol 1986;13(1):38–45.

17. Hochberg FH, Pruitt A. Assumptions in the radiotherapy of glioblastoma. Neurology 1980;30(9):907–11.

18. Choucair AK, Levin VA, Gutin PH, et al. Development of multiple lesions during radiation therapy and chemotherapy in patients with gliomas. J Neurosurg 1986;65(5):654–8.

19. Sharma RR, Singh DP, Pathak A, et al. Local control of high-grade gliomas with limited volume irradiation versus whole brain irradiation. Neurol India 2003; 51(4):512–7.

20. Jansen EP, Dewit LG, van Herk M, et al. Target volumes in radiotherapy for high-grade malignant glioma of the brain. Radiother Oncol 2000;56(2):151–6.
21. Thornton AF Jr, Hegarty TJ, Ten Haken RK, et al. Three-dimensional treatment planning of astrocytomas: a dosimetric study of cerebral irradiation. Int J Radiat Oncol Biol Phys 1991;20(6):1309–15.
22. Narayana A, Yamada J, Berry S, et al. Intensity-modulated radiotherapy in high-grade gliomas: clinical and dosimetric results. Int J Radiat Oncol Biol Phys 2006; 64(3):892–7.
23. Chang CH, Horton J, Schoenfeld D, et al. Comparison of postoperative radiotherapy and combined postoperative radiotherapy and chemotherapy in the multidisciplinary management of malignant gliomas. A joint Radiation Therapy Oncology Group and Eastern Cooperative Oncology Group study. Cancer 1983;52(6):997–1007.
24. Nelson DF, Diener-West M, Horton J, et al. Combined modality approach to treatment of malignant gliomas–re-evaluation of RTOG 7401/ECOG 1374 with long-term follow-up: a joint study of the Radiation Therapy Oncology Group and the Eastern Cooperative Oncology Group. NCI Monogr 1988;6:279–84.
25. Bleehen NM, Stenning SP. A Medical Research Council trial of two radiotherapy doses in the treatment of grades 3 and 4 astrocytoma. The Medical Research Council Brain Tumour Working Party. Br J Cancer 1991;64(4):769–74.
26. Chan JL, Lee SW, Fraass BA, et al. Survival and failure patterns of high-grade gliomas after three-dimensional conformal radiotherapy. J Clin Oncol 2002; 20(6):1635–42.
27. Nelson DF, Curran WJ Jr, Scott C, et al. Hyperfractionated radiation therapy and bis-chlorethyl nitrosourea in the treatment of malignant glioma–possible advantage observed at 72.0 Gy in 1.2 Gy B.I.D. fractions: report of the Radiation Therapy Oncology Group Protocol 8302. Int J Radiat Oncol Biol Phys 1993; 25(2):193–207.
28. Fulton DS, Urtasun RC, Scott-Brown I, et al. Increasing radiation dose intensity using hyperfractionation in patients with malignant glioma. Final report of a prospective phase I-II dose response study. J Neurooncol 1992;14(1): 63–72.
29. Scott CB, Curran WJ, Yung WK, et al. Long term results of RTOG 9006: a randomized trial of hyperfractionated radiotherapy to 72.0 Gy and carmustine versus standard radiotherapy and carmustine for malignant glioma patients with emphasis on anaplastic astrocytoma patients [abstract 401a]. Proc Ann Meet ASCO 1998;17.
30. Nieder C, Andratschke N, Wiedenmann N, et al. Radiotherapy for high-grade gliomas. Does altered fractionation improve the outcome? Strahlenther Onkol 2004;180(7):401–7.
31. Prados M, Rodriguez L, Chamberlain M, et al. Treatment of recurrent gliomas with 1,3-bis(2-chloroethyl)-1-nitrosourea and alpha-difluoromethylornithine. Neurosurgery 1989;24(6):806–9.
32. Levin VA, Hess KR, Choucair A, et al. Phase III randomized study of postradiotherapy chemotherapy with combination alpha-difluoromethylornithine-PCV versus PCV for anaplastic gliomas. Clin Cancer Res 2003;9(3):981–90.
33. Levin VA, Prados MR, Wara WM, et al. Radiation therapy and bromodeoxyuridine chemotherapy followed by procarbazine, lomustine, and vincristine for the treatment of anaplastic gliomas. Int J Radiat Oncol Biol Phys 1995;32(1):75–83.
34. Prados MD, Scott C, Sandler H, et al. A phase 3 randomized study of radiotherapy plus procarbazine, CCNU, and vincristine (PCV) with or without BUdR

for the treatment of anaplastic astrocytoma: a preliminary report of RTOG 9404. Int J Radiat Oncol Biol Phys 1999;45(5):1109–15.

35. Nelson DF, Diener-West M, Weinstein AS, et al. A randomized comparison of misonidazole sensitized radiotherapy plus BCNU and radiotherapy plus BCNU for treatment of malignant glioma after surgery: final report of an RTOG study. Int J Radiat Oncol Biol Phys 1986;12(10):1793–800.

36. Paulino AC, Mai WY, Chintagumpala M, et al. Radiation-induced malignant gliomas: is there a role for reirradiation? Int J Radiat Oncol Biol Phys 2008; 71(5):1381–7.

37. Weller M, Muller B, Koch R, et al. Neuro-Oncology Working Group 01 trial of nimustine plus teniposide versus nimustine plus cytarabine chemotherapy in addition to involved-field radiotherapy in the first-line treatment of malignant glioma. J Clin Oncol 2003;21(17):3276–84.

38. Happold C, Roth P, Wick W, et al. ACNU-based chemotherapy for recurrent glioma in the temozolomide era. J Neurooncol 2009;92(1):45–8.

39. Levin VA, Silver P, Hannigan J, et al. Superiority of post-radiotherapy adjuvant chemotherapy with CCNU, procarbazine, and vincristine (PCV) over BCNU for anaplastic gliomas: NCOG 6G61 final report. Int J Radiat Oncol Biol Phys 1990;18(2):321–4.

40. Cairncross JG, Macdonald DR. Chemotherapy for oligodendroglioma. Progress report. Arch Neurol 1991;48(2):225–7.

41. Macdonald DR, Gaspar LE, Cairncross JG. Successful chemotherapy for newly diagnosed aggressive oligodendroglioma. Ann Neurol 1990;27(5):573–4.

42. van den Bent MJ, Kros JM, Heimans JJ, et al. Response rate and prognostic factors of recurrent oligodendroglioma treated with procarbazine, CCNU, and vincristine chemotherapy. Dutch Neuro-oncology Group. Neurology 1998;51(4):1140–5.

43. Kristof RA, Neuloh G, Hans V, et al. Combined surgery, radiation, and PCV chemotherapy for astrocytomas compared to oligodendrogliomas and oligoastrocytomas WHO grade III. J Neurooncol 2002;59(3):231–7.

44. Postma TJ, van Groeningen CJ, Witjes RJ, et al. Neurotoxicity of combination chemotherapy with procarbazine, CCNU and vincristine (PCV) for recurrent glioma. J Neurooncol 1998;38(1):69–75.

45. Brada M, Stenning S, Gabe R, et al. Temozolomide versus procarbazine, lomustine, and vincristine in recurrent high-grade glioma. J Clin Oncol 2010;28(30):4601–8.

46. Chang SM, Prados MD, Yung WK, et al. Phase II study of neoadjuvant 1, 3-bis (2-chloroethyl)-1-nitrosourea and temozolomide for newly diagnosed anaplastic glioma: a North American Brain Tumor Consortium Trial. Cancer 2004;100(8):1712–6.

47. van den Bent MJ, Taphoorn MJ, Brandes AA, et al. Phase II study of first-line chemotherapy with temozolomide in recurrent oligodendroglial tumors: the European Organization for Research and Treatment of Cancer Brain Tumor Group Study 26971. J Clin Oncol 2003;21(13):2525–8.

48. Brandes AA, Tosoni A, Cavallo G, et al. Correlations between O6-methylguanine DNA methyltransferase promoter methylation status, 1p and 19q deletions, and response to temozolomide in anaplastic and recurrent oligodendroglioma: a prospective GICNO study. J Clin Oncol 2006;24(29):4746–53.

49. Mikkelsen T, Doyle T, Anderson J, et al. Temozolomide single-agent chemotherapy for newly diagnosed anaplastic oligodendroglioma. J Neurooncol 2009; 92(1):57–63.

50. Ducray F, del Rio MS, Carpentier C, et al. Up-front temozolomide in elderly patients with anaplastic oligodendroglioma and oligoastrocytoma. J Neurooncol 2011;101(3):457–62.

51. Chinot OL, Honore S, Dufour H, et al. Safety and efficacy of temozolomide in patients with recurrent anaplastic oligodendrogliomas after standard radiotherapy and chemotherapy. J Clin Oncol 2001;19(9):2449–55.

52. Triebels VH, Taphoorn MJ, Brandes AA, et al. Salvage PCV chemotherapy for temozolomide-resistant oligodendrogliomas. Neurology 2004;63(5):904–6.

53. Chamberlain MC, Johnston S. Bevacizumab for recurrent alkylator-refractory anaplastic oligodendroglioma. Cancer 2009;115(8):1734–43.

54. Medical Research Council Brain Tumor Working Party. Randomized trial of procarbazine, lomustine, and vincristine in the adjuvant treatment of high-grade astrocytoma: a Medical Research Council trial. J Clin Oncol 2001;19(2):509–18.

55. Prados MD, Scott C, Curran WJ Jr, et al. Procarbazine, lomustine, and vincristine (PCV) chemotherapy for anaplastic astrocytoma: a retrospective review of radiation therapy oncology group protocols comparing survival with carmustine or PCV adjuvant chemotherapy. J Clin Oncol 1999;17(11):3389–95.

56. Intergroup Radiation Therapy Oncology Group Trial 9402, Cairncross G, Berkey B, et al. Phase III trial of chemotherapy plus radiotherapy compared with radiotherapy alone for pure and mixed anaplastic oligodendroglioma: Intergroup Radiation Therapy Oncology Group Trial 9402. J Clin Oncol 2006;24(18):2707–14.

57. van den Bent MJ, Carpentier AF, Brandes AA, et al. Adjuvant procarbazine, lomustine, and vincristine improves progression-free survival but not overall survival in newly diagnosed anaplastic oligodendrogliomas and oligoastrocytomas: a randomized European Organisation for Research and Treatment of Cancer phase III trial. J Clin Oncol 2006;24(18):2715–22.

58. van den Bent MJ, Dubbink HJ, Sanson M, et al. MGMT promoter methylation is prognostic but not predictive for outcome to adjuvant PCV chemotherapy in anaplastic oligodendroglial tumors: a report from EORTC Brain Tumor Group Study 26951. J Clin Oncol 2009;27(35):5881–6.

59. Gan HK, Rosenthal MA, Dowling A, et al. A phase II trial of primary temozolomide in patients with grade III oligodendroglial brain tumors. Neuro Oncol 2010;12(5):500–7.

60. Taliansky-Aronov A, Bokstein F, Lavon I, et al. Temozolomide treatment for newly diagnosed anaplastic oligodendrogliomas: a clinical efficacy trial. J Neurooncol 2006;79(2):153–7.

61. Wick W, Hartmann C, Engel C, et al. NOA-04 randomized phase III trial of sequential radiochemotherapy of anaplastic glioma with procarbazine, lomustine, and vincristine or temozolomide. J Clin Oncol 2009;27(35):5874–80.

62. van den Bent MJ, Afra D, de Witte O, et al. Long-term efficacy of early versus delayed radiotherapy for low-grade astrocytoma and oligodendroglioma in adults: the EORTC 22845 randomised trial. Lancet 2005;366(9490):985–90.

63. Irwin C, Hunn M, Purdie G, et al. Delay in radiotherapy shortens survival in patients with high grade glioma. J Neurooncol 2007;85(3):339–43.

64. Do V, Gebski V, Barton MB. The effect of waiting for radiotherapy for grade III/IV gliomas. Radiother Oncol 2000;57(2):131–6.

65. Lassman AB, Iwamoto FM, Cloughesy TF, et al. International retrospective study of over 1000 adults with anaplastic oligodendroglial tumors. Neuro Oncol 2011;13(6):649–59.

66. US National Library of Medicine. ClinicalTrials.gov. Available at: http://www.clinicaltrials.gov/ct2/show/nCT00887146. Accessed November 3, 2011.

67. US National Library of Medicine. ClinicalTrials.gov. Available at: http://clinicaltrials.gov/ct2/show/nCT00626990. Accessed November 3, 2011.

Glioblastoma Multiforme
Overview of Current Treatment and Future Perspectives

Kevin Anton, MD, PhD[a], Joachim M. Baehring, MD, DSc[b],
Tina Mayer, MD[c,d,*]

KEYWORDS

- Glioblastoma multiforme • Glioma • Brain tumor • Chemotherapy • Temozolomide
- Bevacizumab

KEY POINTS

- Current first-line treatment regimens combine surgical resection and chemoradiotherapy, providing a slight increase in overall survival.
- Age on its own should not be used as an exclusion criterion for glioblastoma multiforme (GBM) treatment, but performance status should be factored heavily into the decision-making process for treatment planning.
- Despite aggressive initial treatment, most patients develop recurrent disease, which can be treated with reresection, systemic treatment with targeted agents or cytotoxic chemotherapy, reirradiation, or radiosurgery.
- Research into novel therapies is investigating alternative temozolomide regimens, convection-enhanced delivery, immunotherapy, gene therapy, antiangiogenic agents with and without cytotoxic chemotherapy, poly(adenosine diphosphate-ribose) polymerase-1 inhibitors, and targeting of tumor growth-promoting pathways or cancer stem cell signaling pathways.
- Given the aggressive and resilient nature of GBM, continued efforts to better understand GBM pathophysiology are required to discover novel targets for future therapies.

Disclosures: No potential conflicts of interest.
[a] Department of Pharmacology, Cancer Institute of New Jersey, Robert Wood Johnson Medical School, University of Medicine and Dentistry of New Jersey, 195 Little Albany Street, New Brunswick, NJ 08903, USA; [b] Departments of Neurology, Neurosurgery, and Medicine, Yale University School of Medicine, Yale Brain Tumor Center 15 York Street, New Haven, CT 06510, USA; [c] Department of Medical Oncology, Cancer Institute of New Jersey, Robert Wood Johnson Medical School, University of Medicine and Dentistry of New Jersey, 195 Little Albany Street, New Brunswick, NJ 08903, USA; [d] Department of Medicine, Cancer Institute of New Jersey, Robert Wood Johnson Medical School, University of Medicine and Dentistry of New Jersey, 195 Little Albany Street, New Brunswick, NJ 08903, USA
* Corresponding author. Department of Medical Oncology, Cancer Institute of New Jersey, RWJMS/UMDNJ, 195 Little Albany Street, Room 4555, New Brunswick, NJ 08901.
E-mail address: mayertm@umdnj.edu

Hematol Oncol Clin N Am 26 (2012) 825–853
doi:10.1016/j.hoc.2012.04.006
0889-8588/12/$ – see front matter © 2012 Elsevier Inc. All rights reserved.

INTRODUCTION

Nearly 10,000 cases of glioblastoma multiforme (GBM) are diagnosed annually in the United States,[1] making GBM the most common primary malignant tumor of the central nervous system (CNS). Ongoing research has drastically advanced our understanding of GBM pathophysiology; however, meaningful survival improvement has not occurred.

With near-certain relapse, prognostic factors are important in counseling patients and selecting individual patients for specific treatment modalities. Nomograms can be helpful in predicting the prognosis of individual patients, taking into account pertinent molecular and prognostic factors. Age, performance status, extent of surgical resection, temozolomide (TMZ) treatment, O^6-methylguanine-DNA methyltransferase (MGMT) promoter methylation status, and neurologic functioning as expressed by the Mini-Mental State Examination score are important prognostic factors.[2]

Although no treatment has proved curative and overall mortality remains high, continued research promises to lead to novel individualized and localized therapies.

CURRENT TREATMENTS

Current treatment protocols for GBM combine surgery, chemotherapy, and radiation, providing palliation and moderate survival benefit. For newly diagnosed patients with GBM, standard treatment includes maximal surgical resection followed by combined radiotherapy and chemotherapy.

Surgical Resection

The goal of surgery in GBM treatment is to provide maximal tumor resection, with preservation or restoration of neurologic function. Recent studies have shown gross total resection to enhance the overall survival (OS) in GBM. When maximal total resection is not feasible, near-total and subtotal resection provides additional survival benefit. In a study of 451 patients with GBM undergoing primary resection, the median survival after gross-total resection, near-total resection, and subtotal resection was 13, 11, and 8 months, respectively.[3]

Advances in image-guided surgical techniques, including intraoperative magnetic resonance imaging (MRI), cortical mapping, and stereotactic surgery have assisted in the ability to safely increase the extent of tumor resection. These new modalities have had a significant impact on patients with tumors in eloquent cortical areas where resection is frequently abandoned before total removal to avoid neurologic deficits. A phase III trial of 322 patients showed the benefit of fluorescence-guided tumor resections with 5-aminolevulinic acid.[4] When combined with intraoperative monitoring and cortical and subcortical stimulation, fluorescence guidance provides the surgeon with direct visualization of tumor borders and allows for the largest possible resection with minimal neurologic deficits.[5]

Chemotherapy-Impregnated Wafers

Implantation of biodegradable carmustine (1,2-bis[2-chloreoethyl]-1-nitrosourea, BCNU) wafers (CW) is an approved therapeutic option for patients with newly diagnosed and relapsed glioblastoma. These wafers are placed in the surgical resection site at the time of initial operative debulking. The chemotherapeutic agent is released into surrounding brain tissue beginning immediately after tumor resection and lasting for several weeks. Use of CW results in a statistically significant benefit in the OS of patients undergoing initial surgery for malignant gliomas (13.9

vs 11.6 months).[6] However, subgroup analysis failed to show significant benefit in GBM.

In patients undergoing primary resection and adjuvant radiotherapy, the addition of CW and concomitant TMZ provides significant survival benefit over CW alone. Patients undergoing radiation therapy (XRT) + CW + TMZ compared with patients undergoing XRT + CW alone showed an increase in median OS (21.3 vs 12.4 months).[7] In addition, 2-year survival was found to be 39% of patients undergoing XRT + CW + TMZ therapy versus 18% with XRT + CW. Because this study was underpowered to compare XRT + CW + TMZ cohorts with XRT + TMZ alone, future prospective studies are required to characterize the role of CW in standard of care therapy.

Although integrating CW into the standard adjuvant regimen with concomitant chemotherapy has proved safe and feasible, its use remains physician dependent. In phase III studies, the wafers have been found to delay wound healing and are associated with edema, requiring subsequent steroids, seizures, and blood-brain barrier (BBB) disruption, making the interpretation of follow-up MRI unreliable.[8] Often, the pathologic diagnosis is not known before surgical resection, making CW implantation problematic without proper preparation by the surgeon. In addition, placement of CW can lead to exclusion from enrollment in clinical trials.

Chemoradiotherapy

After maximum surgical resection or biopsy, chemoradiotherapy has been established as the standard treatment administered postoperatively. Radiotherapy uses high-dose volume incorporating the enhancing tumor plus a limited margin to plan the target volume. The total dose delivered is in the range of 50 to 60 Gy in fraction sizes of 1.8 to 2.0 Gy.[9]

Before TMZ therapy, the role of chemotherapy in GBM was controversial. A meta-analysis of 12 randomized trials, which included more than 3000 patients, showed an increase in 1-year survival from 40% to 46% with chemotherapy.[10] One common treatment regimen was PCV (procarbazine, CCNU [lomustine], and vincristine).

In 2005, in an international randomized phase III trial of 573 patients with GBM the European Organization for Research and Treatment of Cancer (EORTC) and National Cancer Institute of Canada (NCIC) reported a significant improvement in survival with the early addition of TMZ to XRT compared with XRT alone.[11] Follow-up results after 5 years showed continued benefit of adjuvant TMZ with XRT with OS of 9.8% compared with 1.9% in the radiotherapy alone group.[12] Median OS rates for radiotherapy + TMZ versus radiotherapy alone were 14.6 months and 12.1 months, respectively. Progression-free survival (PFS) rates for patients receiving radiotherapy + TMZ compared with radiotherapy alone were 11.2% and 1.8% at 2 years, 6.0% and 1.3% at 3 years, 5.6% and 1.3% at 4 years, and 4.1% and 1.3% at 5 years. Treatment is generally well tolerated, with most notable toxicities including myelosuppression, thromboembolic events, fatigue, pneumonia, nausea, vomiting, rash, constipation, and arthralgias.[11,13,14] The dose-limiting toxicity of TMZ is myelosuppression, with any grade 3 or 4 hematologic toxic effect found to affect 14% of patients during adjuvant TMZ therapy. Four percent of patients experienced a grade 3 or 4 neutropenia and 11% experienced a grade 3 or 4 thrombocytopenia.[11]

Standard dosing for concomitant TMZ therapy is 75 mg/m^2/d given daily during XRT followed by 150 to 200 mg/m^2/d for 5 days every 28 days for a total of 6 cycles. Multiple studies are evaluating different dosing protocols as well as the combination of TMZ with other chemotherapeutic and targeted agents in the treatment of GBM. A randomized phase III study (Radiation Therapy Oncology Group [RTOG] 0525) comparing standard adjuvant TMZ and a dose-dense schedule (75–100 mg/m^2 daily, days 1–21) in 833 newly diagnosed patients with GBM found no improvement in OS with dose-dense TMZ regardless of MGMT methylation status.[15]

Treatment of Elderly Patients

The incidence of GBM increases with age, with a median age of onset of 60 years. Patient survival decreases almost linearly beyond the age of 45 years. The median survival times in elderly patients are significantly less than younger patients (4–11 months).[16] Both historical series and clinical trials have found the 2-year survival of less than 5% in patients older than 65 years compared with 26% in patients younger than 50 years.[17] However, poor outcomes and poor response to toxic therapies have resulted in more aggressive treatments being withheld from the elderly population with GBM.

Large population-based studies suggest that nearly 50% of patients with GBM older than 65 years do not receive the standard of care treatment with surgical debulking or radiotherapy.[18,19] A retrospective review of 394 elderly patients with GBM from Memorial Sloan Kettering Cancer Center found significant survival benefit in elderly patients aged 65 years or older undergoing gross total resection compared with subtotal resection or biopsy (60% vs 40% decrease in risk of death).[20] One study found OS increased from 17 to 30 weeks when patients had biopsy and radiation therapy compared with surgical resection of the entire contrast-enhancing lesion and radiation, respectively.[21] Similar studies show the benefit of radiation therapy alone compared with supportive care.[22] A total of 81 patients aged 70 years or older from 10 institutions with GBM had a median OS of 29.1 weeks when treated with supportive care and radiotherapy compared with 16.9 weeks in those patients receiving supportive care alone. Median PFS was 14.9 weeks and 5.4 weeks for radiotherapy and supportive care compared with supportive care alone, respectively.

In an attempt to shorten treatment duration, hypofractionated radiotherapy is often used, which gives larger radiation doses per fraction in fewer total fractions over a shorter period of time. A common regimen of 40 Gy in 15 fractions over 3 weeks has been shown to be equivalent in older patients to the standard 6-week schedule of 60 Gy in 30 fractions.[16] This is a reasonable regimen to consider in older patients with borderline performance status for whom the ability to tolerate a 6-week course of concurrent TMZ and radiation is in question.

A prospective study of 79 elderly patients with GBM older than 65 years investigated the benefit of chemotherapy (PCV or TMZ) in patients undergoing surgery and radiotherapy.[23] Three groups of patients were analyzed after maximal surgical resection. The groups were treated with radiotherapy alone (n = 24), radiotherapy with adjuvant PCV (n = 32), or radiotherapy with adjuvant TMZ (n = 23). The group receiving TMZ had a significant survival benefit compared with those patients receiving radiotherapy alone (14.9 months vs 11.2 months). Whereas OS did not differ between patients receiving adjuvant TMZ or PCV, the PFS was significantly longer in those receiving adjuvant TMZ. The 6-month and 12-month PFS was 56.25% and 15.6% in those patients receiving PCV and 87% and 47.4% in those treated with TMZ. In addition, TMZ therapy was better tolerated, because PCV was associated with more frequent hematologic toxicity.

The 5-year follow-up analysis of the EORTC-NCIC trial published by Stupp and colleagues[12] reported a benefit of concomitant and adjuvant TMZ and radiotherapy in all clinical prognostic subgroups, including patients aged 60 to 70 years. At 2 years, the median OS was 21.8% in those patients receiving combined therapy and 5.7% in those patients receiving radiotherapy alone. This effect was maintained at 5 years with median OS of 6.6% and 0.0%.

A phase II study analyzed the use of TMZ in elderly patients with newly diagnosed GBM and poor performance status.[24] The study, comparing TMZ treatment with supportive care alone, found TMZ to be well tolerated, improve functional status, and increase OS in 70 patients older than 70 years with newly diagnosed GBM and Karnofsky performance score (KPS) less than 70. Furthermore, when patients had a methylated MGMT promoter, TMZ had a more significant impact on PFS and OS.

Age on its own should not be used as an exclusion criterion for GBM treatment, but performance status should be factored heavily into the decision-making process for treatment planning.

RECURRENT DISEASE

Despite aggressive initial treatment with surgical resection, radiotherapy, and chemotherapy virtually all patients with GBM relapse. Unlike newly diagnosed GBM, there is currently no standard of care treatment of GBM relapse. Ongoing clinical trials are investigating targeted agents with various mechanisms of action as salvage therapy for patients with recurrent GBM (**Table 1**).[25–36]

Pseudoprogression

Before initiating treatment of recurrent GBM, true disease progression must be distinguished from pseudoprogression. Pseudoprogression is a treatment-related reaction, occurring frequently with combination radiotherapy + TMZ, which is visualized as increased enhancement or edema on MRI. The reaction is highly suggestive of disease progression but without an increase in tumor activity. This local tissue reaction is triggered by a treatment-induced increase in vessel permeability, inflammatory infiltration, and resulting edema. In most cases, pseudoprogression resolves even without treatment, although with a variable time course, rendering distinction from tumor progression difficult.[37]

An analysis of 85 patients with GBM treated with radiotherapy + TMZ found 21% of patients had pseudoprogression, of whom 67% remained asymptomatic despite the new radiologic changes.[38] Another study found similar results with 31% of 103 patients with GBM undergoing pseudoprogressive changes and 66% remaining asymptomatic.[39] In addition, for those patients with enlarging lesions on first MRI after radiation, Brandes and colleagues found a 91.3% probability of pseudoprogression in patients with methylated MGMT promoter tumors and a 59% probability of early disease progression in unmethylated MGMT promoter tumors.

Current data suggest the need for novel imaging techniques or biochemical markers to better distinguish pseudoprogression from true progression. This strategy prevents patients from undergoing unnecessary surgical interventions and premature discontinuance of adjuvant treatments.

Re-Resection

The US National Institutes of Health (NIH) recurrent GBM scale has been validated for use in identifying patients likely to benefit from repeat surgery.[40] To determine a patient's score, 1 point is assigned for the presence of each of the following factors: KPS score 80 or less, tumor volume 50 cm^3 or greater, and motor-speech-middle cerebral artery score 2 or greater. Patient survival after surgery can be stratified based on their total score, ranging from 0 to 3. Good (0 points), intermediate (1–2 points), and poor (3 points) prognostic groups were found to have postoperative survival times of 10.8, 4.5, and 1.0 months, respectively.

Table 1
Targeted agents in the treatment of recurrent GBM

Drug	Mechanism of Action	Phase	Number of Patients	6-Month PFS (%)	Median OS (wk)	Median PFS (wk)	Reference
Meta-analysis	Various	II	225	15	25	9	Wong et al[25]
Meta-analysis	Various	II	437	16	30		Lamborn et al[26]
BCNU[a]	Alkylating agent	Retrospective	35	13	22	11	Reithmeier et al[27]
Lomustine	Alkylating agent	III	92	19	31	7	Wick et al[28]
Enzastaurin	Protein kinase C β inhibitor	III	174	11	28	6	Wick et al[28]
Temsirolimus (CCI-779)	mTOR inhibitor	II	65	8	19	10	Galanis et al[29]
Erlotinib	EGFR tyrosine kinase inhibitor	II	48	17	43		Cloughesy et al[30]
		II	54	11[b]	33		Van den Bent et al[31]
Erlotinib + sirolimus	EGFR TKI + mTOR inhibitor	II	32	3	34	7	Reardon et al[32]
Vorinostat	Histone deacetylase inhibitor	II	66	17	25		Galanis et al[33]
Imatinib	Multiple TKI, including PDGFR	II	51	16	25	8	Raymond et al[34]
Imatinib + hydroxyurea	Multiple TKI + antimetabolite	II	231	11	26		Reardon et al[35]
		II	33	27	49	14	Reardon et al[36]

Abbreviations: EGFR, epidermal growth factor receptor; mTOR, mammalian target of rapamycin; PDGFR, platelet-derived growth factor receptor; TKI, tyrosine kinase inhibitor.
[a] BCNU was associated with significant toxicity including pulmonary embolism, pulmonary fibrosis, and myelosuppression.
[b] 6-month PFS in control arm of carmustine or TMZ was 24% and erlotinib was believed to have insufficient single-agent activity.

Several case series have shown increased survival periods in patients under-going reoperations. A study of 301 patients, with 46 undergoing re-resection, found a significant increase in survival compared with those treated with the same protocols without reoperations (36 vs 23 weeks).[41] However, most of these studies acknowledge an inherent patient selection bias to perform surgery in patients with high functional status, favorable tumor locations, and minimal medical contraindications.

In a review of studies investigating GBM retreatment strategies, Nieder and colleagues[42] found that median survival in patients undergoing re-resection ranged from 14 to 50 weeks. The role of re-resection by itself remains unclear because most patients receive postoperative radiotherapy or chemotherapy. In a small study of 24 patients undergoing re-resection alone, median survival was 14 weeks.[43] A care-fully selected subgroup of 18 patients underwent reoperation and were compared with 36 patients who did not undergo surgery at the time of tumor recurrence.[44] A median survival time of 5 months in the surgical subgroup was significantly longer than 2 months observed in those patients not undergoing surgical intervention.

Chemotherapy-Impregnated Wafers

In patients undergoing re-resection for GBM relapse, carmustine-impregnated wafers have been investigated in combination with other adjuvant therapies. A double-blind, randomized, placebo-controlled study showed the efficacy of local chemotherapy with CW in patients with recurrent GBM.[45] Six-month survival in patients receiving CW was 64% compared with 44% in patients treated with placebo.

A phase II trial showed that efficacy of implanted CW may be improved with the addition of O^6-benzylguanine, which suppresses tumor O6-alkylguanine-DNA alkyl-transferase levels in patients with recurrent GBM.[46] In the 52 patients studied, the 6-month OS was 82%. The median OS was 50.3 weeks and 1-year and 2-year survival rates were 47% and 10%, respectively. Notable toxicities included grade 3 hydro-cephalus (9.6%), grade 3 cerebrospinal fluid (CSF) leak (19.2%), and grade 3 CSF/brain infection (13.4%).

Overall, CW implantation has been well tolerated and continues to be used in the multimodality treatment protocols required in GBM, although potential toxicities and exclusion from clinical trials remain a concern.

Bevacizumab

Bevacizumab (10 mg/kg intravenously every 2 weeks) received accelerated ap-proval for the treatment of recurrent GBM in May 2009 because of its effectiveness when used alone or in combination with chemotherapy. In a phase II trial of 35 patients with GBM, Vredenburgh and colleagues[47] found 6-month PFS with bevaci-zumab + irinotecan was 46% and 6-month OS was 77%. In a phase II trial evalu-ating the role of bevacizumab alone (n = 85) or in combination with irinotecan (n = 82), the 6-month PFS was 42.6% and 50.3%, respectively.[48] In addition, secondary end points showed OS of 9.2 months for patients treated with bevacizu-mab alone and 8.7 months for those treated with bevacizumab and irinotecan, although the study was not designed to compare efficacy of these 2 arms of treat-ment with each other. The study did show a trend for decreasing steroid dose in patients on therapy.

More recently, a phase II trial of daily TMZ + biweekly bevacizumab found 6-month PFS of 18.8%, 6-month median OS of 37 weeks, and 12-month median OS of 31.3%.[49] Although the results were not as good as results seen in bevacizumab mono-therapy or bevacizumab/irinotecan combination therapy, this study included heavily pretreated patients with 78% having had 2 or more previous chemotherapy regimens and 12% of patients having had previous treatment with bevacizumab. Combination therapy with bevacizumab and etoposide[50] or erlotinib[51] has failed to show a significant difference from other bevacizumab regimens.

A recent meta-analysis reviewed the efficacy of bevacizumab treatment in 548 patients with recurrent GBM, comprising 15 studies published between 2005 and 2009.[52] Median OS, 6-month PFS, and 6-month OS were 9.3 months, 45%, and 76%, respectively. Although requiring confirmation in clinical trial, the analysis found no difference in bevacizumab dose-response benefit between 5, 10, or 15 mg/kg.

Bevacizumab has shown promising results in small cohort studies; however, because of the direct effects of antiangiogenic agents on vessel permeability, the imaging response analyses are difficult to interpret.[53–55] Other reported side effects of bevacizumab therapy include intracranial hemorrhage and thrombotic events, including deep venous thrombosis, pulmonary embolus, and ischemic stroke. A retrospective study of 161 patients with recurrent GBM treated with bevacizumab found an incidence of 1.9% and 1.9% for ischemic stroke and intracranial hemorrhage, respectively.[56] Ischemic stroke appeared to be a complication of prolonged antiangiogenic therapy, whereas intratumoral bleeds occurred more frequently in tumor progression.

Despite its efficacy in the treatment of recurrent GBM, patients inevitably relapse after bevacizumab therapy. A retrospective review of 54 patients with recurrent GBM who progressed on a bevacizumab-containing regimen found that a response was rarely seen when patients were retreated with an alternate bevacizumab-containing regimen.[57] After the second bevacizumab regimen, 6-month PFS was 2% and median PFS was 37.5 days.

An ongoing phase III double-blind, placebo-controlled trial (RTOG 0825) that recently completed accrual with 978 patients is investigating concurrent chemoradiation and adjuvant TMZ with bevacizumab compared with chemoradiation and adjuvant TMZ in newly diagnosed GBM. Results from this study will provide valuable insight into the efficacy of bevacizumab therapy and its ability to provide a clear survival benefit in patients with GBM.

TMZ Rechallenge

TMZ is standard of care therapy in newly diagnosed GBM. However, there is no consensus on optimal therapy for GBM relapse. TMZ rechallenge remains 1 therapeutic option available to patients with recurrent disease.

Studies have shown TMZ rechallenge to be effective when dosed continuously. Perry and colleagues[58] investigated a continuous TMZ dose of 50 mg/m^2 and found 6-month PFS was 57% in patients who relapsed after completing standard concomitant and adjuvant TMZ.

Several dose-intensive schedules have been investigated in recurrent GBM. Twenty-eight patients with GBM were treated with 75 mg/m^2/d for 42 consecutive days in a 70-day cycle. Six-month PFS was 19% and OS was 7.7 months.[59] Brandes and colleagues[60] investigated the 75 mg/m^2/d dose for 21 days every 28 days. Six-month PFS was found to be 30.3%, and OS at 6 months and 1 year was 73% and 38%, respectively. Furthermore, in patients with methylated MGMT, the median survival and percentage of patients alive at 1 year were 48.2 weeks and 50%, respectively. In those patients with unmethylated MGMT, the median survival was 34.7 weeks and 1-year survival was 21.4%. Although prognosis was better in patients with methylated MGMT, there was no clear difference in response and 6-month PFS in relation to MGMT status.

An alternating weekly regimen (1 week on/1 week off) of TMZ was investigated in a randomized, phase II trial of 64 patients with recurrent GBM.[61] TMZ was administered at 150 mg/m^2 on days 1 to 7 and 15 to 21 of 28-day cycles. Six-month and 12-month PFS was 43.8% and 12.5%, respectively. Of the 36 patients with GBM with available tumor specimens, 17 had methylated MGMT and 19 were unmethylated. The median PFS was 19 weeks in patients with unmethylated MGMT and 27 weeks with methylated MGMT; however, these results were not statistically significant. Of the 64 patients with GBM, 22 were chemotherapy naive, whereas 30 had previous nimustine/teniposide therapy, 3 had previous PCV, and 9 had previous lomustine/TMZ. This study is compared with the Brandes and colleagues[60] study in which all patients were chemotherapy naive.

Of importance in recurrent GBM treatment consideration is the expression of the MGMT promoter, which confers resistance to TMZ.[62,63] Continuous suppression of MGMT activity may prove necessary for maximal benefit. The large, multi-center phase II Canadian (RESCUE) study used a continuous dose-intense TMZ regimen of 50 mg/m^2/d[64] in patients who had previous exposure to TMZ. This dosing represented dose intensification from 750 to 1000 mg/m^2/28-d cycle with conventional dosing to 1400 mg/m^2/28-d cycle. Of the 116 patients studied, the median time on continuous TMZ was 2.7 months, with 15 patients completing 12 months of continuous therapy. The overall 6-month PFS for patients with GBM was 23.9% and median survival was 9.3 months. The most significant benefit was shown in patients with GBM who had completed a previous course of concomitant TMZ/radiotherapy with adjuvant TMZ followed by a drug-free period of at least 2 months (6-month PFS of 35.7%). A similar benefit was seen in patients who progressed before completing 6 cycles of adjuvant TMZ with 6-month PFS of 27.3%. However, those patients who progressed while still on extended adjuvant TMZ therapy beyond 6 cycles did significantly worse than the other 2 groups, with a 6-month PFS of 7.4%. The investigators hypothesized that a continuous regimen may lead to a depletion of MGMT and restoration of TMZ sensitivity, as had been previously reported.[65] In addition, the Perry and colleagues study reported similar benefit in patients with or without methylated MGMT, although the methylated group had a longer interval from time of initial surgery to start of therapy for recurrence.

Reirradiation

Investigators have failed to show significant differences between conventional external beam radiotherapy, stereotactic radiotherapy, or brachytherapy. Median survival after various methods of reirradiation was 26 to 60 weeks. In a recent review of more than 300 patients, palliative reirradiation regimens without additional chemotherapy achieved a PFS at 6 months of 28% to 39% and 1-year survival of 18% to 48%, which compares favorably with targeted systemic therapies that have been evaluated for recurrent GBM.[42,66–68]

Given the poor prognosis in patients with GBM, assessment of treatment toxicity and quality of life must be incorporated into therapy decisions. Hypofractionated stereotactic radiotherapy (H-SRT) is able to deliver treatment over a 2-week period compared with the 3-week to 4-week therapy in standard fractionation regimens. A retrospective study of 147 patients between 1994 and 2008 who underwent H-SRT for high-grade gliomas found a significant survival benefit with minimal adverse effects.[69] Using daily fractions of 3.5 Gy with a median dose of 35 Gy, investigators were able to achieve a median survival time of 11 months, comparable with other systemic agents, and minimize toxicities seen at higher doses. The data suggest that higher doses of H-SRT result in improved survival; however, doses greater than 40 Gy have been associated with increased toxicity.

An analysis of 20 patients with recurrent GBM was designed to test the safety and efficacy of H-SRT in combination with bevacizumab treatment.[70] The 6-month PFS for patients with GBM was 65% and median OS was 12.5 months. The overall toxicity in this study was in line with other reports of bevacizumab therapy in patients with malignant glioma. These results suggest that this combination can be evaluated further in the treatment of both newly diagnosed GBM and recurrent GBM.

Radiosurgery

Radiotherapy has shown increasing survival benefit with doses up to 60 Gy, beyond which exposure and toxicity to normal surrounding tissue becomes problematic. Stereotactic radiosurgery (SRS) prevents injury to surrounding normal tissue by producing a sharp radiation decrease outside the target area.

A randomized controlled trial of 203 patients concluded that postoperative SRS followed by external beam radiation therapy (EBRT) and BCNU did not improve the outcome, quality of life, or cognitive functioning of newly diagnosed patients with GBM when compared with EBRT and BCNU alone.[71] Although discouraging for the prospects of SRS in the treatment of GBM, this study analyzed a single timing for SRS therapy and a single combination chemotherapy, leaving room for further investigations.

With the implementation of TMZ into standard GBM therapy, the role of SRS in both newly diagnosed and recurrent GBM continues to be investigated. A retrospective review of 48 patients with GBM treated with SRS between 1991 and 2007, with 22 treated as part of their initial therapy and 26 treated at the time of progression, found an OS benefit in those treated at the time of progression (17.4 vs 15.1 months).[72] In a multivariate analysis, RTOG class III patients, those with more extensive resections, and lack of steroids at the time of SRS had significantly improved OS. The results of this study suggest a role for SRS delivered after radiation therapy in some well-selected patients.

A recent retrospective review analyzed 26 consecutive patients who underwent gamma knife radiosurgery for small recurrent high-grade gliomas (16 with GBM) after radical resection, EBRT, and TMZ between 2004 and 2009. Median OS from SRS was 12.9 months.[73] These results were comparable with the OS from SRS of 13 months found in the prospective cohort of 114 consecutive patients (65 with GBM) published by Kong and colleagues.[74] Several other retrospective studies have reported prolonged survival in patients undergoing SRS for recurrent GBM.[75–77]

The most likely reason why radiotherapy is unable to effectively control long-term disease is the inability to detect the spread pattern of GBM.[78] An area of significant interest is the use of systemic radiosensitizers that may enhance the effect of focal irradiation as well as exert cytotoxic activity on distant cell populations.[79] Many of these agents have failed to show significant benefit and others continue to undergo preclinical investigation.[80,81]

Electrical Fields

The disruption of cancer cell mitosis using a low-intensity, medium frequency, alternating electrical field, called tumor treating fields (TTF), was first described by Kirson and colleagues[82] in 2004. In preclinical studies, tumor cell lines exposed to electrical fields for greater than 24 hours entered a stunned, nonproliferative state, unable to undergo mitosis.

Two single-arm, phase I trials in 2007 (10 patients) and 2009 (20 patients) treated patients with TTF. The median survival in 10 patients with recurrent GBM treated with TTF was 62.2 weeks and no adverse events were noted.[83] A follow-up study studied 10 patients with recurrent GBM treated with TTF alone after TMZ maintenance failure and 10 newly diagnosed patients with GBM treated with postoperative TTF and maintenance TMZ therapy. Patients treated with TTF-TMZ combination therapy showed a median PFS of 155 weeks and a median OS of more than 39 months.[84]

In 2010, the US Food and Drug Administration (FDA) narrowly approved the NovoTTF-100A device for the treatment of GBM despite failure to meet the primary end point (OS) in the pivotal trial comparing the device with salvage chemotherapy. The phase III trial that randomized 237 patients with recurrent GBM to treatment with NovoTTF (20–24 h/d, 7 d/wk) or the best standard chemotherapy (BSC) at each physician's discretion found a median OS of 6.6 months for TTF and 6.0 months for BSC and 6-month PFS of 21% versus 15%.[85] The OS results did not achieve statistical significance. Survey of patients in the study suggested a quality of life benefit with TTF compared with chemotherapy. TTF was well tolerated, with 17% patients experiencing mild to moderate skin rash beneath the electrodes.

FUTURE PERSPECTIVES

Despite recent advances, the prognosis for newly diagnosed patients with GBM remains dismal. Current treatment regimens provide maximal benefit measured in months and virtually all patients relapse, stimulating the need for continued pursuit of novel therapies.

TMZ: Alternate Regimens

Many studies are investigating alternative dosing schedules of TMZ in both newly diagnosed and patients with recurrent GBM. In a randomized phase II study evaluating 2 TMZ regimens in the adjuvant treatment of newly diagnosed GBM, a dose-dense regimen provided a more significant survival benefit than a metronomic regimen.[86] The median OS of the 31 patients assigned to the dose-dense TMZ treatment group was 17.1 months after receiving 150 $mg/m^2/d$ for days 1 to 7 and days 15 to 21 of 28-day cycles. All patients received initial EBRT to approximately 60 Gy with concurrent TMZ at 75 $mg/m^2/d$ through the course of RT. The recently presented results of RTOG 0525, as mentioned earlier, which failed to show a difference between standard and dose-dense TMZ, do raise concerns about efficacy of these alternative regimens.

TMZ rechallenge remains a consideration in recurrent GBM treatment and optional regimens remain under investigation (**Table 2**).[58–61,64,87]

Convection-Enhanced Delivery

A significant challenge in the treatment of CNS disease remains the ability of therapeutic agents to cross the BBB. Convection-enhanced delivery (CED) is a method of infusing agents directly into the CNS parenchyma through stereotactically placed catheters using microinfusion pumps. Initial studies of CED infused radiolabeled transferrin and sucrose into the CNS of cats using a needle.[88] In the ensuing 17 years of investigation, chemotherapeutics, nanoparticles, toxins, liposomes, antibodies, viruses, proteins, and growth factors have all been shown to be deliverable using CED.[89–93]

Table 2
Alternative teniozolomide dosing regimens for recurrent GBM

Regimen	Dosage	# of Patients with GBM	Results in GBM Patients	Additional Findings	Comments	Reference
1 week on/1 week off	150 mg/m² on days 1 to 7 and 15 to 21 of 28-day cycles	64	6-month PFS 43.8%; 12-month PFS 12.5%; Median PFS 24 weeks	Potential benefit with unmethylated MGMT (not stat. significant)	Of 64 GBM patients, 22 were chemo naïve, 9 had prior TMZ, 33 had other prior chemotherapy	Wick et al[61]
3 weeks on/1 week off	75 mg/m2 on days 1-21 of 28-day cycles	33	6-month PFS 30.6%; 6- and 12-month median OS 73% and 38%; Median PFS 16.1 weeks	No difference in median PFS and 6-month PFS between methylated and unmethylated MGMT	No prior TMZ therapy; 2nd-line treatments included nitrosourea-based regimens (n=12). carboplatin and etoposide (n=3), and 3 experimental drugs (n=3)	Brandes et al[60]
Twice daily for days 1 to 5	200 mg/m² initial dose then 90 mg/m² every 12 hours for 9 doses	68	6-month PFS 35%; 6- and 12-month median OS 71% and 35%; Median PFS 4 months	Did not assess MGMT status	No prior TMZ therapy	Balmaceda et al[87]
42 days on/28 days off	75 mg/m2 on days 1 to 42 of 70-day cycles	28	6-month PFS 19%; 6-month median OS 60%; Median survival 7.7 months	Did not assess MGMT status	Of the 35 total patients, 27 had received prior chemotherapy with 23/27 being nitrosourea-based	Khan et al[59]
Continuous	50 mg/m²/day; Group 1 (n=21) dosed at 2nd relapse on conventional 5/28 TMZ; Group 2 (n=14) dosed at 1st progression after concurrent chemoradiation with TMZ	35	Group 1: 6-month PFS from 2nd relapse 17% Group 2: 6-month PFS from 1st relapse 57%	Did not assess MGMT status	All patients had prior TMZ therapy	Perry et al[58]
	50 mg/m²/day for up to 1 year; Group 1 progressed on adjuvant TMZ prior to completing 6 cycles; Group 2 progressed on extended adjuvant TMZ; Group 3 progressed after completing adjuvant TMZ and a > 2 month treatment-free period	88	Group 1: 6-month PFS 273% Group 2: 6-month PFS 7.4% Group 3: 6-month PFS 35.7%	6-month PFS in methylated MGMT 40% vs. 36.4% in unmethylated MGMT	All patients had prior TMZ therapy	Perry et al[64]

A randomized phase III trial compared CED of IL13-PE38QQR with CW in the treatment of patients with recurrent GBM at first recurrence.[94] IL13-PE38QQR, also known as cintredekin besudotox (CB), is a recombinant cytotoxin composed of human interleukin-13 (IL-13) fused to a truncated, mutated form of *Pseudomonas aeruginosa* exotoxin A (PE38QQR). The agent targets tumor cells expressing the IL-13 receptor, binds the receptor, and facilitates the entry of exotoxin, inducing caspase-mediated apoptosis. Of the 276 randomized patients (183 received CB and 93 received CW) who underwent resection and had histopathologically proved GBM, median survival was 36.4 weeks and 35.3 weeks for the CB and CW groups, respectively. CB treatment was associated with a significantly higher number of thromboembolic events; however, no statistically significant survival benefit was noted.

The efficacy of trabedersen, a transforming growth factor β_2 inhibitor, was evaluated in a randomized, open-label, dose-finding phase IIb study of recurrent high-grade gliomas using CED.[95] Two doses of trabedersen (10 and 80 μM) were compared with standard chemotherapy consisting of either TMZ (150–200 mg/m^2 on days 1–5 in 28-day cycles) or PCV (lomustine 110 mg/m^2 on day 1, procarbazine 60 mg/m^2 on days 8–21, and vincristine 1.4 mg/m^2 on days 8 and 29 in 56-day cycles). The GBM subgroup consisted of 28 patients treated with 10-μM trabedersen, 34 with 80 μM trabedersen, and 33 with standard chemotherapy. The median survival with 10-μM trabedersen, 80-μM trabedersen, and standard chemotherapy were 7.3, 10.9, and 10.0 months, respectively.

Despite the lack of significant survival benefit in patients treated with CED technology, the pressure gradient-assisted slow infusion of therapeutic agents remains an area of clinical interest. The ability to bypass the BBB and deliver local therapies to the tumor site may prove beneficial in future trials.

Immunotherapy

Standard chemotherapeutic agents are limited by their lack of specificity and resulting damage to normal tissue. The ability to recognize tumor-specific mutations for targeted elimination of neoplastic cells is the key concept behind immunotherapy.

One tumor-specific cell surface marker is epidermal growth factor receptor variant III (EGFRvIII), which is not found in normal tissue[96] but expressed in approximately one-third of GBMs.[97,98] An EGFRvIII vaccine named PEPvIII was tested in a multicenter phase II trial of 18 patients with newly diagnosed EGFRvIII-expressing GBM. Patients had undergone gross total resection, had a KPS score 80% or greater, and had no progression after standard EBRT with concurrent TMZ. The median OS in vaccinated patients was 26 months compared with 15 months in a TMZ-treated matched, historical cohort (n = 17). PFS was also increased in the vaccine-treated group (14.4 vs 6.3 months). The best outcomes were seen in patients with unmethylated MGMT. In addition, the 6 patients who developed an EGFRvIII-specific antibody response had a median OS of 47.7 months, whereas the 8 patients who did not develop a response had a median OS of 22.8 months.

A follow-up phase II trial of EGFRvIII vaccine investigated the efficacy of EGFRvIII vaccine in patients receiving either standard dosing TMZ or dose-intense TMZ therapy.[99] The data suggest that EGFRvIII vaccination induces immune responses despite TMZ-induced lymphopenia and eradicates EGFRvIII-expressing tumor cells without autoimmunity. A phase III study of the EGFRvIII vaccine is in progress.

Investigations into other methods of inducing glioma-specific immune responses including preparations of autologous dendritic-cell–based tumor vaccines[100] are ongoing (**Table 3**).[100–110]

Table 3
Immunotherapeutic agents in the treatment of GBM

Drug	Mechanism of Action	Type of GBM	Phase	Dosage	Number of Patients with GBM	Median OS	Median PFS	Comments	Reference
CDX-110 (Rindopepimut)	EGFRvIII vaccine	Newly diagnosed	II	Vaccine administered biweekly ×3, then monthly with TMZ until progression	65	21.3 mo	—	Median OS for unmethylated MGMT was 17.9 mo; median OS for methylated MGMT was 37 mo	Lai et al[101]
DC-based vaccine	Induction of glioma-specific immune response	Newly diagnosed (n = 8) + Recurrent (n = 8)	I/II	1.07–6.17 DC/dose; 6 to 10 total doses	16	520 d	—	5-year survival 18.8%; survival of newly diagnosed patients (median survival 381 d, 5-y survival 12.5%) was lower than recurrent patients with GBM (median survival 966 d, 5-y survival 25%)	Chang et al[100]
		Newly diagnosed (n = 15) + Recurrent (n = 8)	I	3 biweekly intradermal DC vaccinations	23	31.4 mo; newly diagnosed 35.9 mo; Recurrent 17.9 mo	—	Newly diagnosed patients received DC vaccine after standard chemo radiotherapy and before adjuvant TMZ; recurrent patients 7–30 wk after surgery	Prins et al[102]
		Recurrent	II	Intradermal DC vaccine injections: Cohort A: wk 1 and 3, then every 4 wk Cohort B: 5 vaccinations at 2-w interval then every 4 wk Cohort C: 4-weekly vaccinations	56	9.6 mo	3 mo	1-y, 2-y, and 3-y OS 37.4%, 14.8%, 11.1%, respectively; 12-mo PFS 10.7%; trend for improved survival in cohort C	De Vleeschouwer et al[103]
		Recurrent	Single-institution analysis of 4 trials	3–4 intradermal doses	39	10.9 mo	2.8 mo	32 patients at first recurrence, 4 at second recurrence, 3 at third recurrence; 12-mo survival, 43.2%; 6-mo PFS, 17.1%	Hu et al[104]

AdV-tk + valacyclovir	Viral delivery of antiherpetic prodrug (valacyclovir)	Newly diagnosed	Ib	3×10^{10} to 3×10^{11} vp	10	12.4 mo[a]	9.1 mo[a]	AdV-tk administered in tumor bed during surgery; valacyclovir × 14 d starting on day 1–3; RT starting 3–7 d after AdV-tk injection	Chiocca et al[105]
		Newly diagnosed	II	3×10^{11} vp	36	15.8 mo	8 mo	2-y survival 37.5%; survival was not significantly different between methylated (n = 12) and unmethylated (n = 9) MGMT	Chiocca et al[106]
Autologous heat shock protein vaccine (HSPPC-96)	Activation of T-cell–mediated immunity	Recurrent	II	25 µg given intradermally weekly ×4, followed by biweekly injections	33	11 mo	9.1 wk	30 of 33 patients were evaluable, having received a minimum of 4 injections; median of 6 injections	Parsa et al[107]
ICT-107	Vaccine targeting cancer stem cell antigens	Newly diagnosed	I	Administered intradermally 3× at 2-wk intervals	16	Not reached	16.9 mo[b]	2-y OS = 80.2%; 2-y PFS 43.75%; expression of MAGE1, AIM2, gp100, and HER2 associated with increased PFS	Phuphanich et al[108]
Oligodeoxy-nucleotides containing unmethylated cytosine-guanine motifs (CpG-ODNs)	Activation of toll-like receptor 9 (TLR9)	Recurrent	II	20 mg CpG-28 injected in 2 mL through intracerebral catheters	31	6.4 mo	9.1 wk	Median survival with methylated MGMT (n = 3) was 7.1 mo and unmethylated MGMT (n = 5) was 5.7 mo	Carpentier et al[109]
Wilms tumor 1 (WT1) peptide vaccine	Induction of immune response to WT1 tumor-associated antigen	Recurrent	II	Weekly intradermal injections of 3.0 mg for 12 total vaccinations	21	36.7 wk	20 wk	6-month PFS 33.3%; Overall response rate 9.5%; Disease control rate 57.1%	Izumoto et al[110]

Abbreviations: AdV-tk, adenovirus-mediated herpes simplex virus thymidine kinase; DC, dendritic cell; tk, tyrosine kinase; vp, vector particles.

[a] Results are for 12 total patients (10 GBM and 2 anaplastic astrocytoma).

[b] Results are for newly diagnosed GBM subset of patients.

Gene Therapy

A randomized phase III study of herpes simplex virus type 1 thymidine kinase and ganciclovir gene therapy was investigated as adjuvant therapy to surgical resection and radiotherapy in 248 patients with newly diagnosed GBM.[111] The 12-month OS was 50% and 55% in the gene therapy and standard therapy groups, respectively. The lack of benefit for gene therapy shown in this study and the limited number of large trials have made the interpretation of gene therapy efficacy difficult. Delivery and transfection efficiency remain the biggest challenges.

A candidate undergoing phase I/II testing in recurrent high-grade glioma patients is Toca 511 and Toca FC (Tocagen, San Diego, CA, USA). Toca 511 is a replication-competent retroviral vector engineered to efficiently deliver a modified cytosine deaminase (CD) prodrug-activating gene to glioma cells. Toca FC is an extended-release tablet containing flucytosine (5-FC), an antifungal drug. CD catalyzes the conversion of 5-FC to the anticancer agent, 5-fluorouracil (5-FU) within the tumor cells. The concept hypothesizes the use of higher local concentrations of 5-FU in the tumor cells that would otherwise be unattainable given the narrow therapeutic index of 5-FU. A preclinical study in a GBM mouse model reported a doubling in the median survival time in mice treated with a single cycle of 5-FC when compared with a saline vehicle control.[112] Treatment was administered for 15 days after intratumoral injection of CD. When treated with multiple cycles of 5-FC, mice showed 100% survival for more than 100 days, which was significantly longer than the median survival of 30 days seen in the placebo group.

Antiangiogenic Agents

Bevacizumab was approved for the treatment of glioblastoma in 2009, leading to a major interest in the development of antiangiogenic therapies for use in neuro-oncology. Glioblastoma is a highly vascularized tumor and GBM tumor cells are known secretors of the proangiogenic factors, vascular endothelial growth factor (VEGF) and basic fibroblast growth factor.

As discussed earlier, bevacizumab has shown promising results in clinical trials. Additional antiangiogenic agents, including cediranib, cilengitide, lenalidomide, and vandetanib are under investigation (**Table 4**).[49,51,52,113–123]

Randomized phase II trials of cilengitide, an integrin receptor inhibitor, in recurrent GBM found cilengitide monotherapy to be well tolerated and show modest antitumor activity with a 6-month PFS of 12% to 15% and median OS of 9.9 months.[116,117] These results support the continued investigation of antiangiogenic agents in combination with other therapies.

There are major differences between the functionality and morphology of tumor vasculature and normal blood vessels. GBM vasculature is composed of disorganized, tortuous, and highly permeable vessels, leading to an abnormal BBB.[124] The 30% to 50% of patients with GBM responding to bevacizumab or cediranib treatment suggests that not all GBM vessel formation is solely dependent on VEGF.[48,125–127] In addition, although GBMs often have a response to anti-VEGF therapy, they develop resistance to this form of therapy. Hypothesized mechanisms of resistance include activation of parallel proangiogenic signaling pathways, recruitment of bone marrow-derived myeloid cells for the support and protection of vascular cells, increasing pericyte coverage of blood vessels, and stimulation of tumor invasion.[128,129]

Recent evidence suggests vasculogenic mimicry, whereby gliomas form vessel-like structures by the transformation of tumor cells.[130,131] The vessels, lined

Table 4
Antiangiogenic agents in the treatment of GBM

Drug	Mechanism of Action	Type of GBM	Phase	Dosage	Number of Patients	6-Mo PFS (%)	Median OS	Median PFS	Reference
ABT-510 + TMZ	Thrombospondin mimetic agent + alkylating agent	Newly diagnosed	I	20–200 mg/d	23	—	64.4 wk	—	Nabors et al[113]
Bevacizumab	VEGF-A inhibitor	Recurrent	Meta-analysis of phase II	5–15 mg/kg	548	45	9.3 mo	—	Wong et al[52]
Bevacizumab + erlotinib	VEGF-A Inhibitor + TKI	Recurrent	II	10 mg/kg every 14 d	25	28	42 wk	—	Sathornsumetee et al[51]
Bevacizumab + TMZ	VEGF-A inhibitor + alkylating agent	Recurrent	II	10 mg/kg every 14 d	32	18.8	37.1 wk	15.8 wk	Desjardins et al[49]
		Newly diagnosed	II	10 mg/kg every 14 d	70	88	19.6 mo	13.6 mo	Lai et al[114]
Cediranib (AZD2171)	VEGF receptor TKI	Recurrent	II	45 mg/d	31	26	32 wk	17 wk	Batchelor et al[115]
Cilengitide	Integrin inhibitor	Recurrent	II	2000 mg 2×/wk	40	15	43 wk	8 wk	Reardon et al[116]
		Recurrent	II	2000 mg 2×/wk	26	12		8 wk	Gilbert et al[117]
Cilengitide + TMZ	Integrin inhibitor + alkylating agent	Newly diagnosed	I/IIa	500 mg 2×/wk	50	69	16.1 mo	8 mo	Stupp et al[118]
Sorafenib + TMZ	PDGFR/VEGFR-2 inhibitor + alkylating agent	Newly diagnosed	II	400 mg 2×/d	28	—	12 mo	6 mo	Hainsworth et al[119]
Sunitinib	Multi-TKI targeting PDGFR and VEGFR-2	Recurrent	II	37.5 mg/d	21	—	3.8 mo	1.6 mo	Neyns et al[120]
Sunitinib + irinotecan	Multi-TKI + topoisomerase 1 inhibitor	Recurrent	I	50 mg/d	15	24[a]	53.1 wk[a]	6.9 wk[a]	Reardon et al[121]
Thalidomide	Antiangiogenic	Recurrent	II	100–500 mg/d	42	18	31 wk	—	Marx et al[122]
Vandetanib + TMZ	VEGFR/EGFR TKI + alkylating agent	Newly diagnosed	I	100 mg/d as MTD	13	—	11 mo	8 mo	Drappatz et al[123]

Abbreviations: MTD, maximum tolerated dose; TKI, tyrosine kinase inhibitor; VEGFR, vascular endothelial growth factor receptor.
[a] Results are for 25 total patients (15 GBM, 8 anaplastic astrocytoma, and 2 anaplastic oligodendroglioma).

by nonendothelial cells, allow gliomas to maintain vascular perfusion. This study provides further evidence for the refractory nature of GBM to anti-VEGF therapy.

Targeting of Growth-Promoting Pathways

Another compelling molecular target in the treatment of GBM is mammalian target of rapamycin (mTOR), a mediator of phosphatidylinositol-3-kinase (PI3K) signaling.[132] Essential for normal development, tightly regulated PI3K signaling is important in cell growth, metabolism, proliferation, and survival.[133,134] The association with cancer development is through mutation and the persistent activation of PI3K.[135] Nearly all patients with GBM harbor PI3K-activating mutations.[136,137]

A phase II trial of temsirolimus (CCI-779) in 64 patients with recurrent GBM showed a 6-month PFS of 7.8% and median OS of 4.4 months.[29] Another phase II study of CCI-779 in 41 patients with recurrent GBM found 1 patient to be progression-free at 6 months.[138] The median time to progression was 9 weeks. A study of 32 patients with recurrent GBM treated with erlotinib, an EGFR tyrosine kinase inhibitor, and sirolimus, an mTOR inhibitor, found median PFS and 6-month PFS of 6.9 weeks and 3.1%, respectively.[32] Median OS was 33.8 weeks. This study included patients treated with previous bevacizumab (n = 9). A pilot subset of a larger phase I/II trial of everolimus and gefitinib in 20 patients with recurrent GBM found median PFS and median OS of 2.6 months and 5.8 months, respectively.[139] One patient was progression-free after 6 months. A previous retrospective review of 22 heavily pretreated patients with recurrent GBM receiving sirolimus plus gefitinib or erlotinib found a 6-month PFS of 25%.[140]

Preclinical mouse models of GBM have resulted in promising results with mTOR inhibitor treatment; however, several phase I/II single-agent trials with the rapamycin analogue CCI-779 have failed to provide clinical benefit in humans.[138,141] Further clinical studies are required to address the future of mTOR treatment in GBM. Ongoing clinical trials investigating the role of mTOR inhibitors, including the RTOG 0913 study investigating everolimus in combination with RT/TMZ as initial treatment in newly diagnosed GBM, are described in **Table 5**.

Additional agents and pathways representing potential targets include histone deacetylase inhibitors, such as valproic acid,[142] hedgehog, and modulators for the Ras/Raf/MAPK signaling pathway.[143] These pathways are known to play a role in the sustained growth, migration, and local invasion of brain tumor-initiating cells, resistance to therapies, and relapse of disease. These targets are of great clinical interest because of the potential for brain tumor-initiating cell eradication and improved efficacy of current therapies.[144]

Poly(Adenosine Diphosphate-Ribose) Polymerase-1 Inhibitors

Ionizing radiation elicits its cytotoxicity by inducing single-strand and double-strand breaks in the DNA of proliferating cells. Radiation-induced single-strand breaks are primarily repaired using base excision repair, of which poly(adenosine diphosphate-ribose) polymerase-1 (PARP-1) is an essential factor.[145] Preclinical studies have suggested that inhibition or downregulation of PARP-1 increases sensitivity to ionizing radiation.[146,147]

Breast cancer-associated (BRCA) protein 1-deficient and 2-deficient cells are sensitive to PARP inhibition.[148] A phase II study of patients with ovarian cancer associated with BRCA-1 and BRCA-2 confirmed the effectiveness of the PARP inhibitor olaparib.[149] There are no published data confirming the effectiveness of PARP inhibition in patients with glioblastoma. Given the success seen in preclinical models, ongoing

Table 5
Ongoing clinical trials of mTOR inhibitors in the treatment of GBM

Drug	Trial Identifier	Type of GBM	Phase	Combination Therapies	Status on October 11, 2011	Target Number of Patients	Purpose/Treatment Groups
Sirolimus	NCT00509431	Recurrent	I/II	Erlotinib	Active, not recruiting	99	Investigate continuous, daily doses of erlotinib in combination with sirolimus
	NCT00821080	Recurrent	I	Vandetanib	Recruiting	33	Analyze combination sirolimus + vandetanib therapy and define MTD
Temsirolimus	NCT01019434	Newly diagnosed	I/II	RT	Recruiting	108	Arm 1: RT + TMZ followed by adjuvant TMZ; Arm 2: RT + temsirolimus followed by adjuvant temsirolimus
	NCT00329719	Recurrent	I/II	Sorafenib	Recruiting	144	Arm 1: Temsirolimus + sorafenib without surgery; Arm 2: Temsirolimus on day 1, sorafenib 2×/d days 1–8; surgical intervention on day 8 followed by temsirolimus + sorafenib
	NCT00112736	Recurrent	I/II	Erlotinib	Active, not recruiting	74	Arm 1: Temsirolimus + erlotinib; Arm 2: Temsirolimus + erlotinib followed by surgery and adjuvant temsirolimus + erlotinib
	NCT01051557	Recurrent	I/II	Perifosine	Recruiting	92	Evaluate combination therapy of temsirolimus + perifosine
	NCT00335764	Recurrent	I/II	Sorafenib	Active, not recruiting	183	Arm 1: Erlotinib + sorafenib; Arm 2: Temsirolimus + sorafenib; Arm 3: Sorafenib + tipafarnib
Everolimus	NCT00553150	Newly diagnosed	I/II	RT + TMZ	Recruiting	138	Evaluate everolimus, RT, and TMZ followed by adjuvant TMZ
	NCT01062399 (RTOG 0913)	Newly diagnosed	I/II	RT + TMZ	Recruiting	246	Arm 1: RT + TMZ followed by adjuvant TMZ; Arm 2: RT + TMZ + everolimus followed by adjuvant TMZ + everolimus
	NCT01434602	Recurrent	I/II	Sorafenib	Not yet recruiting	118	Evaluate the combination of everolimus and sorafenib in the treatment of recurrent GBM
	NCT00805961	Newly diagnosed	II	RT + TMZ + bevacizumab	Active, not recruiting	60	RT + TMZ + bevacizumab followed by adjuvant bevacizumab + everolimus

Abbreviations: MTD, maximum tolerated dose; RT, radiotherapy.

Table 6
Ongoing clinical trials of PARP inhibitors in the treatment of GBM

Drug	Trial Identifier	Type of GBM	Phase	Combination Therapies	Status on October 11, 2011	Target Number of Patients	Purpose/Treatment Groups
ABT-888 (veliparib)	NCT00770471	Newly diagnosed	I/II	RT + TMZ	Recruiting	126	Investigate the efficacy of RT + TMZ + ABT-888 combination therapy in patients with newly diagnosed GBM
	NCT01026493 (RTOG 0929)	Recurrent	I/II	TMZ	Phase I accrual met, phase II recruiting in 2012	240	Define the MTD and efficacy of ABT-888 + TMZ in patients with recurrent GBM
AZD2281 (olaparib)	NCT01390571	Recurrent	I	TMZ	Recruiting	34	Assess the best dose of olaparib + extended low-dose TMZ in patients with relapsed GBM
BSI-201 (iniparib)	NCT00687765	Newly diagnosed	I/II	RT + TMZ	Recruiting	100	Analyze the efficacy of RT + TMZ + BSI-201 combination therapy in patients with newly diagnosed GBM
MK-4827	NCT01294735	Recurrent	I	TMZ	Recruiting	54	Evaluate MK-4827 + TMZ therapy in patients with advanced cancer (GBM and melanoma). Patients treated with up to 2 previous treatment regimens (not including TMZ or bevacizumab) will be included

Abbreviations: MTD, maximum tolerated dose; RT, radiotherapy.

early-phase clinical trials are investigating the role of PARP inhibition in GBM treatment (**Table 6**).

SUMMARY

Historically, 3-year survival in GBM was 2% to 5%. The most recent analysis of 17 SEER (Surveillance Epidemiology and End Results) registries between 1995 and 2007 found 3-year survival of 7.31% in patients with GBM (Central Brain Tumor Registry of the United States Statistical Report, February 2011). After approval by the FDA on March 15, 2005 of TMZ for the treatment of adult patients with newly diagnosed GBM, several promising therapies, including bevacizumab, have come under investigation. Data from trials using alternative regimens and combination therapies with treatments already in clinical practice have provided limited benefit, and further trials are ongoing.

Irrespective of the selected treatment regimen, patients with GBM inevitably relapse. Bevacizumab-containing regimens, despite their clinical effectiveness, are no exception. Clinical trials are actively seeking therapies effective in patients who progress on bevacizumab therapy.

Ongoing trials evaluating new treatment modalities such as inhibition of angiogenesis, mTOR inhibition, PARP inhibition, gene therapy, and several novel inhibitors targeting cancer stem cell signaling pathways such as notch and hedgehog may prove efficacious. Results from these studies are highly anticipated. However, given the aggressive and resilient nature of GBM, continued efforts to better understand GBM pathophysiology are required to discover novel targets for future therapies. Combinations of targeted drugs may prove beneficial when single-agent therapy fails to show benefit.

In addition to the development of broad-based drug therapy, recognition of individualized variations in tumor histopathology or genetics may provide invaluable insight into the most effective treatment regimen for specific patients.[136,150]

REFERENCES

1. Wen PY, Kesari S. Malignant gliomas in adults. N Engl J Med 2008;359(5): 492–507.
2. Gorlia T, van den Bent MJ, Hegi ME, et al. Nomograms for predicting survival of patients with newly diagnosed glioblastoma: prognostic factor analysis of EORTC and NCIC trial 26981-22981/CE.3. Lancet Oncol 2008;9(1):29–38.
3. McGirt MJ, Chaichana KL, Gathinji M, et al. Independent association of extent of resection with survival in patients with malignant brain astrocytoma. J Neurosurg 2009;110(1):156–62.
4. Stummer W, Pichlmeier U, Meinel T, et al. Fluorescence-guided surgery with 5-aminolevulinic acid for resection of malignant glioma: a randomised controlled multicentre phase III trial. Lancet Oncol 2006;7(5):392–401.
5. Feigl GC, Ritz R, Moraes M, et al. Resection of malignant brain tumors in eloquent cortical areas: a new multimodal approach combining 5-aminolevulinic acid and intraoperative monitoring. J Neurosurg 2010;113(2):352–7.
6. Westphal M, Hilt DC, Bortey E, et al. A phase 3 trial of local chemotherapy with biodegradable carmustine (BCNU) wafers (Gliadel wafers) in patients with primary malignant glioma. Neuro Oncol 2003;5(2):79–88.
7. McGirt MJ, Than KD, Weingart JD, et al. Gliadel (BCNU) wafer plus concomitant temozolomide therapy after primary resection of glioblastoma multiforme. J Neurosurg 2009;110(3):583–8.

8. Sabel M, Giese A. Safety profile of carmustine wafers in malignant glioma: a review of controlled trials and a decade of clinical experience. Curr Med Res Opin 2008;24(11):3239–57.
9. Laperriere N, Zuraw L, Cairncross G. Radiotherapy for newly diagnosed malignant glioma in adults: a systematic review. Radiother Oncol 2002;64(3):259–73.
10. Stewart LA. Chemotherapy in adult high-grade glioma: a systematic review and meta-analysis of individual patient data from 12 randomised trials. Lancet 2002; 359(9311):1011–8.
11. Stupp R, Mason WP, van den Bent MJ, et al. Radiotherapy plus concomitant and adjuvant temozolomide for glioblastoma. N Engl J Med 2005;352(10): 987–96.
12. Stupp R, Hegi ME, Mason WP, et al. Effects of radiotherapy with concomitant and adjuvant temozolomide versus radiotherapy alone on survival in glioblastoma in a randomised phase III study: 5-year analysis of the EORTC-NCIC trial. Lancet Oncol 2009;10(5):459–66.
13. Combs SE, Wagner J, Bischof M, et al. Radiochemotherapy in patients with primary glioblastoma comparing two temozolomide dose regimens. Int J Radiat Oncol Biol Phys 2008;71(4):999–1005.
14. Athanassiou H, Synodinou M, Maragoudakis E, et al. Randomized phase II study of temozolomide and radiotherapy compared with radiotherapy alone in newly diagnosed glioblastoma multiforme. J Clin Oncol 2005;23(10):2372–7.
15. Gilbert M, Wang M, Aldape K, et al. RTOG 0525: a randomized phase III trial comparing standard adjuvant temozolomide (TMZ) with a dose-dense (dd) schedule in newly diagnosed glioblastoma (GBM) [meeting abstracts]. J Clin Oncol 2011;29(Suppl 15).
16. Roa W, Brasher PM, Bauman G, et al. Abbreviated course of radiation therapy in older patients with glioblastoma multiforme: a prospective randomized clinical trial. J Clin Oncol 2004;22(9):1583–8.
17. Yovino S, Grossman SA. Treatment of glioblastoma in "elderly" patients. Curr Treat Options Oncol 2011;12(3):253–62.
18. Iwamoto FM, Reiner AS, Panageas KS, et al. Patterns of care in elderly glioblastoma patients. Ann Neurol 2008;64(6):628–34.
19. Scott J, Tsai YY, Chinnaiyan P, et al. Effectiveness of radiotherapy for elderly patients with glioblastoma. Int J Radiat Oncol Biol Phys 2011;81(1):206–10.
20. Iwamoto FM, Cooper AR, Reiner AS, et al. Glioblastoma in the elderly: the Memorial Sloan-Kettering Cancer Center Experience (1997-2007). Cancer 2009;115(16):3758–66.
21. Kelly PJ, Hunt C. The limited value of cytoreductive surgery in elderly patients with malignant gliomas. Neurosurgery 1994;34(1):62–6 [discussion: 66–7].
22. Keime-Guibert F, Chinot O, Taillandier L, et al. Radiotherapy for glioblastoma in the elderly. N Engl J Med 2007;356(15):1527–35.
23. Brandes AA, Vastola F, Basso U, et al. A prospective study on glioblastoma in the elderly. Cancer 2003;97(3):657–62.
24. Gallego Perez-Larraya J, Ducray F, Chinot O, et al. Temozolomide in elderly patients with newly diagnosed glioblastoma and poor performance status: an ANOCEF phase II trial. J Clin Oncol 2011;29(22):3050–5.
25. Wong ET, Hess KR, Gleason MJ, et al. Outcomes and prognostic factors in recurrent glioma patients enrolled onto phase II clinical trials. J Clin Oncol 1999;17(8):2572–8.
26. Lamborn KR, Yung WK, Chang SM, et al. Progression-free survival: an important end point in evaluating therapy for recurrent high-grade gliomas. Neuro Oncol 2008;10(2):162–70.

27. Reithmeier T, Graf E, Piroth T, et al. BCNU for recurrent glioblastoma multiforme: efficacy, toxicity and prognostic factors. BMC Cancer 2010;10:30.
28. Wick W, Puduvalli VK, Chamberlain MC, et al. Phase III study of enzastaurin compared with lomustine in the treatment of recurrent intracranial glioblastoma. J Clin Oncol 2010;28(7):1168–74.
29. Galanis E, Buckner JC, Maurer MJ, et al. Phase II trial of temsirolimus (CCI-779) in recurrent glioblastoma multiforme: a North Central Cancer Treatment Group Study. J Clin Oncol 2005;23(23):5294–304.
30. Cloughesy T, Yung A, Vredenburgh J, et al. Phase II study of erlotinib in recurrent GBM: molecular predictors of outcome. ASCO Annual Meeting Proceedings. J Clin Oncol 2005;23(16 Suppl Pt I–II):1507.
31. van den Bent MJ, Brandes AA, Rampling R, et al. Randomized phase II trial of erlotinib versus temozolomide or carmustine in recurrent glioblastoma: EORTC brain tumor group study 26034. J Clin Oncol 2009;27(8):1268–74.
32. Reardon DA, Desjardins A, Vredenburgh JJ, et al. Phase 2 trial of erlotinib plus sirolimus in adults with recurrent glioblastoma. J Neurooncol 2010;96(2):219–30.
33. Galanis E, Jaeckle KA, Maurer MJ, et al. Phase II trial of vorinostat in recurrent glioblastoma multiforme: a North Central Cancer Treatment Group Study. J Clin Oncol 2009;27(12):2052–8.
34. Raymond E, Brandes A, Van Oosterom A, et al. Multicentre phase II study of imatinib mesylate in patients with recurrent glioblastoma: an EORTC: NDDG/ BTG Intergroup Study. J Clin Oncol 2004;22(Suppl 14).
35. Reardon DA, Dresemann G, Taillibert S, et al. Multicentre phase II studies evaluating imatinib plus hydroxyurea in patients with progressive glioblastoma. Br J Cancer 2009;101(12):1995–2004.
36. Reardon DA, Egorin MJ, Quinn JA, et al. Phase II study of imatinib mesylate plus hydroxyurea in adults with recurrent glioblastoma multiforme. J Clin Oncol 2005;23(36):9359–68.
37. Giglio P, Gilbert MR. Cerebral radiation necrosis. Neurologist 2003;9(4):180–8.
38. Taal W, Brandsma D, de Bruin HG, et al. Incidence of early pseudo-progression in a cohort of malignant glioma patients treated with chemoirradiation with temozolomide. Cancer 2008;113(2):405–10.
39. Brandes AA, Franceschi E, Tosoni A, et al. MGMT promoter methylation status can predict the incidence and outcome of pseudoprogression after concomitant radiochemotherapy in newly diagnosed glioblastoma patients. J Clin Oncol 2008;26(13):2192–7.
40. Park JK, Hodges T, Arko L, et al. Scale to predict survival after surgery for recurrent glioblastoma multiforme. J Clin Oncol 2010;28(24):3838–43.
41. Barker FG 2nd, Chang SM, Gutin PH, et al. Survival and functional status after resection of recurrent glioblastoma multiforme. Neurosurgery 1998;42(4):709–20 [discussion: 720–3].
42. Nieder C, Grosu AL, Molls M. A comparison of treatment results for recurrent malignant gliomas. Cancer Treat Rev 2000;26(6):397–409.
43. Young B, Oldfield EH, Markesbery WR, et al. Reoperation for glioblastoma. J Neurosurg 1981;55(6):917–21.
44. Guyotat J, Signorelli F, Frappaz D, et al. Is reoperation for recurrence of glioblastoma justified? Oncol Rep 2000;7(4):899–904.
45. Brem H, Piantadosi S, Burger PC, et al. Placebo-controlled trial of safety and efficacy of intraoperative controlled delivery by biodegradable polymers of

chemotherapy for recurrent gliomas. The Polymer-brain Tumor Treatment Group. Lancet 1995;345(8956):1008–12.

46. Quinn JA, Jiang SX, Carter J, et al. Phase II trial of Gliadel plus O6-benzylguanine in adults with recurrent glioblastoma multiforme. Clin Cancer Res 2009;15(3): 1064–8.

47. Vredenburgh JJ, Desjardins A, Herndon JE 2nd, et al. Bevacizumab plus irinotecan in recurrent glioblastoma multiforme. J Clin Oncol 2007;25(30):4722–9.

48. Friedman HS, Prados MD, Wen PY, et al. Bevacizumab alone and in combination with irinotecan in recurrent glioblastoma. J Clin Oncol 2009;27(28):4733–40.

49. Desjardins A, Reardon DA, Coan A, et al. Bevacizumab and daily temozolomide for recurrent glioblastoma. Cancer 2012;118(5):1302–12.

50. Reardon DA, Desjardins A, Vredenburgh JJ, et al. Metronomic chemotherapy with daily, oral etoposide plus bevacizumab for recurrent malignant glioma: a phase II study. Br J Cancer 2009;101(12):1986–94.

51. Sathornsumetee S, Desjardins A, Vredenburgh JJ, et al. Phase II trial of bevacizumab and erlotinib in patients with recurrent malignant glioma. Neuro Oncol 2010;12(12):1300–10.

52. Wong ET, Gautam S, Malchow C, et al. Bevacizumab for recurrent glioblastoma multiforme: a meta-analysis. J Natl Compr Canc Netw 2011;9(4):403–7.

53. van den Bent MJ, Vogelbaum MA, Wen PY, et al. End point assessment in gliomas: novel treatments limit usefulness of classical Macdonald's Criteria. J Clin Oncol 2009;27(18):2905–8.

54. Abrey LE. Bevacizumab in recurrent malignant glioma. Curr Neurol Neurosci Rep 2008;8(3):233–4.

55. Wen PY, Macdonald DR, Reardon DA, et al. Updated response assessment criteria for high-grade gliomas: response assessment in neuro-oncology working group. J Clin Oncol 2010;28(11):1963–72.

56. Fraum TJ, Kreisl TN, Sul J, et al. Ischemic stroke and intracranial hemorrhage in glioma patients on antiangiogenic therapy. J Neurooncol 2011;105(2):281–9.

57. Quant EC, Norden AD, Drappatz J, et al. Role of a second chemotherapy in recurrent malignant glioma patients who progress on bevacizumab. Neuro Oncol 2009;11(5):550–5.

58. Perry JR, Rizek P, Cashman R, et al. Temozolomide rechallenge in recurrent malignant glioma by using a continuous temozolomide schedule: the "rescue" approach. Cancer 2008;113(8):2152–7.

59. Khan RB, Raizer JJ, Malkin MG, et al. A phase II study of extended low-dose temozolomide in recurrent malignant gliomas. Neuro Oncol 2002;4(1):39–43.

60. Brandes AA, Tosoni A, Cavallo G, et al. Temozolomide 3 weeks on and 1 week off as first-line therapy for recurrent glioblastoma: phase II study from gruppo italiano cooperativo di neuro-oncologia (GICNO). Br J Cancer 2006;95(9):1155–60.

61. Wick A, Felsberg J, Steinbach JP, et al. Efficacy and tolerability of temozolomide in an alternating weekly regimen in patients with recurrent glioma. J Clin Oncol 2007;25(22):3357–61.

62. Pegg AE. Methylation of the O6 position of guanine in DNA is the most likely initiating event in carcinogenesis by methylating agents. Cancer Invest 1984;2(3): 223–31.

63. Gerson SL. Clinical relevance of MGMT in the treatment of cancer. J Clin Oncol 2002;20(9):2388–99.

64. Perry JR, Belanger K, Mason WP, et al. Phase II trial of continuous dose-intense temozolomide in recurrent malignant glioma: RESCUE study. J Clin Oncol 2010; 28(12):2051–7.

65. Tolcher AW, Gerson SL, Denis L, et al. Marked inactivation of O6-alkylguanine-DNA alkyltransferase activity with protracted temozolomide schedules. Br J Cancer 2003;88(7):1004–11.
66. Combs SE, Gutwein S, Thilmann C, et al. Stereotactically guided fractionated re-irradiation in recurrent glioblastoma multiforme. J Neurooncol 2005;74(2): 167–71.
67. Nieder C, Astner ST, Mehta MP, et al. Improvement, clinical course, and quality of life after palliative radiotherapy for recurrent glioblastoma. Am J Clin Oncol 2008;31(3):300–5.
68. Combs SE, Widmer V, Thilmann C, et al. Stereotactic radiosurgery (SRS): treatment option for recurrent glioblastoma multiforme (GBM). Cancer 2005;104(10): 2168–73.
69. Fogh SE, Andrews DW, Glass J, et al. Hypofractionated stereotactic radiation therapy: an effective therapy for recurrent high-grade gliomas. J Clin Oncol 2010;28(18):3048–53.
70. Gutin PH, Iwamoto FM, Beal K, et al. Safety and efficacy of bevacizumab with hypofractionated stereotactic irradiation for recurrent malignant gliomas. Int J Radiat Oncol Biol Phys 2009;75(1):156–63.
71. Souhami L, Seiferheld W, Brachman D, et al. Randomized comparison of stereotactic radiosurgery followed by conventional radiotherapy with carmustine to conventional radiotherapy with carmustine for patients with glioblastoma multiforme: report of Radiation Therapy Oncology Group 93-05 protocol. Int J Radiat Oncol Biol Phys 2004;60(3):853–60.
72. Pouratian N, Crowley RW, Sherman JH, et al. Gamma Knife radiosurgery after radiation therapy as an adjunctive treatment for glioblastoma. J Neurooncol 2009;94(3):409–18.
73. Elliott RE, Parker EC, Rush SC, et al. Efficacy of gamma knife radiosurgery for small-volume recurrent malignant gliomas after initial radical resection. World Neurosurg 2011;76(1–2):128–40 [discussion: 161–2].
74. Kong DS, Lee JI, Park K, et al. Efficacy of stereotactic radiosurgery as a salvage treatment for recurrent malignant gliomas. Cancer 2008;112(9):2046–51.
75. Hsieh PC, Chandler JP, Bhangoo S, et al. Adjuvant gamma knife stereotactic radiosurgery at the time of tumor progression potentially improves survival for patients with glioblastoma multiforme. Neurosurgery 2005;57(4):684–92 [discussion: 684–92].
76. Larson DA, Gutin PH, McDermott M, et al. Gamma knife for glioma: selection factors and survival. Int J Radiat Oncol Biol Phys 1996;36(5):1045–53.
77. Shrieve DC, Alexander E 3rd, Wen PY, et al. Comparison of stereotactic radiosurgery and brachytherapy in the treatment of recurrent glioblastoma multiforme. Neurosurgery 1995;36(2):275–82 [discussion: 282–4].
78. Romanelli P, Conti A, Pontoriero A, et al. Role of stereotactic radiosurgery and fractionated stereotactic radiotherapy for the treatment of recurrent glioblastoma multiforme. Neurosurg Focus 2009;27(6):E8.
79. Chang JE, Khuntia D, Robins HI, et al. Radiotherapy and radiosensitizers in the treatment of glioblastoma multiforme. Clin Adv Hematol Oncol 2007;5(11): 894–902, 907–15.
80. Sheehan J, Ionescu A, Pouratian N, et al. Use of trans sodium crocetinate for sensitizing glioblastoma multiforme to radiation: laboratory investigation. J Neurosurg 2008;108(5):972–8.
81. Sheehan J, Sherman J, Cifarelli C, et al. Effect of trans sodium crocetinate on brain tumor oxygenation. Laboratory investigation. J Neurosurg 2009;111(2):226–9.

82. Kirson ED, Gurvich Z, Schneiderman R, et al. Disruption of cancer cell replication by alternating electric fields. Cancer Res 2004;64(9):3288–95.

83. Kirson ED, Dbaly V, Tovarys F, et al. Alternating electric fields arrest cell proliferation in animal tumor models and human brain tumors. Proc Natl Acad Sci U S A 2007;104(24):10152–7.

84. Kirson ED, Schneiderman RS, Dbaly V, et al. Chemotherapeutic treatment efficacy and sensitivity are increased by adjuvant alternating electric fields (TTFields). BMC Med Phys 2009;9:1.

85. Stupp R, Kanner A, Engelhard H, et al. A prospective, randomized, open-label, phase III clinical trial of NovoTTF-100A versus best standard of care chemotherapy in patients with recurrent glioblastoma [meeting abstract]. J Clin Oncol 2010;28(Suppl 18):LBA2007.

86. Clarke JL, Iwamoto FM, Sul J, et al. Randomized phase II trial of chemoradiotherapy followed by either dose-dense or metronomic temozolomide for newly diagnosed glioblastoma. J Clin Oncol 2009;27(23):3861–7.

87. Balmaceda C, Peereboom D, Pannullo S, et al. Multi-institutional phase II study of temozolomide administered twice daily in the treatment of recurrent high-grade gliomas. Cancer 2008;112(5):1139–46.

88. Bobo RH, Laske DW, Akbasak A, et al. Convection-enhanced delivery of macromolecules in the brain. Proc Natl Acad Sci U S A 1994;91(6):2076–80.

89. Debinski W, Tatter SB. Convection-enhanced delivery for the treatment of brain tumors. Expert Rev Neurother 2009;9(10):1519–27.

90. Vogelbaum MA, Sampson JH, Kunwar S, et al. Convection-enhanced delivery of cintredekin besudotox (interleukin-13-PE38QQR) followed by radiation therapy with and without temozolomide in newly diagnosed malignant gliomas: phase 1 study of final safety results. Neurosurgery 2007;61(5):1031–7 [discussion: 1037–8].

91. Sampson JH, Akabani G, Archer GE, et al. Intracerebral infusion of an EGFR-targeted toxin in recurrent malignant brain tumors. Neuro Oncol 2008;10(3):320–9.

92. Kunwar S, Prados MD, Chang SM, et al. Direct intracerebral delivery of cintredekin besudotox (IL13-PE38QQR) in recurrent malignant glioma: a report by the Cintredekin Besudotox Intraparenchymal Study Group. J Clin Oncol 2007; 25(7):837–44.

93. Carpentier A, Laigle-Donadey F, Zohar S, et al. Phase 1 trial of a CpG oligodeoxynucleotide for patients with recurrent glioblastoma. Neuro Oncol 2006;8(1): 60–6.

94. Kunwar S, Chang S, Westphal M, et al. Phase III randomized trial of CED of IL13-PE38QQR vs Gliadel wafers for recurrent glioblastoma. Neuro Oncol 2010; 12(8):871–81.

95. Bogdahn U, Hau P, Stockhammer G, et al. Targeted therapy for high-grade glioma with the TGF-beta2 inhibitor trabedersen: results of a randomized and controlled phase IIb study. Neuro Oncol 2011;13(1):132–42.

96. Humphrey PA, Wong AJ, Vogelstein B, et al. Anti-synthetic peptide antibody reacting at the fusion junction of deletion-mutant epidermal growth factor receptors in human glioblastoma. Proc Natl Acad Sci U S A 1990;87(11):4207–11.

97. Wong AJ, Ruppert JM, Bigner SH, et al. Structural alterations of the epidermal growth factor receptor gene in human gliomas. Proc Natl Acad Sci U S A 1992;89(7):2965–9.

98. Heimberger AB, Hlatky R, Suki D, et al. Prognostic effect of epidermal growth factor receptor and EGFRvIII in glioblastoma multiforme patients. Clin Cancer Res 2005;11(4):1462–6.

99. Sampson JH, Aldape KD, Archer GE, et al. Greater chemotherapy-induced lymphopenia enhances tumor-specific immune responses that eliminate EGFRvIII-expressing tumor cells in patients with glioblastoma. Neuro Oncol 2011;13(3): 324–33.

100. Chang CN, Huang YC, Yang DM, et al. A phase I/II clinical trial investigating the adverse and therapeutic effects of a postoperative autologous dendritic cell tumor vaccine in patients with malignant glioma. J Clin Neurosci 2011;18(8): 1048–54.

101. Lai R, Recht L, Reardon DA, et al. Long-term follow-up of ACT III: a phase II trial of rindopepimut (CDX-110) in newly diagnosed glioblastoma. Neuro Oncol 2011;13(Suppl 3):iii34–40.

102. Prins RM, Soto H, Konkankit V, et al. Gene expression profile correlates with T-cell infiltration and relative survival in glioblastoma patients vaccinated with dendritic cell immunotherapy. Clin Cancer Res 2011;17(6):1603–15.

103. De Vleeschouwer S, Fieuws S, Rutkowski S, et al. Postoperative adjuvant dendritic cell-based immunotherapy in patients with relapsed glioblastoma multiforme. Clin Cancer Res 2008;14(10):3098–104.

104. Hu J, Patil C, Nuno M, et al. Dendritic cell vaccine therapy for patients with recurrent glioblastoma: a single-institution pooled analysis of four trials. Neuro Oncol 2011;13(Suppl 3):iii34–40.

105. Chiocca EA, Aguilar LK, Bell SD, et al. Phase IB study of gene-mediated cytotoxic immunotherapy adjuvant to up-front surgery and intensive timing radiation for malignant glioma. J Clin Oncol 2011;29(27):3611–9.

106. Chiocca EA, Aguilar LK, Aguilar-Cordova E, et al. Phase 2 study of gene-mediated cytotoxic immunotherapy adjuvant to up-front surgery and intensive timing radiation for malignant glioma. Neuro Oncol 2011;13(Suppl 3): iii34–40.

107. Parsa A, Crane C, Han S, et al. Autologous heat shock protein vaccine (HSPPC-96) for patients with recurrent glioblastoma (GBM): results of a phase II multicenter clinical trial with immunological assessments [meeting abstracts]. J Clin Oncol 2011;29(Suppl 15):2565.

108. Phuphanich S, Wheeler C, Rudnick J, et al. Glioma-associated antigens associated with prolonged survival in a phase I study of ICT-107 for patients with newly diagnosed glioblastoma [meeting abstracts]. J Clin Oncol 2011;29(Suppl 15): 2042.

109. Carpentier A, Metellus P, Ursu R, et al. Intracerebral administration of CpG oligonucleotide for patients with recurrent glioblastoma: a phase II study. Neuro Oncol 2010;12(4):401–8.

110. Izumoto S, Tsuboi A, Oka Y, et al. Phase II clinical trial of Wilms tumor 1 peptide vaccination for patients with recurrent glioblastoma multiforme. J Neurosurg 2008;108(5):963–71.

111. Rainov NG. A phase III clinical evaluation of herpes simplex virus type 1 thymidine kinase and ganciclovir gene therapy as an adjuvant to surgical resection and radiation in adults with previously untreated glioblastoma multiforme. Hum Gene Ther 2000;11(17):2389–401.

112. Tai CK, Wang WJ, Chen TC, et al. Single-shot, multicycle suicide gene therapy by replication-competent retrovirus vectors achieves long-term survival benefit in experimental glioma. Mol Ther 2005;12(5):842–51.

113. Nabors LB, Fiveash JB, Markert JM, et al. A phase 1 trial of ABT-510 concurrent with standard chemoradiation for patients with newly diagnosed glioblastoma. Arch Neurol 2010;67(3):313–9.

114. Lai A, Tran A, Nghiemphu PL, et al. Phase II study of bevacizumab plus temozolomide during and after radiation therapy for patients with newly diagnosed glioblastoma multiforme. J Clin Oncol 2011;29(2):142–8.
115. Batchelor TT, Duda DG, di Tomaso E, et al. Phase II study of cediranib, an oral pan-vascular endothelial growth factor receptor tyrosine kinase inhibitor, in patients with recurrent glioblastoma. J Clin Oncol 2010;28(17):2817–23.
116. Reardon DA, Fink KL, Mikkelsen T, et al. Randomized phase II study of cilengitide, an integrin-targeting arginine-glycine-aspartic acid peptide, in recurrent glioblastoma multiforme. J Clin Oncol 2008;26(34):5610–7.
117. Gilbert MR, Kuhn J, Lamborn KR, et al. Cilengitide in patients with recurrent glioblastoma: the results of NABTC 03-02, a phase II trial with measures of treatment delivery. J Neurooncol 2012;106(1):147–53.
118. Stupp R, Hegi ME, Neyns B, et al. Phase I/IIa study of cilengitide and temozolomide with concomitant radiotherapy followed by cilengitide and temozolomide maintenance therapy in patients with newly diagnosed glioblastoma. J Clin Oncol 2010;28(16):2712–8.
119. Hainsworth JD, Ervin T, Friedman E, et al. Concurrent radiotherapy and temozolomide followed by temozolomide and sorafenib in the first-line treatment of patients with glioblastoma multiforme. Cancer 2010;116(15):3663–9.
120. Neyns B, Chaskis C, Dujardin M, et al. Phase II trial of sunitinib malate in patients with temozolomide refractory recurrent high-grade glioma [meeting abstracts]. J Clin Oncol 2009;27(15 Suppl):2038.
121. Reardon DA, Vredenburgh JJ, Coan A, et al. Phase I study of sunitinib and irinotecan for patients with recurrent malignant glioma. J Neurooncol 2011; 105(3):621–7.
122. Marx GM, Pavlakis N, McCowatt S, et al. Phase II study of thalidomide in the treatment of recurrent glioblastoma multiforme. J Neurooncol 2001;54(1): 31–8.
123. Drappatz J, Norden AD, Wong ET, et al. Phase I study of vandetanib with radiotherapy and temozolomide for newly diagnosed glioblastoma. Int J Radiat Oncol Biol Phys 2010;78(1):85–90.
124. Jain RK, di Tomaso E, Duda DG, et al. Angiogenesis in brain tumours. Nat Rev Neurosci 2007;8(8):610–22.
125. Batchelor TT, Sorensen AG, di Tomaso E, et al. AZD2171, a pan-VEGF receptor tyrosine kinase inhibitor, normalizes tumor vasculature and alleviates edema in glioblastoma patients. Cancer Cell 2007;11(1):83–95.
126. Kreisl TN, Kim L, Moore K, et al. Phase II trial of single-agent bevacizumab followed by bevacizumab plus irinotecan at tumor progression in recurrent glioblastoma. J Clin Oncol 2009;27(5):740–5.
127. Weller M. Angiogenesis in glioblastoma: just another moving target? Brain 2010; 133(Pt 4):955–6.
128. Bergers G, Hanahan D. Modes of resistance to anti-angiogenic therapy. Nat Rev Cancer 2008;8(8):592–603.
129. Shojaei F, Ferrara N. Refractoriness to antivascular endothelial growth factor treatment: role of myeloid cells. Cancer Res 2008;68(14):5501–4.
130. El Hallani S, Boisselier B, Peglion F, et al. A new alternative mechanism in glioblastoma vascularization: tubular vasculogenic mimicry. Brain 2010;133(Pt 4): 973–82.
131. Soda Y, Marumoto T, Friedmann-Morvinski D, et al. Transdifferentiation of glioblastoma cells into vascular endothelial cells. Proc Natl Acad Sci U S A 2011; 108(11):4274–80.

132. Akhavan D, Cloughesy TF, Mischel PS. mTOR signaling in glioblastoma: lessons learned from bench to bedside. Neuro Oncol 2010;12(8):882–9.
133. Engelman JA, Luo J, Cantley LC. The evolution of phosphatidylinositol 3-kinases as regulators of growth and metabolism. Nat Rev Genet 2006;7(8):606–19.
134. Chalhoub N, Zhu G, Zhu X, et al. Cell type specificity of PI3K signaling in Pdk1- and Pten-deficient brains. Genes Dev 2009;23(14):1619–24.
135. Vivanco I, Sawyers CL. The phosphatidylinositol 3-Kinase AKT pathway in human cancer. Nat Rev Cancer 2002;2(7):489–501.
136. Cancer Genome Atlas Research Network. Comprehensive genomic characterization defines human glioblastoma genes and core pathways. Nature 2008; 455(7216):1061–8.
137. Parsons DW, Jones S, Zhang X, et al. An integrated genomic analysis of human glioblastoma multiforme. Science 2008;321(5897):1807–12.
138. Chang SM, Wen P, Cloughesy T, et al. Phase II study of CCI-779 in patients with recurrent glioblastoma multiforme. Invest New Drugs 2005;23(4):357–61.
139. Kreisl TN, Lassman AB, Mischel PS, et al. A pilot study of everolimus and gefitinib in the treatment of recurrent glioblastoma (GBM). J Neurooncol 2009;92(1): 99–105.
140. Doherty L, Gigas DC, Kesari S, et al. Pilot study of the combination of EGFR and mTOR inhibitors in recurrent malignant gliomas. Neurology 2006;67(1):156–8.
141. Sarkaria JN, Galanis E, Wu W, et al. Combination of temsirolimus (CCI-779) with chemoradiation in newly diagnosed glioblastoma multiforme (GBM) (NCCTG trial N027D) is associated with increased infectious risks. Clin Cancer Res 2010;16(22):5573–80.
142. Weller M, Gorlia T, Cairncross JG, et al. Prolonged survival with valproic acid use in the EORTC/NCIC temozolomide trial for glioblastoma. Neurology 2011; 77(12):1156–64.
143. Kondo Y, Hollingsworth EF, Kondo S. Molecular targeting for malignant gliomas (Review). Int J Oncol 2004;24(5):1101–9.
144. Mimeault M, Batra SK. Complex oncogenic signaling networks regulate brain tumor-initiating cells and their progenies: pivotal roles of wild-type EGFR, EGFR-vIII mutant and hedgehog cascades and novel multitargeted therapies. Brain Pathol 2011;21(5):479–500.
145. Dantzer F, de La Rubia G, Menissier-De Murcia J, et al. Base excision repair is impaired in mammalian cells lacking Poly(ADP-ribose) polymerase-1. Biochemistry 2000;39(25):7559–69.
146. Dungey FA, Loser DA, Chalmers AJ. Replication-dependent radiosensitization of human glioma cells by inhibition of poly(ADP-Ribose) polymerase: mechanisms and therapeutic potential. Int J Radiat Oncol Biol Phys 2008;72(4): 1188–97.
147. Shall S, de Murcia G. Poly(ADP-ribose) polymerase-1: what have we learned from the deficient mouse model? Mutat Res 2000;460(1):1–15.
148. Farmer H, McCabe N, Lord CJ, et al. Targeting the DNA repair defect in BRCA mutant cells as a therapeutic strategy. Nature 2005;434(7035):917–21.
149. Audeh MW, Carmichael J, Penson RT, et al. Oral poly(ADP-ribose) polymerase inhibitor olaparib in patients with BRCA1 or BRCA2 mutations and recurrent ovarian cancer: a proof-of-concept trial. Lancet 2010;376(9737):245–51.
150. Knisely JP, Baehring JM. A silver lining on the horizon for glioblastoma. Lancet Oncol 2009;10(5):434–5.

Meningiomas, Nerve Sheath Tumors, and Pituitary Tumors
Diagnosis and Treatment

Florian Roser, MD*, Jürgen Honegger, MD,
Martin U. Schuhmann, MD, Marcos S. Tatagiba, MD

KEYWORDS

- Meningioma • Nerve sheath tumor • Pituitary tumor

KEY POINTS

- Microsurgical removal remains the mainstay of therapy for meningiomas and intracranial schwannomas.
- If risk of morbidity is increased through, for example, skull base infiltration, multimorbidity, or age, subtotal resection and/or adjuvant radiosurgery is a valuable option.
- Even today there is no standard systemic therapeutic option for recurrent tumors, but individual applied therapy regimes are promising.
- For nonfunctioning pituitary adenomas, acromegaly, and Cushing disease, transsphenoidal surgery is the treatment of first choice.
- Today both microscopic and endoscopic techniques are well established in transnasal surgery. Extended transsphenoidal approaches are increasingly applied in pituitary surgery.

MENINGIOMAS
Biology

Meningiomas represent the most important group of intracranial mesodermal tumors. Harvey Cushing coined the term meningioma in 1922, and it is still the commonly used medical designation for a tumor arising from the meninges,[1] despite the fact that meningiomas actually arise from arachnoid epithelial cells, which are a highly metabolically active subgroup of arachnoid cells involved in the reabsorption of cerebrospinal fluid. However, meningiomas almost always grow in the meninges or, more rarely, in the overlying bone, which they may destroy. Thus, in terms of their manifestations, the term meningioma is completely justified. Meningiomas account for 13% to 26% of all intracranial tumors and are very often benign, indolent, and slow growing, yet quite

Department of Neurosurgery, University of Tuebingen, Hoppe-Seyler Strasse 3, 72076 Tuebingen, Germany
* Corresponding author.
E-mail address: f.roser@gmx.de

Hematol Oncol Clin N Am 26 (2012) 855–879
doi:10.1016/j.hoc.2012.04.005
0889-8588/12/$ – see front matter © 2012 Elsevier Inc. All rights reserved.

heterogeneous; as a result their clinical pattern, spontaneous course, and treatment options all differ for each individual case.[2,3] About 6 of every 100,000 individuals present with a meningioma each year, and 2% of meningiomas are diagnosed in children and adolescents.[4] Peak incidence occurs in the fifth to the seventh decades of life. Women are 2 to 3 times more likely than men to develop a meningioma, whereas malignant meningiomas occur more frequently in men and children.[5,6] The incidence has increased in recent decades, primarily as a result of increased imaging procedures and rising life expectancy.

Ionizing radiation is a proven risk factor for the occurrence of meningiomas, even at low dose (eg, 8 Gy for the treatment of tinea capitis in Israel during the 1950s), with a latency period of 35 years,[7] and radiation often causes atypical meningiomas with high proliferation indices.[8] Although meningiomas very often express progesterone and estrogen receptors and women develop meningiomas 3 times more frequently than men, and the coincidental occurrence of breast cancer and meningiomas has been accepted, no connection has been demonstrated to date, beyond basic research, between the occurrence of meningiomas and hormonal stimulation.[9,10] No proof of more frequent occurrence of meningiomas related to increased use of mobile communication devices or as late sequelae of head trauma has been shown in large cross-sectional epidemiologic studies.[11,12]

The subtype classification established in 2007 includes 9 types of low-grade meningiomas (meningothelial, fibrous, transitional, psammomatous, angiomatous, microcytic, secretory, metaplastic, and lymphoplastic), 3 atypical World Health Organization class II (WHO-II) subtypes (atypical, clear-cell, and chordoid), and 3 malignant types of meningiomas (rhabdoid, papillary, and anaplastic).[3] Atypical and anaplastic meningiomas are more frequently found in men, in whom anaplastic meningiomas occur more often as primary growths, and atypical meningiomas are frequently a manifestation of recurrence in WHO-I tumors.[13] Grade III meningiomas represent about 1% to 3% of all meningiomas, characterized by their high rates of mitosis and nuclear polymorphism. These tumors often infiltrate the brain parenchyma and show signs of tumor necrosis. Typical genetic aberrations found in meningiomas are monosomy 22 and mutations in the neurofibromatosis type 2 gene (NF2), which is localized on chromosome 22.[14] The NF2 gene mutation leads to a defect in the gene product, merlin.[15] Loss of alleles at additional sites can contribute to tumor progression, and lead to the development of atypical and anaplastic meningiomas.[16] The occurrence of a 1p deletion is especially associated with an increased risk of relapse, malignant transformation, and tumor progression.[17–19]

Most meningiomas have a good prognosis, with the 5-year survival rate more than 80% and the 10-year survival rate 74% to 79%.[20] The spontaneous course involves growth for all meningiomas, but in very different bandwidths (tumor doubling time between 0.5 and 100 years).[21] Calcified, larger, and spinal meningiomas tend to grow more slowly, and tumors in younger people grow more rapidly. The combination of negative progesterone receptor status and a high proliferation index (Ki-67) is considered to have adverse prognostic significance and, despite radical resection, is associated with relapse.[22] Because of their tendency to recur, atypical meningiomas have a 5-year survival rate of 57%.[23] Higher recurrence rates are also associated with incomplete resection (here the Simpson classification developed in 1957 is still the standard[24]) as well as a higher WHO rating, hemangiopericytic histology, larger tumors, higher mitosis and apoptosis rates, and chromosomal aberrations.

Meningiomas are not characterized by any specific symptoms, and because of their slow and indolent pattern of growth may remain asymptomatic for long periods. Seizures are the most frequent clinical manifestation, occurring in 25% to 40% of cases.[25] A meningioma may become clinically apparent through compression, irritation, or invasion of neighboring brain areas, resulting in symptoms that vary according to the localization and size of the tumor; in addition, they may become symptomatic by causing perifocal edema around the tumor. Increased expression of vascular endothelial growth factor (VEGF) leads to enhanced vascularization and abnormal increases in vascular permeability, which result in edema.[26] Especially in small-sized tumors, it is peritumor edema that may be responsible for the clinical symptoms.[27–29]

Thus, a parasagittal meningioma in the middle fossa may manifest as disturbances in motor function (parasagittal cortical syndrome, contralateral hemiparesis) which, depending on which brain area is compressed, can result in disturbances of speech, focal seizures, or pareses. Loss of the sense of smell and visual disturbances occur as the result of olfactory meningiomas or tuberculum sellae meningiomas, respectively. Depending on their location, meningiomas of the sphenoid wing may surround the internal carotid artery, the optic nerve, or the oculomotor nerve, and thereby cause deterioration of vision. Cavernous sinus meningiomas affect cranial nerves III, IV, and VI. Occipital headaches with disturbances of gait and dizziness may be a manifestation of a meningioma located at the craniocervical junction. Isolated cranial nerve disturbances (loss of hearing, dizziness, double vision, facial paresis) are often the first symptoms of meningiomas located at the base of the skull.

Diagnosis

Today, magnetic resonance imaging (MRI) represents the most sensitive method for diagnosing and interpreting the differential diagnosis of meningiomas, because in comparison with computed tomography (CT) examination it provides significantly better soft-tissue imaging. Modern MRI sequencing includes special applications for specific issues regarding venous drainage (susceptibility-weighted imaging), MR angiography, MR spectroscopy for the differential diagnosis of metastases or intrinsic brain processes, and diffusion tensor image sequencing for the imaging of possible deviations in the course of the pyramidal tract. However, CT examination can provide essential information about bony infiltration of the meningioma, especially in the area of the sphenoid wing.[30,31] In addition, demonstration of calcifications on CT may affect the treatment strategy. Angiography is reserved for specific situations, and can provide dynamic information about vascular supply and drainage. If there is a strong tumor blush shown on angiography, selective embolization may make subsequent surgery easier and contribute to improved postoperative outcome.[32–34] Most meningiomas receive their blood supply from meningeal arteries, but collateral supply through pial vessels may be seen in infiltrative meningiomas with perifocal edema. Using modern nuclear medicine examinations such as positron emission tomography combined with MRI, infiltrative zones can be better represented, thereby optimizing preoperative planning as well as volume planning for radiation therapy.[35]

Surgical Therapy

The treatment regimen for meningiomas must be individualized and interdisciplinary (Fig. 1). As recently as 20 years ago, maximally radical surgery was the preferred treatment option for all meningiomas. However, today the preservation of quality of life stands alongside maximizing life expectancy as the main focus of treatment. Therefore, multimodal treatment programs, with design based on localization, tumor characteristics, and various individual factors such as age, comorbidities, and so forth, have proved to be most effective. Most patients with meningiomas can be cured through surgical resection of their tumors. The urgency of intervention depends on

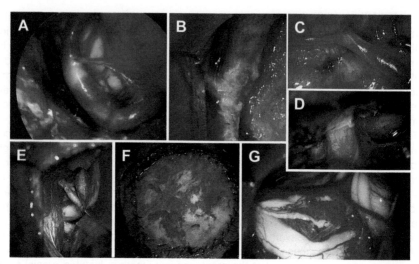

Fig. 1. Intraoperative appearance of meningiomas. (*A*) Endoscopic control in foramen magnum meningioma. (*B*) Tumor infiltration of adventitia of carotid artery. (*C*) Pial infiltration. (*D*) Decompression of the optic canal in clinoid meningioma. (*E*) Dural en plaque infiltration at petrous apex meningioma. (*F*) Dural reconstruction after complete resection of a convexity meningioma. (*G*) Cerebellopontine angle meningioma with displacement of vestibulocochlear nerve group.

size, localization, and clinical presentation. A regimen of "wait-and-scan" can be justified for asymptomatic tumors regardless of their localization and size, to enable estimation of the dynamics of the process. Meningiomas most frequently occur in the cerebral convexities and the falx cerebri. Less often they arise in the frontal base, the region of the sphenoid wing, the cerebellopontine angle and, least often, in the spinal canal.[36] Interventricular and orbital meningiomas are also very rare.[37,38] The proportion of the most aggressive and largest tumors is greatest in the cerebral convexity and lowest in the spinal canal.[39]

Technical and methodologic innovations in neurosurgery may also be used to provide support in the treatment of meningiomas. Navigational assistance may provide help with minimally invasive procedures and limit the extent of the bony resection required at the base of the skull,[40] while fluorescence-based resections can be helpful in the case of infiltrating recurrent meningiomas[41] and modern ultrasound equipment and neuroendoscopy help visualize the tumor bed.[42]

Because of their surgical accessibility, convexity meningiomas have the highest rate of radical resection. Concomitant resection of the involved dura is critical for preventing recurrence; the question of whether the dural tail demonstrated on MRI represents tumor or reactive dural thickening has not been definitely answered.[43] Infiltration of the venous sinus can be a limiting factor in the extent of the resection. If preoperative imaging (CT angiography, MR angiography) shows a blocked sagittal sinus with the presence of venous collateral circulation, an en bloc resection is possible. Because of the relatively silent brain areas in the frontal cortex, frontobasal meningiomas often remain asymptomatic for long periods of time and are only detected relatively late, when there is loss of the sense of smell or increasing apathy on the part of the patient. Frequently there is transosseous penetration of the tumor through the base of the skull into the sinuses, which necessitates reconstruction of the frontal base after resection of the tumor. Typically it is not possible to preserve the olfactory nerves when treating such tumors. Meningiomas of the cavernous sinus or portions of tumors that infiltrate the cavernous sinus are generally reserved for treatment by radiosurgical procedures, because resection in this area leads to permanent cranial nerve deficits.[44,45] Maintenance of vital cranial nerve functions is of critical importance in surgery at the base of the skull. Here, intraoperative monitoring plays a key role. Monitoring should include not only surveillance of long tracts (somatosensory-evoked potential, motor-evoked potentials) but also of the cranial nerves in the operative area (N. II–XII), to provide early warning of impending functional disturbances.[46,47] Spinal meningiomas are a special case. Because of their proximity to the spinal cord, these meningiomas are symptomatic at an early stage and thus are almost always benign (psammomatous), and have a tendency to calcify. Because of their extremely slow growth, even in comparison with intracranial tumors, their size in relation to the spinal cord can be enormous.[39,48] There is no alternative to surgical resection for spinal meningiomas. Electrophysiologic neuromonitoring for preservation of spinal cord function has proved to be prognostically favorable. Ventral meningiomas growing en plaque cannot be radically resected, and often their dural portion also remains in situ.[49] However, recurrence rates are not any higher, and the Simpson classification does not prove useful here (**Fig. 2**).

Surgical morbidity rates in the elderly are not significantly increased, and even surgical interventions at the base of the skull can be performed with relative safety.[50] However, careful preoperative assessment is necessary.[51] Serendipitous findings of meningiomas in elderly patients should initially be observed and treated with antiseizure medication, if necessary. Should there be a definite tendency for growth, treatment can be initiated according to the size of the tumor. Radiosurgery is the therapy of choice in patients with multiple morbidities.[52] The treatment regimen for young patients with neurofibromatosis, who often suffer from massive meningiomatosis, should be adapted individually to the patient's overall clinical status. Radical resections requiring acceptance of a high morbidity risk have just as small a place as primary radiation treatments of meningiomas in very young patients.[53] Because the issue in neurofibromatosis patients is maintenance of quality of life, given their high tumor burden, surgical decompression under continuous electrophysiologic monitoring has proved to be an effective strategy. In the absence of radical treatment, extremely close monitoring of the course of the entire neuroaxis is necessary to detect recurrences.[54]

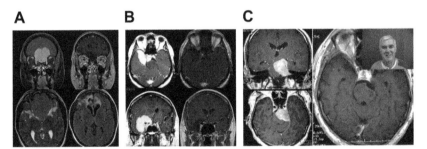

Fig. 2. Case descriptions. (*A*) Large bihemispheric olfactory-groove meningioma with perifocal edema (T2-weighted axial and T1-weighted coronal magnetic resonance imaging [MRI]). Preoperative symptoms were anosmia and lethargy (frontal lobe syndrome). Resection was over a 3 × 2-cm small craniotomy via eyebrow incision. (*B*) Sphenopetroclival meningioma. Pterional approach and subtotal resection with remnants at cavernous sinus wall with endoscopic-assisted resection of posterior fossa tumor parts. (*C*) Large sphenopetroclival meningioma. Complete resection via retrosigmoid approach. Loss of trochlear nerve function, otherwise with preservation of all involved cranial nerves (N. III–XII).

Radiation Therapy

The focus of therapeutic measures is primarily based on the surgical removal of the tumor, because this is the best way to accomplish immediate reduction in volume. Conventional, fractionated-radiation therapy represents a noninvasive measure primarily used for the subsequent treatment of partially resected tumors. Tumor-conformal irradiation with a sharp fall in the dosage curve at the edge of the tumor, and the low degree of invasiveness of the procedure are critically important. Indications for postoperative radiation are the presence of a malignant or anaplastic meningioma or atypical meningiomas independent of their resection status, and incompletely resected benign meningiomas that show recurrent growth during postoperative follow-up.[55] The recommended total dose is 54 Gy, divided in individual doses of 1.8 Gy 5 times weekly. The target volume includes the tumor (or residual tumor) area plus a safety margin of 2 to 3 cm. For optic sheath and cavernous sinus meningiomas as well as inoperable sphenoid wing meningiomas, fractionated 3-dimensional conformation irradiation is indicated. Malignant meningiomas are irradiated using a total dosage of 60 Gy in 1.8- to 2-Gy individual doses, with the safety margin extended to beyond 2 cm.

Small and well-circumscribed meningiomas with a maximum diameter of 3.5 cm are well suited for stereotactic single-dose radiosurgery using a linear accelerator or Gamma Knife, provided they are located at a sufficient distance from sensitive structures, especially the visual system.[56] The average dose level is about 15 Gy (the minimum dose corresponding to the target volume). Radiosurgery is useful as primary treatment of tumors in a difficult location, in patients with elevated surgical risks, or for meningiomatosis.[57–60] It is also used as adjuvant treatment after microsurgical partial resection. In individual cases, treatment may be repeated in the event of recurrence or further progression of the tumor.

Chemotherapy

Chemotherapeutic approaches have not shown clear benefit to date.[61] Treatments have been restricted thus far to isolated cases.[61] Experimental approaches using hormone preparations or hydroxyurea (20 mg/kg/d in ongoing treatment over 1 to 2 years) have not yet established a routine place in clinical practice, and their effectiveness still needs to be proved.[62,63] Antibody-based treatments, including those with platelet-derived growth factor receptor inhibitors (imatinib),[64] somatostatins,[65] temozolomide,[66] and calcium antagonists[67] have not yet been proved as being effective. For anaplastic meningiomas, a therapeutic regimen similar to that used for soft-tissue sarcomas or treatment with an anti-VEGF agent (bevacizumab) may be used as a compassionate intervention.[68]

Despite all of the advances in diagnosis, microsurgical techniques, radiosurgical treatment procedures, and neuropathologic diagnostic methods, many meningiomas continue to present a great challenge that can only be managed through an interdisciplinary approach. There is a persistent conflict between retaining functionality with the aim of a better quality of life, the necessity of treating the tumor, and problems with long-term control of incompletely resected, atypical, or anaplastic meningiomas. These decisions are based on the assessment of the risks and benefits of microsurgical treatment and radiation therapy as well as their long-term consequences, especially regarding the occurrence of secondary tumors and necrosis resulting from radiosurgical procedures.[69,70] The hope remains that targeted therapy consisting of individualized chemotherapy based on molecular genetic testing of the tumor, will one day be able to resolve the problem of meningiomas that recur despite multiple operations and radiation therapies.[71]

PITUITARY TUMORS
Epidemiology

The prevalence of pituitary adenomas is very high, with 14.4% in autopsy series and 22.5% in radiologic studies.[72] Usually these are asymptomatic microadenomas (<10 mm). A clinically relevant pituitary adenoma requiring treatment occurs in only a small percentage of afflicted patients. A cross-sectional study in the province of Liège (Belgium) revealed 940 clinically relevant pituitary adenomas per 1 million inhabitants.[73] Histologically, pituitary adenomas are usually benign tumors, for which differentiation is made between the frequent, typical pituitary adenomas and the atypical adenomas that show histologic signs of increased proliferation activity.[74] Pituitary carcinomas, defined by cerebrospinal or systemic metastatic spread, are very rare.

Clinically, nonfunctioning pituitary adenomas without hormone secretion are differentiated from functioning pituitary adenomas by the overproduction of a pituitary hormone. A characteristic clinical entity develops in functioning adenomas depending on the pituitary hormone being produced in excess. More than 80% of symptomatic pituitary tumors are pituitary adenomas and a further 10% are craniopharyngiomas. A considerable number of other rare tumor entities are encountered in the pituitary area.[75] This article focuses on the predominant pituitary adenomas.

Clinical Symptoms

Nonfunctioning pituitary adenomas
Nonfunctioning pituitary adenomas may be inconspicuous for a long time. Clinical symptoms appear first as a macroadenoma (>10 mm) caused by a local mass effect (**Fig. 3**). Most often, nonfunctioning pituitary adenomas become clinically manifest with visual impairment (so-called chiasmal syndrome) and symptoms of hypopituitarism. Headache is also often observed as an unspecific symptom. Pituitary apoplexy, caused by a hemorrhagic infarction of a pituitary adenoma, is a dramatic clinical manifestation. Pituitary apoplexy typically leads to acute headache and may be accompanied by nausea, vomiting, meningism, acute visual impairment, pareses of the oculomotor nerves, and high-grade hypopituitarism.

Prolactinoma
Prolactin-producing pituitary adenomas (so-called prolactinomas) are the most common functioning adenomas. Women of child-bearing age are frequently affected. The clinical manifestation is an amenorrhea-galactorrhea syndrome predominantly caused by a microprolactinoma. In men, prolactinoma leads to hypogonadism with impaired libido and sexual potency, as well as infertility.

Acromegaly, gigantism
Growth hormone (GH)-producing adenomas lead to acromegaly with overall increased tissue growth. Externally the typical signs occur, with coarsened facial features, prominent supraorbital ridge, enlarged nose, prognathism, and enlargement of hands and feet; visceromegaly also arises. Other important associated conditions are arterial hypertension, diabetes mellitus, congestive heart failure, arthropathy, goiter, macroglossia, sleep apnea, carpal tunnel syndrome, excessive sweating, and swelling of soft tissue. The increased mortality is mainly due to cardiovascular disease.[76]

Gigantism is the juvenile presentation of a GH-secreting pituitary adenoma. Increased body height results from excessive GH exposure before epiphyseal fusion.

Cushing disease
Corticotropin-producing pituitary adenomas cause excessive cortisol release in the adrenal cortex, which elicits the clinical entity of Cushing disease. The term Cushing

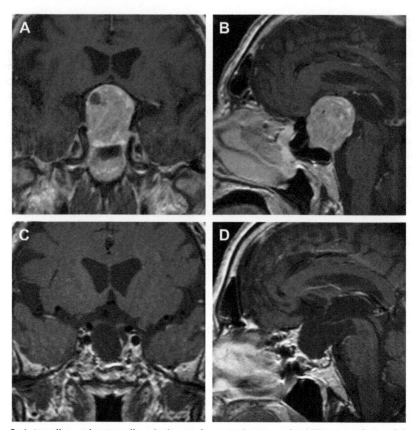

Fig. 3. Intrasellar and suprasellar pituitary adenoma. Preoperative MRI: coronal view (*A*) and sagittal view (*B*). MRI following transsphenoidal microsurgery demonstrates complete adenoma resection: coronal view (*C*) and sagittal view (*D*).

disease is used if the cause of hypercortisolism is a pituitary adenoma. Characteristic external stigmata are plethoric moonface, buffalo hump, purple striae, truncal obesity, excessive bruising, and leathery skin. Excess glucocorticoid causes progressive obesity, myopathy, osteoporosis, depression, glucose intolerance, hypercholesterinemia, arterial hypertension, immunosuppression, and hypogonadism.[77] Left untreated, Cushing disease results in death.

Other functioning pituitary adenomas
Other characteristic clinical entities are thyroid-stimulating hormone (TSH)-producing pituitary adenomas and follicle-stimulating hormone (FSH)-producing pituitary adenomas. Thee lesions, however, are much less frequent than the aforementioned entities.

Endocrinologic Diagnostics

The aim of endocrinologic evaluation is to examine pituitary function on the one hand and to prove any hormone oversecretion by the pituitary adenoma.

Anterior pituitary function
Examination of hormones formed in the pituitary gland and of subsequent peripheral hormones is part of basic endocrinologic evaluation. The following hormones are

determined in the baseline diagnostics: adrenocorticotropic hormone (corticotropin; ACTH), cortisol, GH, insulin-like growth factor (IGF-1), FSH, luteinizing hormone (LH), estradiol (in women), testosterone (in men), TSH, free triiodothyronine (T3), free thyroxine (T4), and prolactin. Perioperative examination of the adrenal axis is particularly important, because the integrity is essential for a physiologic stress response. If adrenal insufficiency is present, perioperative hydrocortisone replacement is vital. The gold standard for examination of the adrenal axis is the insulin tolerance test. The corticotropin-releasing hormone (CRH) test and the ACTH test are also used as alternatives.

Hormone excess due to functioning adenomas

Prolactinomas Diagnosis of prolactinomas requires examination of the prolactin level. A 10-fold elevated prolactin level is diagnostic for the presence of a prolactinoma. However, the prolactin level may be lower in the presence of smaller prolactinomas.

Attention must be paid especially to the following in interpreting the prolactin level:

1. The prolactin level can be increased by medication (eg, neuroleptics)
2. Compression of the pituitary stalk by other pituitary tumors leads to a usually mild functional hyperprolactinemia, which should not be confused with the prolactin excess of prolactinomas.

Acromegaly Two diagnostic criteria are used for proof of acromegaly[76]:

Elevated IGF-1 level as matched for age and gender
Failure to suppress GH in response to an oral glucose tolerance test usually to a level of less than 1 ng/mL; with sensitive GH assays, a threshold of 0.4 ng/mL is suggested.

Cushing disease The endocrinologic diagnostics of Cushing disease is particularly complicated. First, the presence of a Cushing syndrome must be endocrinologically proven. If the plasma ACTH level is normal or elevated, additional endocrinologic examinations must differentiate between pituitary-dependent Cushing syndrome attributable to an ACTH-producing adenoma (ie, Cushing disease) and ectopic Cushing syndrome. Stimulation of the plasma ACTH and cortisol levels in the CRH-stimulation test and/or suppression of the cortisol level in the high-dose dexamethasone suppression test indicate Cushing disease.[78] If the source of ACTH is unclear, bilateral petrosal sinus sampling is performed. A central/peripheral ACTH gradient greater than 3 after CRH stimulation is proof of pituitary-dependent Cushing syndrome.

Radiologic Diagnostics

The method of choice for neuroradiologic examination is MRI. MRI shows displacement of the pituitary gland and stalk, and the extent of chiasma compression by the pituitary adenoma. About 25% of clinically relevant pituitary adenomas invade the cavernous sinus. Invasive growth can be evaluated using the Knosp criteria.[79]

MRI usually enables a differential-diagnostic categorization of the pituitary tumors. Using MRI, a decision concerning the appropriate surgical approach can be made based on the size and configuration of the tumor. Postoperatively, MRI demonstrates the completeness of surgical resection (see **Fig. 3**).

Ophthalmologic Diagnostics

With suprasellar adenoma extension, the optic chiasm is elevated and compressed, which results in visual dysfunction called chiasmal syndrome with the typical finding of bitemporal hemianopia. Ikeda and Yoshimoto[80] have shown that chiasmal syndrome occurs with a suprasellar displacement of the optic chiasm of more than 8 mm on sagittal MRI.

Thorough ophthalmologic examination is obligatory in all suprasellar pituitary adenomas. The ophthalmologic diagnostics include determination of visual acuity and examination of visual fields. In addition, examination must be made as to whether papillary atrophy is present as an expression of irreversible damage to optic nerve fibers. A complete ophthalmologic status is required to recognize independent ocular diseases.

Operative Treatment

Transsphenoidal operation

More than 90% of all pituitary adenomas can be operated on using a transsphenoidal approach.[81] Since Jules Hardy introduced the surgical microscope in the late 1960s, selective adenomectomy with preservation of the pituitary became possible.[82] Classically the microsurgical technique is performed. In 1987, Griffith and Veerapen[83] described the direct perinasal approach, whereby the preparation begins deep in the nose, after which the bony nasal septum is separated from the rostrum of the sphenoid sinus and displaced to the opposite side using a speculum. The minimally invasive septum-pushover technique, which is based on the technical innovation by Griffith and Veerapen, is widely used today. After the sphenoid sinus is opened and the sellar floor is resected, the adenoma is excised using microinstruments and curettes.

Endoscopy has become established as an alternative operation technique. The purely endoscopic technique was first described by Jho and Carrau,[84] and has continued to gain popularity. Because the optic in the endoscopic technique is placed in the sphenoid sinus, the surgeon has a panoramic overview of the surgical field. The microsurgical technique, on the other hand, provides manual freedom of movement, a 3-dimensional view, and no smearing of the optic system in the case of bleeding, because the microscope is positioned externally. The dispute among experts about which surgical technique is better does not seem justified, because microsurgery and endoscopy differ only in the visualization instrument used.

Extended transnasal approaches

Extended transnasal approaches are increasingly applied in pituitary surgery.[85] The transtuberculum sellae approach enables an intracranial view by removal of the tuberculum sellae.[86] Thus, adenomas attached in the suprasellar space or localized at the pituitary stalk can also be excised. Extended approaches also allow removal of larger adenomas that have developed well beyond the borders of the sella turcica, for example into the cavernosus sinus and the clivus.[87]

Technical support

The use of neuronavigation is very common in neurosurgery today. In transsphenoidal surgery, the authors use neuronavigation in reoperations and in children with non-pneumatized sphenoid sinus as an orientation during the surgical approach. Neuronavigation improves the radicality of the procedure and reduces the surgical risk, because the borders of the tumor and the position of important anatomic structures (eg, the carotid artery) can be identified intraoperatively based on preoperative MRI data. In some neurosurgical centers, such as the authors' in Tuebingen, intraoperative MRI is available, which allows intraoperative control of the completeness of resection and, if required, further more radical resection during the same surgical procedure.[88]

Results of the transsphenoidal operation

The complication rate of transsphenoidal surgery is low. Typical complications are meningitis and cerebrospinal fluid rhinorrhea. In experienced hands, these 2 complications are in a range of 1% or even less.[89] Life-threatening injury to the carotid artery is very rare. With selective adenomectomy, pituitary function can usually be preserved. New hormone deficits are found in only about 5% of the patients, and a preoperative hypopituitarism may recover at least partially after the operation in up to 50% of the cases.[90] A chiasmal syndrome regresses postoperatively in about 75% of the patients. Postoperative deterioration of vision is rarely encountered. The recurrence rate of nonfunctioning adenomas is low with total resection. However, if adenoma remnants remain, renewed growth must be expected with relatively high probability of recurrence during the further course.[91]

Prolactinomas Whereas surgery is the initial therapy of first choice in nonfunctioning adenomas, acromegaly, and Cushing disease, medical therapy is usually the initial treatment in prolactinomas (**Fig. 4**). However, transsphenoidal surgery has regained recognition in the treatment of prolactinomas in the past years. Long-term remission can be achieved in more than 90% of microprolactinomas,[92] whereas dopamine agonist (DA) therapy must often be continued for life. For this reason, an increasing number of those affected choose the surgical option. The operation is often performed before family planning, because the female patients can then become pregnant without medical treatment. Surgical treatment can also be offered to very young patients and children to avoid the risks of medical therapy over decades. Further indications for the operation are acute visual loss in macroadenomas, nonresponsiveness to DA therapy, or intolerance to DA.

Acromegaly For complete remission a postoperative GH level of less than 2.5 ng/mL, suppression of growth hormone to less than 1 ng/mL during a glucose tolerance test, and an IGF-1 level within the normal range are required. The largest published operative study described an overall remission rate of 57.3%, but the chance of remission depends in great measure on the size and invasive behavior of the pituitary adenoma. The remission rates for microadenomas were 75%, and 74% for intrasellar macroadenomas.[93]

Regarding Cushing disease, in the literature the initial success rate of transsphenoidal operation is between 70% and 90%.[94] Because of the severity of the disease, the authors favor early reoperation following failure of the first operation.[75]

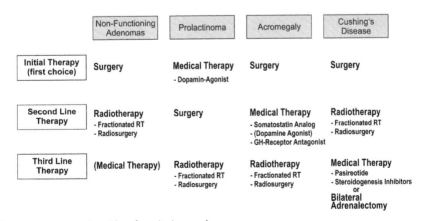

Fig. 4. Treatment algorithm for pituitary adenomas.

Transcranial operation

Transcranial operation is indicated if the adenoma configuration suggests low chance for removal of the suprasellar adenoma.[81,95] This is the case in adenomas with multi-lobulated suprasellar extension, which indicates a perforation of the diaphragma sellae. A small sella turcica and a narrow sellar entrance may also make craniotomy necessary for the resection of an adenoma with suprasellar growth.

Medical Therapy

Nonfunctioning adenomas

No established medical treatment is available for nonfunctioning adenomas.

Prolactinomas

The prolactinoma is the best example of a tumor that responds to medical treatment (see **Fig. 4**). With the second-generation DAs such as cabergolin, treatment is more effective and has fewer side effects than the classic DA bromocriptine.[96] The excellent results are, however, relativized by a current study, which revealed side effects in 42% of patients during the long-term course.[97] The DA therapy even had to be withdrawn in 18% of patients because of side effects. At present, there are also reservations concerning drug therapy, due to more recent knowledge that long-term administration of DAs may lead to restrictive cardiac valvulopathy.[98]

A meta-analysis revealed a pooled proportion of patients with persisting normoprolactinemia after DA withdrawal of only 21%.[99]

Acromegaly

The most important indication for medical therapy is a postoperative persistence of GH excess (see **Fig. 4**). Somatostatin analogues are the drug-treatment option of first choice. These agents develop their effect via somatostatin receptors directly on the adenoma and, in addition to decreasing GH, may also effect tumor shrinkage. The currently used somatostatin analogues are lanreotide and octreotide. A meta-analysis showed IGF-1 normalization in 47% of the patients under treatment with lanreotide and in 67% of those under treatment with octreotide.[100] DAs can be tried if GH is only slightly increased, but they are less effective in eradicating the GH excess and normalizing IGF-1. Some years ago, the GH-receptor antagonist pegvisomant became available for the treatment of acromegaly.[101] Pegvisomant acts in the periphery and blocks IGF-1 production, and is used if the response to somatostatin analogues is insufficient. Normalization of IGF-1 can be achieved in 62% to 78% of the patients.

Cushing disease

It is difficult to achieve long-term control of hypercortisolism with medical treatment. Medical treatment can be applied for acute treatment of severe Cushing syndrome. Medical therapy is also suitable for patients awaiting a response to radiation therapy and whenever a palliative treatment is needed (see **Fig. 4**).[102] Steroidogenesis inhibitors, which act on the adrenal gland, can be used for medical therapy.[102] The most experience with this drug group has been acquired with metyrapone and ketoconazole.

Other medicaments develop their effect centrally on the adenoma. The somatostatin analogues octreotide and lanreotide have generally been found to be ineffective. Encouraging results have been obtained with the novel somatostatin analogue pasireotide.[103] Pasireotide has a particularly high affinity to the somatostatin receptor subtype 5, which predominates in ACTH-producing pituitary adenomas.[103]

Aggressive pituitary adenomas
Successful treatment of aggressive pituitary adenomas and pituitary carcinomas with the chemotherapeutic temozolomide was recently reported.[104] This result opens a perspective for treatment of functioning and nonfunctioning adenomas that no longer respond to conventional therapy.

Radiotherapy

In nonfunctioning pituitary adenomas, radiotherapy (RT) is usually performed in residual or recurrent adenomas that cannot be surgically removed (see **Fig. 4**). In the case of small residual adenomas, RT can be postponed until there is proof of adenoma progression. In Cushing disease, RT can be used as second-line treatment if surgery fails to cure the patient (see **Fig. 4**). In prolactinomas and acromegaly, RT is the third-line treatment and is indicated when surgical and medical options have been exhausted. Two principal radiotherapeutic techniques are available: fractionated RT and stereotactic singe-fraction radiotherapy (ie, radiosurgery).

Fractionated radiotherapy
Today, conventional fractionated RT is performed with mask-fixing and has been refined to tumor-conformal delivery. Fractionated RT is performed in adenomas in the immediate vicinity of the optic pathway and in large-irradiation volumes. The usual radiation doses are 45 to 54 Gy, applied in fractions of 1.8 (to 2) Gy. The risk of delayed-onset hypopituitarism is more than 50%. Infrequent complications are optic neuropathy, secondary malignoma, and cerebrovascular insults.

In nonfunctioning adenomas, the rate of recurrence-free survival 10 years following surgery and fractionated RT is 80% to 97%.[105] Remission rates for Cushing disease reported in the literature range from 10% to 83%.[106] The UK National Acromegaly Register Study Group reported on 884 acromegalic patients who received conventional pituitary irradiation and found a normalization rate of 63% for IGF-1 at 10 years' follow-up.[107] However, the withdrawal of suppressive medications is not specified. The remission rates are lower in prolactinomas than in Cushing disease and acromegaly.

Radiosurgery
Single-fraction radiosurgery is particularly indicated for small invasive residual adenomas in the cavernous sinus that are not amenable to surgery. The following modalities are available for radiosurgery: Gamma Knife radiosurgery, linear accelerator (LINAC)-based radiosurgery, Cyberknife radiosurgery, and proton-beam radiation. To prevent optic neuropathy, the dose delivered to the optic apparatus should not exceed 10 to 12 Gy. Advantages of radiosurgery over fractionated RT are the lower rate of hypopituitarism and, in cases of functioning adenomas, the more rapid decrease of the hormone excess,[108] which usually starts within a few months. A comprehensive review of the literature revealed a tumor control rate greater than 90% for nonfunctioning pituitary adenomas with tumor margin doses of 14 to 25 Gy,[109] but the data on long-term follow-up are sparse. Higher radiation doses are required to correct hormone excess than are required to prevent tumor growth. Tumor-margin doses from 15 to 32 Gy are usually reported for functioning adenomas. In large contemporary series, the rates of biochemical remission are approximately 50% for Cushing disease,[110,111] 35% for acromegaly, and 25% for prolactinoma.[111]

INTRACRANIAL NERVE SHEATH TUMORS

Almost all intracranial nerve sheath tumors are schwannomas or synonymously termed neurinomas. These tumors originate from the Schwann cells of those 9 cranial nerves belonging to the peripheral nervous system; thus olfactory, optic, and cochlear nerve are excluded. Because cranial nerves III to XII originate within the posterior fossa, the vast majority of schwannomas occur and extend at the skull base of the posterior fossa, with the exception of those rare trigeminal schwannomas that grow predominantly into the middle fossa or from the cavernous sinus outward to the infratemporal region.

Schwannomas account for 8% of all intracranial tumors.[112] About 90% are sporadic and solitary while 4% occur in patients with neurofibromatosis type 2 (NF2), for which bilateral vestibular schwannomas are diagnostic. Because schwannomas usually occur in sensory cranial nerves, by far the most common intracranial schwannoma is the vestibular schwannoma (VS), originating from the vestibular nerve but often misnamed as acoustic neurinoma, comprising about 90% of all intracranial schwannomas. The second most common schwannoma originates from the trigeminal nerve, accounting for up to 8% of all schwannomas.[113] Schwannomas of the jugular foramen, the hypoglossal nerve, the oculomotor nerve, or the facial nerve are rare, and often occur in the context of NF2.

Schwannomas are benign tumors assigned to WHO-I. Derived from Schwann cells, they are histologically dominated by spindle cells that form 2 characteristic histopathologic patterns: Antoni A type with compact areas of spindle cells with pink cytoplasm, and occasional occurrence of nuclear palisading. The Antoni B type has looser characteristics with cells showing clear, vacuolated cytoplasm caused by lipid accumulation.[114] Further characteristics in histology are thick-walled blood vessels within the tumor and a strong and diffuse staining for S100 protein.

Because of the dominance of VS intracranial nerve sheath tumors, the following focuses primarily on this entity. The general rules and principles, however, do apply to other schwannomas in a comparable fashion. VS account for about 8% to 10% of the primary intracranial tumors, and 80% to 90% of those are located within the cerebellopontine angle.[112] In children they constitute less than 1% of all primary pediatric brain tumors and even less than 1% of all posterior fossa tumors.[115] In most cases the presence of VSs in childhood and adolescence is connected to the coexistence of NF2. The overall incidence of VS is estimated to be 1 in 100,000 per year, cumulating to a lifetime risk of 1:1000 in the general population.[116,117] Most patients with unilateral sporadic VS present at an age beyond 40 years.[117] In a large series of 1000 surgically treated symptomatic VS the mean age at surgery was 46.3 years, with an inverse linear correlation of tumor size and age: the largest tumors were symptomatic at the earliest age.[118] Around 5% to 7% of all VSs are due to NF2, an autosomal dominant inherited disease, which has an estimated incidence of 1:25,000 at birth.[119] Although NF2 is characterized by bilateral VSs at the time of presentation, up to 10% to 25% of NF2-associated VSs might initially present unilaterally.[120] The average age of clinical onset in NF2 patients is 18 to 24 years, thus just beyond adolescence.[121] Of 1000 surgically treated VSs, 120 were operated on in 82 NF2 patients of mean age 27.5 years.[118,122]

Symptomatology and Establishment of Diagnosis

Symptomatic cochlear nerve involvement occurs in 95% of patients. Hearing loss, which is usually chronic, is found in 95%, with an average duration of about 4 years, tinnitus is present in 63% with an average duration of 3 years; vestibular nerve affection occurs in 61%, mostly manifesting as unsteadiness while walking and frequently fluctuating in severity. Trigeminal nerve disturbances occur in 17%. A primary facial nerve involvement is rare (6%). Large tumors might cause ataxia as a result of severe cerebellar or brainstem compression or occlusive hydrocephalus. An affection of lower cranial nerve function is extremely rare. In cases of unclear eighth-nerve symp-tomatology, MRI should be performed, and is the procedure of choice to diagnose intracranial schwannomas.

Typical MRI features of VSs are the presence of an isointense to (rarely) mixed iso-hypointense mass in T1-weighted images showing a rather homogeneous enhance-ment (two-thirds homogeneous, one-third inhomogeneous) after contrast application. Central slightly irregular hypointensities in postcontrast images of larger tumors extending into the cerebellopontine angle are common, corresponding to circum-scribed degenerative cystic and necrotic areas.[123] Lesions are slightly hyperintense in T2-weighted images. High-resolution constructive interference in steady-state images often allow to delineate, especially in smaller tumors, the course of the neigh-boring cochlear and facial nerve within the cistern or even within the internal auditory canal. In all cases for which surgery is planned, a thin-slice (2 mm) bone-window CT scan with reduced radiation dose should be performed, to provide the surgeon with crucial information such as position of emissary veins and the jugular bulb, and topo-graphic orientation of the semicircular canals in relation to the planned opening of the internal auditory canal, so as to avoid injury to the former.

Tumor extension is best described according to the Hannover classification, to provide a uniform anatomic basis for the process of decision making in the later course of the disease: T1, purely intrameatal; T2, intrameatal and limited extrameatal exten-sion; T3A; filling the cerebellopontine cistern, not reaching the brainstem; T3B; filling the cerebellopontine cistern and reaching the brainstem; T4A; compressing the brain-stem; T4B; hydrocephalus secondary to compression of the fourth ventricle.[118]

Treatment Options

Sporadic VSs will most likely be diagnosed at a time of beginning hearing loss when the tumor often has grown to a considerable size of at least T3. The widespread use of MRI, however, also leads to an increasing number of incidentally discovered smaller VSs. Multiple management strategies are at hand. Already the question of timing of an intervention ranges from prophylactic treatment despite unimpaired hearing at the time of proven growth, to intervention at the time of beginning hearing loss, to treatment after loss of functional hearing to, finally, treatment only at the time of brainstem compression.

Because schwannomas are benign and slow-growing tumors, conservative management (wait and see) has also been used. In a meta-analysis on conservative management, 43% of tumors showed growth, 51% remained stable, and 6% regressed without treatment during an average follow-up of 3.2 years. However, hearing loss occurred in one-half of 347 individuals in whom it was assessed longitu-dinally.[124] In the authors' opinion an observational approach is only appropriate in elderly patients with significant treatment risks and tumor size of T3A or smaller.

In patients younger than 60 to 65 years, progression is likely and treatment is war-ranted. The 2 basic treatment options are neurosurgical resection and radiosurgery. Purely from the point of tumor biology, gross total surgical resection is the treatment of choice because it carries the strongest potential for cure. However, in VS surgery functionality of the involved cochlear nerve and facial nerve are very important cofac-tors. The rate of functional preservation is on the one hand strongly dependent on the experience of the surgeon and the microsurgical technique used; on the other hand, it depends on tumor-associated factors such as adherence/infiltration, tumor size, and the level of preoperative hearing.[125,126] In case of bilateral VS in NF2, a long-term threat of bilateral deafness and facial nerve paralysis exists. Therefore, the avoidance of functional deficits has even higher priority.

Surgical Technique

Three possible surgical routes exist with which to approach a VS. The retromastoid suboccipital (retrosigmoid) approach can be used for any tumor size, with an attempt to preserve hearing. Facial nerve preservation rates are high. This approach is as well suited for almost all other posterior fossa schwannomas and constitutes the authors' preferred option. Another advantage is the straightforwardness of the procedure, with a usual skin to tumor time of 30 minutes in experienced hands. The translabyrinthine approach has been developed mainly by ear/nose/throat surgeons for VS when hearing preservation is not an issue; however, the approach per se is rather time consuming. The epidural middle fossa approach is suitable only for small tumors (T1, T2) when hearing preservation is the goal. However, it requires elevation of the temporal lobe, which can be problematic especially on the left side when the Labbé vein is at risk.

For small VSs the authors perform surgery with the patient in supine position with the head turned to the contralateral side, the same positioning as used for vascular decompression procedures in the cerebellopontine angle. A park-bench position is the alternative option. In larger tumors a semisitting position is preferred, under permanent surveillance of the right atrium via transesophageal ultrasound for early and highly sensitive detection of air embolism. The semisitting position combines an upright head position with intrathoracic and cervical venous pressure higher than in the sitting position, a fact that reduces the risk of air embolism significantly. The major surgical advantage of the vertical head position is that irrigation replaces suction to keep the operating field clear of blood and that bimanual dissection by the surgeon is enabled, which in the authors' experience is the key feature for preservation of function (**Fig. 5**).

In all cases of functional hearing, the goal is to perform a decompression of the cochlear nerve by (1) partially opening the bony internal auditory canal and (2) resection of the tumor under control of the integrity of brainstem auditory evoked potentials (BAEP). The quality of preoperative BAEP and tumor size is essential for the rate of hearing preservation, because the smaller the tumor and the better the preoperative BAEP, the higher the rate of hearing preservation that can be achieved. Functional hearing rates do vary between 47% and 88%, depending on the coexistence of one or several advantageous factors.[126]

Extensive intraoperative neurophysiologic monitoring (IOM) is also, however, the "conditio sine qua non" in all other cases of schwannoma surgery where hearing

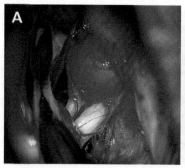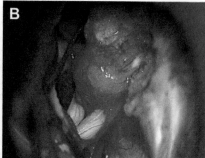

Fig. 5. (*A*) Cerebellopontine angle (*right*) seen from semisitting position. (*B*) Internal auditory canal drilled open to expose the intracanalicular portion of vestibular schwannoma (classification T2).

preservation is not an issue, because functional outcome of the facial nerve but also of trigeminal and caudal cranial nerves is decisively influenced by the IOM guidance of the surgeon.[127]

In the case of nonfunctional hearing preoperatively, which is often found in larger tumors greater than T3A, the limitation regarding total tumor removal is the preservation of the facial nerve function. Facial nerve motor-evoked potentials provide additional information about the nerve integrity before the facial nerve is identified and exposed for direct stimulation. The rate of long-term preservation of facial nerve function is in the 90% range in sporadic VS.[125,128]

Patients are followed postoperatively with MRI surveillance scans. Imaging is usually done for the first time at 3 months postoperatively, then every year for about 5 years in non-NF2 cases (**Fig. 6**). There are few, if any, recurrences when the removal of surgical tumor is complete.[129,130] However, in patients who undergo subtotal removal in an attempt to preserve anatomic continuity of the facial or cochlear nerves, regrowth and/or recurrence occurs in up to 15%.[131,132]

Radiosurgery and Stereotactic Radiotherapy

In sporadic unilateral VS in adults, radiosurgery is a firmly established alternative treatment option for smaller to medium-sized tumors, with a large body of available literature suggesting good tumor control rates in the 90% range, preservation rate for serviceable hearing of 50% to 80%, and long-term facial nerve injury rate of 1%.[133–135] Long-term outcome analysis beyond 15 years, however, is still rare in the literature. Experiences with radiosurgery in NF2 patients is less promising, with lower control rates in younger patients, rather rapid decrease of hearing function over the first 5 years, and a considerable risk for induction of new schwannomas or malignant transformation.[136,137]

An experimental chemotherapeutic approach with bevacizumab has shown some promising results recently in selected NF2 patients regarding tumor response and hearing improvement.[138] However, it could be shown that this effect is only sustained under continued therapy and that rebound occurs after therapy is stopped.[139]

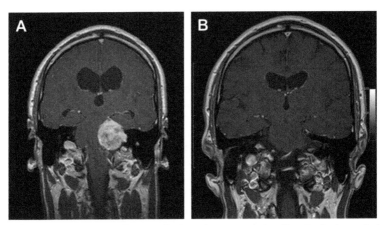

Fig. 6. (A) Brainstem-compressing vestibular schwannoma leading to hydrocephalus. (B) Postoperative coronal T1-weighted MR images.

REFERENCES

1. Eisenhardt L, Cushing H. Diagnosis of intracranial tumors by supravital technique. Am J Pathol 1930;6(5):541–52.
2. Claus EB, Bondy ML, Schildkraut JM, et al. Epidemiology of intracranial meningioma. Neurosurgery 2005;57(6):1088–95 [discussion: 1088–95].
3. Louis DN, Ohgaki H, Wiestler OD, et al. The 2007 WHO classification of tumours of the central nervous system. Acta Neuropathol 2007;114(2):97–109.
4. DeAngelis LM. Brain tumors. N Engl J Med 2001;344(2):114–23.
5. Jaaskelainen J, Haltia M, Servo A. Atypical and anaplastic meningiomas: radiology, surgery, radiotherapy, and outcome. Surg Neurol 1986;25(3):233–42.
6. Matsuno A, Fujimaki T, Sasaki T, et al. Clinical and histopathological analysis of proliferative potentials of recurrent and non-recurrent meningiomas. Acta Neuropathol (Berl) 1996;91(5):504–10.
7. Albrecht S, Goodman JC, Rajagopolan S, et al. Malignant meningioma in Gorlin's syndrome: cytogenetic and p53 gene analysis. Case report. J Neurosurg 1994;81(3):466–71.
8. Lindboe CF, Helseth E, Myhr G. Lhermitte-Duclos disease and giant meningioma as manifestations of Cowden's disease. Clin Neuropathol 1995;14(6):327–30.
9. Baheti AD, Mahore AS, Zade BP, et al. Meningioma and cavernous angioma following childhood radiotherapy. J Cancer Res Ther 2010;6(3):333–5.
10. Sadetzki S, Flint-Richter P, Ben Tal T, et al. Radiation-induced meningioma: a descriptive study of 253 cases. J Neurosurg 2002;97(5):1078–82.
11. Bondy M, Ligon BL. Epidemiology and etiology of intracranial meningiomas: a review. J Neurooncol 1996;29(3):197–205.
12. Schuz J, Bohler E, Berg G, et al. Cellular phones, cordless phones, and the risks of glioma and meningioma (Interphone Study Group, Germany). Am J Epidemiol 2006;163(6):512–20.
13. Roser F, Nakamura M, Ritz R, et al. Proliferation and progesterone receptor status in benign meningiomas are not age dependent. Cancer 2005;104(3):598–601.
14. Fredman P, Dumanski J, Davidsson P, et al. Expression of the ganglioside GD3 in human meningiomas is associated with monosomy of chromosome 22. J Neurochem 1990;55(6):1838–40.
15. Gusella JF, Ramesh V, MacCollin M, et al. Merlin: the neurofibromatosis 2 tumor suppressor. Biochim Biophys Acta 1999;1423(2):M29–36.
16. Rempel SA, Schwechheimer K, Davis RL, et al. Loss of heterozygosity for loci on chromosome 10 is associated with morphologically malignant meningioma progression. Cancer Res 1993;53(Suppl 10):2386–92.
17. Ketter R, Henn W, Niedermayer I, et al. Predictive value of progression-associated chromosomal aberrations for the prognosis of meningiomas: a retrospective study of 198 cases. J Neurosurg 2001;95(4):601–7.
18. Simon M, von Deimling A, Larson JJ, et al. Allelic losses on chromosomes 14, 10, and 1 in atypical and malignant meningiomas: a genetic model of meningioma progression. Cancer Res 1995;55(20):4696–701.
19. Weber RG, Bostrom J, Wolter M, et al. Analysis of genomic alterations in benign, atypical, and anaplastic meningiomas: toward a genetic model of meningioma progression. Proc Natl Acad Sci U S A 1997;94(26):14719–24.
20. Talback M, Stenbeck M, Rosen M. Up-to-date long-term survival of cancer patients: an evaluation of period analysis on Swedish Cancer Registry data. Eur J Cancer 2004;40(9):1361–72.

21. Nakamura M, Roser F, Michel J, et al. The natural history of incidental meningiomas. Neurosurgery 2003;53(1):62–70.
22. Roser F, Nakamura M, Bellinzona M, et al. The prognostic value of progesterone receptor status in meningiomas. J Clin Pathol 2004;57:1033–7.
23. Goyal LK, Suh JH, Mohan DS, et al. Local control and overall survival in atypical meningioma: a retrospective study. Int J Radiat Oncol Biol Phys 2000;46(1): 57–61.
24. Simpson D. The recurrence of intracranial meningiomas after surgical treatment. J Neurol Neurosurg Psychiatry 1957;20:22–39.
25. Chozick BS, Reinert SE, Greenblatt SH. Incidence of seizures after surgery for supratentorial meningiomas: a modern analysis. J Neurosurg 1996;84(3):382–6.
26. Goldman CK, Bharara S, Palmer CA, et al. Brain edema in meningiomas is associated with increased vascular endothelial growth factor expression. Neurosurgery 1997;40(6):1269–77.
27. Bitzer M, Opitz H, Popp J, et al. Angiogenesis and brain oedema in intracranial meningiomas: influence of vascular endothelial growth factor. Acta Neurochir (Wien) 1998;140(4):333–40.
28. Bitzer M, Wockel L, Morgalla M, et al. Peritumoural brain oedema in intracranial meningiomas: influence of tumour size, location and histology. Acta Neurochir (Wien) 1997;139(12):1136–42.
29. de Vries J, Wakhloo AK. Cerebral oedema associated with WHO-I, WHO-II, and WHO-III-meningiomas: correlation of clinical, computed tomographic, operative and histological findings. Acta Neurochir (Wien) 1993;125(1–4):34–40.
30. Roser F, Nakamura M, Jacobs C, et al. Sphenoid wing meningiomas with osseous involvement. Surg Neurol 2005;64(1):37–43 [discussion: 43].
31. Tokgoz N, Oner YA, Kaymaz M, et al. Primary intraosseous meningioma: CT and MRI appearance. AJNR Am J Neuroradiol 2005;26(8):2053–6.
32. Bendszus M, Rao G, Burger R, et al. Is there a benefit of preoperative meningioma embolization? Neurosurgery 2000;47(6):1306–11.
33. Gruber A, Killer M, Mazal P, et al. Preoperative embolization of intracranial meningiomas: a 17-years single center experience. Minim Invasive Neurosurg 2000;43(1):18–29.
34. Kaji T, Hama Y, Iwasaki Y, et al. Preoperative embolization of meningiomas with pial supply: successful treatment of two cases. Surg Neurol 1999;52(3):270–3.
35. Thorwarth D, Henke G, Muller AC, et al. Simultaneous (68)Ga-DOTATOC-PET/ MRI for IMRT treatment planning for meningioma: first experience. Int J Radiat Oncol Biol Phys 2011;81(1):277–83.
36. Solero CL, Fornari M, Giombini S, et al. Spinal meningiomas: review of 174 operated cases. Neurosurgery 1989;25(2):153–60.
37. Nakamura M, Roser F, Bundschuh O, et al. Intraventricular meningiomas: a review of 16 cases with reference to the literature. Surg Neurol 2003;59(6): 491–503.
38. Roser F, Nakamura M, Martini-Thomas R, et al. The role of surgery in meningiomas involving the optic nerve sheath. Clin Neurol Neurosurg 2006;108(5): 470–6.
39. Roser F, Nakamura M, Bellinzona M, et al. Proliferation potential of spinal meningiomas. Eur Spine J 2006;15(2):211–5.
40. Omay SB, Barnett GH. Surgical navigation for meningioma surgery. J Neurooncol 2010;99(3):357–64.
41. Hefti M. Comment concerning: intraoperative 5-aminolevulinic-acid-induced fluorescence in meningiomas, Acta Neurochir DOI:10.1007/s00701-010-0708-4,

Intratumoral heterogeneity and fluorescence intensity in meningioma after 5-ALA pretreatment. Acta Neurochir (Wien) 2011;153(4):959–60.

42. Chen TC, Rabb C, Apuzzo ML. Complex technical methodologies and their applications in the surgery of intracranial meningiomas. Neurosurg Clin N Am 1994;5(2):261–81.

43. Wallace EW. The dural tail sign. Radiology 2004;233(1):56–7.

44. Brell M, Villa S, Teixidor P, et al. Fractionated stereotactic radiotherapy in the treatment of exclusive cavernous sinus meningioma: functional outcome, local control, and tolerance. Surg Neurol 2006;65(1):28–33 [discussion: 33–4].

45. Dufour H, Muracciole X, Metellus P, et al. Long-term tumor control and functional outcome in patients with cavernous sinus meningiomas treated by radiotherapy with or without previous surgery: is there an alternative to aggressive tumor removal? Neurosurgery 2001;48(2):285–94.

46. Nakamura M, Roser F, Dormiani M, et al. Facial and cochlear nerve function after surgery of cerebellopontine angle meningiomas. Neurosurgery 2005;57(1): 77–90 [discussion: 77–90].

47. Nakamura M, Roser F, Dormiani M, et al. Intraoperative auditory brainstem responses in patients with cerebellopontine angle meningiomas involving the inner auditory canal: analysis of the predictive value of the responses. J Neurosurg 2005;102(4):637–42.

48. Cavanaugh DA, Jawahar A, Lee JA, et al. Intraspinal meningioma in a 101-year old: should age determine the aggressiveness of intervention? Surg Neurol 2008;69(2):130–4.

49. Caroli E, Acqui M, Roperto R, et al. Spinal en plaque meningiomas: a contemporary experience. Neurosurgery 2004;55(6):1275–9.

50. Roser F, Ebner FH, Ritz R, et al. Management of skull based meningiomas in the elderly patient. J Clin Neurosci 2007;14(3):224–8.

51. Cornu P, Chatellier G, Dagreou F, et al. Intracranial meningiomas in elderly patients. Postoperative morbidity and mortality. Factors predictive of outcome. Acta Neurochir (Wien) 1990;102(3–4):98–102.

52. Bateman BT, Pile-Spellman J, Gutin PH, et al. Meningioma resection in the elderly: nationwide inpatient sample, 1998-2002. Neurosurgery 2005;57(5): 866–72 [discussion: 866–72].

53. Moffat DA, Quaranta N, Baguley DM, et al. Management strategies in neurofibromatosis type 2. Eur Arch Otorhinolaryngol 2003;260(1):12–8.

54. Baser ME, Dg RE, Gutmann DH. Neurofibromatosis 2. Curr Opin Neurol 2003; 16(1):27–33.

55. Milker-Zabel S, Zabel A, Schulz-Ertner D, et al. Fractionated stereotactic radiotherapy in patients with benign or atypical intracranial meningioma: long-term experience and prognostic factors. Int J Radiat Oncol Biol Phys 2005;61(3): 809–16.

56. Chuang CC, Chang CN, Tsang NM, et al. Linear accelerator-based radiosurgery in the management of skull base meningiomas. J Neurooncol 2004;66(1–2): 241–9.

57. Iwai Y, Yamanaka K, Ishiguro T. Gamma knife radiosurgery for the treatment of cavernous sinus meningiomas. Neurosurgery 2003;52(3):517–24.

58. Kondziolka D, Lunsford LD, Coffey RJ, et al. Gamma knife radiosurgery of meningiomas. Stereotact Funct Neurosurg 1991;57(1–2):11–21.

59. Lunsford LD. Contemporary management of meningiomas: radiation therapy as an adjuvant and radiosurgery as an alternative to surgical removal? [editorial]. J Neurosurg 1994;80(2):187–90.

60. Ojemann SG, Sneed PK, Larson DA, et al. Radiosurgery for malignant meningioma: results in 22 patients. J Neurosurg 2000;93(Suppl 3):62–7.
61. Crocker D, Murtagh FR, Phuphanich S. Multiple malignant meningiomas following systemic chemotherapy for Hodgkin's lymphoma: a three-dimensional magnetic resonance imaging analysis [letter]. J Neuroimaging 1995;5(1):51–3.
62. Newton HB, Slivka MA, Stevens C. Hydroxyurea chemotherapy for unresectable or residual meningioma. J Neurooncol 2001;49(2):165–70.
63. Schrell UM, Rittig MG, Anders M, et al. Hydroxyurea for treatment of unresectable and recurrent meningiomas. II. Decrease in the size of meningiomas in patients treated with hydroxyurea [see comments]. J Neurosurg 1997;86(5):840–4.
64. Wen PY, Yung WK, Lamborn KR, et al. Phase II study of imatinib mesylate for recurrent meningiomas (North American Brain Tumor Consortium study 01-08). Neuro Oncol 2009;11(6):853–60.
65. Chamberlain MC, Glantz MJ, Fadul CE. Recurrent meningioma: salvage therapy with long-acting somatostatin analogue. Neurology 2007;69(10):969–73.
66. Chamberlain MC, Tsao-Wei DD, Groshen S. Temozolomide for treatment-resistant recurrent meningioma. Neurology 2004;62(7):1210–2.
67. Ragel BT, Gillespie DL, Kushnir V, et al. Calcium channel antagonists augment hydroxyurea- and ru486-induced inhibition of meningioma growth in vivo and in vitro. Neurosurgery 2006;59(5):1109–20 [discussion: 1120–1].
68. Puchner MJ, Hans VH, Harati A, et al. Bevacizumab-induced regression of anaplastic meningioma. Ann Oncol 2010;21(12):2445–6.
69. Kantar M, Cetingul N, Kansoy S, et al. Radiotherapy-induced secondary cranial neoplasms in children. Childs Nerv Syst 2004;20(1):46–9.
70. Mikulec AA, Kinsella LJ. Subacute brainstem necrosis: a complication of stereotactic radiotherapy for skull base meningioma. Otol Neurotol 2011;32(7):e50–1.
71. Norden AD, Drappatz J, Wen PY. Targeted drug therapy for meningiomas. Neurosurg Focus 2007;23(4):E12.
72. Ezzat S, Asa SL, Couldwell WT, et al. The prevalence of pituitary adenomas: a systematic review. Cancer 2004;101(3):613–9.
73. Daly AF, Rixhon M, Adam C, et al. High prevalence of pituitary adenomas: a cross-sectional study in the province of Liege, Belgium. J Clin Endocrinol Metab 2006;91(12):4769–75.
74. DeLellis RA, Lloyd RV, Heitz PU, et al. Tumours of endocrine organs. World Health Organization classification of tumours. Lyon (France): IARC; 2004.
75. Honegger J, Beschorner R, Ernemann U. Perisellar tumours including cysts, hamartomas, and vascular tumours. In: Wass JA, Stewart PM, editors. Oxford textbook of endocrinology and diabetes. Oxford (NY): Oxford University Press; 2011. p. 246–59.
76. Wass JA, Trainer PJ, Korbonits M. Acromegaly. In: Wass JA, Stewart PM, editors. Oxford textbook of endocrinology and diabetes. Oxford (NY): Oxford University Press; 2011. p. 197–209.
77. Yanovski JA, Cutler GB Jr. Glucocorticoid action and the clinical features of Cushing's syndrome. Endocrinol Metab Clin North Am 1994;23(3):487–509.
78. Arnaldi G, Angeli A, Atkinson AB, et al. Diagnosis and complications of Cushing's syndrome: a consensus statement. J Clin Endocrinol Metab 2003;88(12): 5593–602.
79. Knosp E, Steiner E, Kitz K, et al. Pituitary adenomas with invasion of the cavernous sinus space: a magnetic resonance imaging classification compared with surgical findings. Neurosurgery 1993;33(4):610–7 [discussion: 617–8].

80. Ikeda H, Yoshimoto T. Visual disturbances in patients with pituitary adenoma. Acta Neurol Scand 1995;92(2):157–60.
81. Honegger J, Ernemann U, Psaras T, et al. Objective criteria for successful transsphenoidal removal of suprasellar nonfunctioning pituitary adenomas. A prospective study. Acta Neurochir (Wien) 2007;149(1):21–9 [discussion: 29].
82. Hardy J. Transphenoidal microsurgery of the normal and pathological pituitary. Clin Neurosurg 1969;16:185–217.
83. Griffith HB, Veerapen R. A direct transnasal approach to the sphenoid sinus. Technical note. J Neurosurg 1987;66(1):140–2.
84. Jho HD, Carrau RL. Endoscopic endonasal transsphenoidal surgery: experience with 50 patients. J Neurosurg 1997;87(1):44–51.
85. Weiss MH. Transnasal transsphenoidal approach. In: Apuzzo ML, editor. Surgery of the third ventricle. Baltimore (MD): Williams & Wilkins; 1987. p. 476–94.
86. Mason RB, Nieman LK, Doppman JL, et al. Selective excision of adenomas originating in or extending into the pituitary stalk with preservation of pituitary function. J Neurosurg 1997;87(3):343–51.
87. Zhao B, Wei YK, Li GL, et al. Extended transsphenoidal approach for pituitary adenomas invading the anterior cranial base, cavernous sinus, and clivus: a single-center experience with 126 consecutive cases. J Neurosurg 2010;112(1):108–17.
88. Nimsky C, von Keller B, Ganslandt O, et al. Intraoperative high-field magnetic resonance imaging in transsphenoidal surgery of hormonally inactive pituitary macroadenomas. Neurosurgery 2006;59(1):105–14 [discussion: 105–14].
89. Ciric I, Ragin A, Baumgartner C, et al. Complications of transsphenoidal surgery: results of a national survey, review of the literature, and personal experience. Neurosurgery 1997;40(2):225–36 [discussion: 236–7].
90. Fatemi N, Dusick JR, Mattozo C, et al. Pituitary hormonal loss and recovery after transsphenoidal adenoma removal. Neurosurgery 2008;63(4):709–18 [discussion: 718–9].
91. O'Sullivan EP, Woods C, Glynn N, et al. The natural history of surgically treated but radiotherapy-naive nonfunctioning pituitary adenomas. Clin Endocrinol (Oxf) 2009;71(5):709–14.
92. Amar AP, Couldwell WT, Chen JC, et al. Predictive value of serum prolactin levels measured immediately after transsphenoidal surgery. J Neurosurg 2002;97(2):307–14.
93. Nomikos P, Buchfelder M, Fahlbusch R. The outcome of surgery in 668 patients with acromegaly using current criteria of biochemical 'cure'. Eur J Endocrinol 2005;152(3):379–87.
94. Hammer GD, Tyrrell JB, Lamborn KR, et al. Transsphenoidal microsurgery for Cushing's disease: initial outcome and long-term results. J Clin Endocrinol Metab 2004;89(12):6348–57.
95. Buchfelder M, Kreutzer J. Transcranial surgery for pituitary adenomas. Pituitary 2008;11(4):375–84.
96. Webster J, Piscitelli G, Polli A, et al. A comparison of cabergoline and bromocriptine in the treatment of hyperprolactinemic amenorrhea. Cabergoline Comparative Study Group. N Engl J Med 1994;331(14):904–9.
97. Kars M, Pereira AM, Smit JW, et al. Long-term outcome of patients with macroprolactinomas initially treated with dopamine agonists. Eur J Intern Med 2009;20(4):387–93.
98. Valassi E, Klibanski A, Biller BM. Clinical review: potential cardiac valve effects of dopamine agonists in hyperprolactinemia. J Clin Endocrinol Metab 2010;95(3):1025–33.

99. Dekkers OM, Lagro J, Burman P, et al. Recurrence of hyperprolactinemia after withdrawal of dopamine agonists: systematic review and meta-analysis. J Clin Endocrinol Metab 2010;95(1):43–51.
100. Freda PU, Katznelson L, van der Lely AJ, et al. Long-acting somatostatin analog therapy of acromegaly: a meta-analysis. J Clin Endocrinol Metab 2005;90(8):4465–73.
101. Brue T. ACROSTUDY: status update on 469 patients. Horm Res 2009;71(Suppl 1):34–8.
102. Biller BM, Grossman AB, Stewart PM, et al. Treatment of adrenocorticotropin-dependent Cushing's syndrome: a consensus statement. J Clin Endocrinol Metab 2008;93(7):2454–62.
103. Boscaro M, Ludlam WH, Atkinson B, et al. Treatment of pituitary-dependent Cushing's disease with the multireceptor ligand somatostatin analog pasireotide (SOM230): a multicenter, phase II trial. J Clin Endocrinol Metab 2009;94(1):115–22.
104. Raverot G, Sturm N, de Fraipont F, et al. Temozolomide treatment in aggressive pituitary tumors and pituitary carcinomas: a French multicenter experience. J Clin Endocrinol Metab 2010;95(10):4592–9.
105. Brada M, Rajan B, Traish D, et al. The long-term efficacy of conservative surgery and radiotherapy in the control of pituitary adenomas. Clin Endocrinol (Oxf) 1993;38(6):571–8.
106. Estrada J, Boronat M, Mielgo M, et al. The long-term outcome of pituitary irradiation after unsuccessful transsphenoidal surgery in Cushing's disease. N Engl J Med 1997;336(3):172–7.
107. Jenkins PJ, Bates P, Carson MN, et al. Conventional pituitary irradiation is effective in lowering serum growth hormone and insulin-like growth factor-I in patients with acromegaly. J Clin Endocrinol Metab 2006;91(4):1239–45.
108. Landolt AM, Haller D, Lomax N, et al. Stereotactic radiosurgery for recurrent surgically treated acromegaly: comparison with fractionated radiotherapy. J Neurosurg 1998;88(6):1002–8.
109. Sheehan JP, Niranjan A, Sheehan JM, et al. Stereotactic radiosurgery for pituitary adenomas: an intermediate review of its safety, efficacy, and role in the neurosurgical treatment armamentarium. J Neurosurg 2005;102(4):678–91.
110. Jagannathan J, Sheehan JP, Pouratian N, et al. Gamma Knife surgery for Cushing's disease. J Neurosurg 2007;106(6):980–7.
111. Pollock BE, Brown PD, Nippoldt TB, et al. Pituitary tumor type affects the chance of biochemical remission after radiosurgery of hormone-secreting pituitary adenomas. Neurosurgery 2008;62(6):1271–6 [discussion: 1276–8].
112. Antonescu CR, Woodruff JM. Primary tumors of cranial, spinal and peripheral nerve. In: McLendon RE, Rosenblum MK, Bigner DD, editors. Russell and Rubinstein's pathology of tumors of the nervous system. London: Oxford University Press; 2006. p. 787–836. Chapter 56.
113. Samii M, Migliori MM, Tatagiba M, et al. Surgical treatment of trigeminal schwannomas. J Neurosurg 1995;82(5):711–8.
114. Vogel H. Nervous system. New York: Cambridge University Press; 2009.
115. Pollack IF. Brain tumors in children. N Engl J Med 1994;331(22):1500–7.
116. Propp JM, McCarthy BJ, Davis FG, et al. Descriptive epidemiology of vestibular schwannomas. Neuro Oncol 2006;8(1):1–11.
117. Tos M, Charabi S, Thomsen J. Incidence of vestibular schwannomas. Laryngoscope 1999;109(5):736–40.
118. Matthies C, Samii M. Management of 1000 vestibular schwannomas (acoustic neuromas): clinical presentation. Neurosurgery 1997;40(1):1–9 [discussion: 9–10].

119. Evans DG, Moran A, King A, et al. Incidence of vestibular schwannoma and neurofibromatosis 2 in the North West of England over a 10-year period: higher incidence than previously thought. Otol Neurotol 2005;26(1):93–7.

120. Evans DG, Lye R, Neary W, et al. Probability of bilateral disease in people presenting with a unilateral vestibular schwannoma. J Neurol Neurosurg Psychiatry 1999;66(6):764–7.

121. Evans DG, Huson SM, Donnai D, et al. A clinical study of type 2 neurofibromatosis. Q J Med 1992;84(304):603–18.

122. Samii M, Matthies C, Tatagiba M. Management of vestibular schwannomas (acoustic neuromas): auditory and facial nerve function after resection of 120 vestibular schwannomas in patients with neurofibromatosis 2. Neurosurgery 1997;40(4):696–705 [discussion: 705–6].

123. Duvoisin B, Fernandes J, Doyon D, et al. Magnetic resonance findings in 92 acoustic neuromas. Eur J Radiol 1991;13(2):96–102.

124. Smouha EE, Yoo M, Mohr K, et al. Conservative management of acoustic neuroma: a meta-analysis and proposed treatment algorithm. Laryngoscope 2005;115(3):450–4.

125. Samii M, Matthies C. Management of 1000 vestibular schwannomas (acoustic neuromas): the facial nerve–preservation and restitution of function. Neurosurgery 1997;40(4):684–94 [discussion: 694–5].

126. Samii M, Matthies C. Management of 1000 vestibular schwannomas (acoustic neuromas): hearing function in 1000 tumor resections. Neurosurgery 1997; 40(2):248–60 [discussion: 260–2].

127. Matthies C, Samii M. Management of vestibular schwannomas (acoustic neuromas): the value of neurophysiology for evaluation and prediction of auditory function in 420 cases. Neurosurgery 1997;40(5):919–29 [discussion: 929–30].

128. Anderson DE, Leonetti J, Wind JJ, et al. Resection of large vestibular schwannomas: facial nerve preservation in the context of surgical approach and patient-assessed outcome. J Neurosurg 2005;102(4):643–9.

129. Darrouzet V, Martel J, Enee V, et al. Vestibular schwannoma surgery outcomes: our multidisciplinary experience in 400 cases over 17 years. Laryngoscope 2004;114(4):681–8.

130. Samii M, Matthies C. Management of 1000 vestibular schwannomas (acoustic neuromas): surgical management and results with an emphasis on complications and how to avoid them. Neurosurgery 1997;40(1):11–21 [discussion: 21–3].

131. Cerullo L, Grutsch J, Osterdock R. Recurrence of vestibular (acoustic) schwannomas in surgical patients where preservation of facial and cochlear nerve is the priority. Br J Neurosurg 1998;12(6):547–52.

132. Ohta S, Yokoyama T, Nishizawa S, et al. Regrowth of the residual tumour after acoustic neurinoma surgery. Br J Neurosurg 1998;12(5):419–22.

133. Hasegawa T, Fujitani S, Katsumata S, et al. Stereotactic radiosurgery for vestibular schwannomas: analysis of 317 patients followed more than 5 years. Neurosurgery 2005;57(2):257–65 [discussion: 257–65].

134. Lunsford LD, Niranjan A, Flickinger JC, et al. Radiosurgery of vestibular schwannomas: summary of experience in 829 cases. J Neurosurg 2005;102(Suppl): 195–9.

135. Paek SH, Chung HT, Jeong SS, et al. Hearing preservation after gamma knife stereotactic radiosurgery of vestibular schwannoma. Cancer 2005;104(3): 580–90.

136. Evans DG, Birch JM, Ramsden RT, et al. Malignant transformation and new primary tumours after therapeutic radiation for benign disease: substantial risks in certain tumour prone syndromes. J Med Genet 2006;43(4):289–94.
137. Mathieu D, Kondziolka D, Flickinger JC, et al. Stereotactic radiosurgery for vestibular schwannomas in patients with neurofibromatosis type 2: an analysis of tumor control, complications, and hearing preservation rates. Neurosurgery 2007;60(3):460–8 [discussion: 468–70].
138. Plotkin SR, Stemmer-Rachamimov AO, Barker FG 2nd, et al. Hearing improvement after bevacizumab in patients with neurofibromatosis type 2. N Engl J Med 2009;361(4):358–67.
139. Mautner VF, Nguyen R, Knecht R, et al. Radiographic regression of vestibular schwannomas induced by bevacizumab treatment: sustain under continuous drug application and rebound after drug discontinuation. Ann Oncol 2010; 21(11):2294–5.

Medulloblastoma/Primitive Neuroectodermal Tumor and Germ Cell Tumors

The Uncommon but Potentially Curable Primary Brain Tumors

Ayman Samkari, MD[a,b,c], Eugene Hwang, MD[a,b,c], Roger J. Packer, MD[a,c,d,e],*

KEYWORDS

- Medulloblastoma • Primitive neuroectodermal tumor • Pineoblastoma
- Germ cell tumor

KEY POINTS

- Brain tumors are the most common solid tumors during childhood. Treatment of central nervous system (CNS) germ cell tumors and embryonal brain tumors is complex; however, survival rates have improved.
- Medulloblastoma is the most common malignant brain tumor in children. Neither clinical stratification nor pathologic classification has been fully adequate in predicting outcomes. The presence of certain molecular markers has been shown to impact survival. Molecular stratification will guide future therapeutic approaches.
- CNS primitive neuroectodermal tumors (PNETs) have worse outcomes when compared with medulloblastoma. Supratentorial PNETs are characterized by multiple genetic alterations, which are different from pineoblastomas and medulloblastomas.
- There is no standard therapy for relapsed CNS PNETs and medulloblastoma.
- CNS germ cell tumors are classified into pure germinomas and nongerminomatous germ cell tumors. The treatment approach is dependent on the subtype, but usually combines radiotherapy and chemotherapy.

The authors have nothing to disclose.
[a] The Brain Tumor Institute, Division of Neurology, Children's National Medical Center, 111 Michigan Avenue, Washington, DC 20010, USA; [b] Division of Hematology and Oncology, Center for Cancer and Blood Disorders, Children's National Medical Center, 111 Michigan Avenue Northwest, Washington, DC 20010, USA; [c] School of Medicine and Health Sciences, The George Washington University, Washington, 2300 Eye Street, NW Washington, DC 20037, USA; [d] Center for Neuroscience and Behavioral Medicine, Division of Neurology, Children's National Medical Center, 111 Michigan Avenue Northwest, Washington, DC 20010, USA; [e] Division of Neurology, Children's National Medical Center, 111 Michigan Avenue, Washington, DC 20010, USA
* Corresponding author. Center for Neuroscience and Behavioral Medicine, Division of Neurology, Children's National Medical Center, 111 Michigan Avenue Northwest, Washington, DC 20010.
E-mail address: rpacker@childrensnational.org

Hematol Oncol Clin N Am 26 (2012) 881–895
doi:10.1016/j.hoc.2012.04.002
0889-8588/12/$ – see front matter © 2012 Elsevier Inc. All rights reserved.

INTRODUCTION

Brain tumors are the most common solid tumors and the second most common malignancy during childhood. The overall annual incidence in the United States is estimated to be 33 per million children younger than 14 years. Major advances in neurosurgery, chemotherapy, and radiation techniques have led to a decline in mortality rate in the last 2 decades.[1,2]

Treatment of brain tumors including central nervous system (CNS) germ cell tumors and embryonal brain tumors is complex, and although survival rates have improved for some subtypes of these lesions,[1] the treatment-related morbidity remains high.[3,4] Novel diagnostic and treatment strategies are essential to selectively target these tumors without affecting the normal tissue. The evolution of and current approaches in both diagnosis and treatment of germ cell and medulloblastoma/primitive neuroectodermal tumors (PNETs) in children are reviewed in this article.

MEDULLOBLASTOMA

Medulloblastoma is a malignant embryonal (World Health Organization [WHO] grade IV) tumor that affects the cerebellum, comprises approximately 17% of all pediatric brain tumors, and is the most common malignant brain tumor in children. Studies have shown a bimodal peak distribution with maximum incidence between age 3 to 5 and 8 to 9 years.[5] The etiology of some medulloblastomas has been linked to certain genetic disorders, including Gorlin syndrome (patched homolog 1 [PTCH1] mutation)[6] and Turcot syndrome (adenomatous polyposis coli [APC] mutation).[7] Overall survival for children with average-risk disease (to be defined later in this article) now exceeds 80%, but remains lower in infants and for those with high-risk disease. In addition, treatment-related long-term side effects are considerable; examples include neurocognitive impairment; endocrine abnormalities; hearing loss; and secondary malignancy.[8,9] Evolution of treatment approaches seeks to improve survival rates while decreasing toxicity through developing targeted molecular therapy, as well as improving radiation techniques and reduction of radiotherapy doses.

Histologic Features of Medulloblastoma

Histopathologically, classical medulloblastoma consists of densely packed cells with immunopositivity for neuronal markers such as synaptophysin and neuron-specific enolase. Glial differentiation denoted by immunopositivity to glial fibrillary acidic protein may occur. Other histologic subtypes include: (1) desmoplastic/nodular medulloblastoma characterized by nodular reticulin-free zones surrounded by densely packed cells, this type being more common in infants and adults[10]; (2) medulloblastoma with extensive nodularity, similar to the desmoplastic variant but with more expanded lobular architecture; (3) anaplastic medulloblastoma characterized by high mitotic activity with marked nuclear pleomorphisim and atypical forms; and (4) large-cell medulloblastoma characterized by a monomorphic large round cell with variable amounts of eosinophilic cytoplasm. Any of these types can present histologically with myogenic differentiation (medullomyoblastoma) or melanotic differentiation (melanocytic medulloblastoma).[11,12]

Risk Stratification of Medulloblastoma

Current clinical and radiographic disease stratification uses patient age, extent of tumor resection, pathologic subtype, and metastatic (M) status.[13] Previous studies showed that children younger than 3 years had inferior 5-year progression-free survival (PFS) when compared with children 3 years or older (32% vs 58%, respectively).[14] The extent of surgical excision was found in early series to be a statistically significant prognostic factor, as M0 patients in whom less than 1.5 cm^2 residual tumor was evident experienced a better 5-year PFS when compared with those with residual tumor of 1.5 cm^2 or greater (78% vs 54%)[14]; more recent studies have questioned the significance of the relatively arbitrary 1.5 cm^2 criteria. Infants with desmoplastic medulloblastomas had better outcomes than infants with classic medulloblastomas, with reported 3-year event-free survival (EFS) of 73%,[15] and tumors with diffuse anaplasia have been associated with a poorer prognosis than classic tumors.[14] Patients are considered high risk if they have more than 1.5 cm^2 of residual tumor postresection, have large-cell or anaplastic histology, and/or have evidence of metastatic disease,[16,17] as shown in **Table 1**.

Neither the clinical stratification nor the pathologic classification has been fully adequate in predicting outcomes. Subsets of children with average-risk medulloblastoma may still do very poorly, with resistance to treatment, early relapse, and dissemination.

Molecular Stratification

The presence of certain molecular markers has been shown to affect survival. Studies showed that nuclear immunoreactivity for β-catenin, CTNNB1 mutation, overexpression of neurotrophin-3 receptor (TRKC3), and monosomy 6 were associated with improved survival, whereas ERBB2 expression and MYCC or OTX2 amplification were associated with poorer outcomes.[18–20] However, the clinical utility of some of these markers remains limited given conflicting conclusions in reports.[21] Recently, multiple molecular pathways have been implicated in the pathogenesis of medulloblastoma. For example, in some tumors the sonic hedgehog (Shh) pathway is activated and mediates tumorigenesis via the activation of glioma-associated homolog 1 (Gli1); this activation may be through modification of any component of the Shh pathway, including elements such as patched, suppressor of fused (SUFU), and smoothened (SMO) proteins.[22] Gli1 is a transcription factor that promotes proliferation through activation of various oncogenes including cyclinD1 and cyclinD2.[23] In other medulloblastomas, the wingless type (Wnt) pathway seems to mediate activation of several oncogenes that promote tumorigenesis and inhibit apoptosis such as MYC, cyclinD1, and RE1-silencing transcription factor (REST).[23] Using high-density microarrays, recent analysis led to the discovery of other genes altered in 16% of children with medulloblastoma, including histone-lysine N-methyl transferase genes (MLL2 or MLL3).[24]

Multiple independent groups have further used gene and mRNA profiling to discover the presence of at least 4 molecular subtypes of medulloblastoma. The subtypes include tumors associated with: (1) Wnt pathway activation; (2) Shh pathway activation; (3) c-MYC activation (labeled group C); and (4) high levels of the orthodenticle homeobox 2 (OTX2) and forkhead box protein G1b (FOXG1B), but lacking high expression of MYC (group D). These groups seem to predict outcome more accurately than historical staging criteria.[23,25] In one study, when outcomes for children with metastatic disease were controlled for molecular tumor subtype, overall survival was similar in those with or without metastatic disease.[26] The Wnt pathway subtype

Table 1 Medulloblastoma risk stratification		
	Average-Risk Disease	**High-Risk Disease**
Extent of resection	Near total and total	Biopsy and subtotal
M status	M0	M1–M4
Histology	Classic/desmoplastic	Anaplastic/large cell

is associated with excellent prognosis,[10,18,27] and to a lesser extent so are tumors with Shh activation.[10,27] Group C tumors (c-MYC amplified) have poor outcomes.[10] Group D patients have increased heterogeneity in their outcomes, implying that additional factors are needed to differentiate this group. Reports have demonstrated that immunopositivity for follistatin-like 5 (FSTL5) identified a cohort of patients at high risk for relapse and death. As greater than 50% of non-Wnt/non-Shh tumors displayed FSTL5 negativity, some group D tumors may potentially carry a better prognosis.[28]

Treatment of Medulloblastoma

The treatment of medulloblastoma is complex and usually involves a combination of surgery, radiation therapy, and chemotherapy.[16] The role of surgery was recognized in the early 1900s by Harvey Cushing,[17,29] and studies subsequently demonstrated that residual tumor bulk is one of the most important predictors for PFS in medulloblastoma.[14] Surgery can be complicated in up to 20% of posterior fossa tumors by cerebellar mutism or posterior fossa syndrome, which typically arises hours to 1 to 2 days after resection. This condition is characterized by speech impairment progressing to significant mutism, hypotonia, ataxia, and emotional lability.[30] It is thought to be due to an injury in the dentate nuclei and their efferent pathways.[31] However, Cushing recognized that tumor resection alone was inadequate, as most of his surgically treated patients suffered relapse. Focal radiotherapy was thus used as adjuvant therapy, and evolved to encompass the posterior fossa. After poor survival rates were noted with focal radiotherapy alone, craniospinal irradiation (CSI) was used with resultant improved survival. Current standard radiotherapy is, therefore, CSI with a focal boost to the posterior fossa and other areas of disease.[32] Standard doses were historically 36 Gy of CSI for both average-risk and high-risk patients, with a focal boost to 54 Gy.

Radiation to the developing brain is fraught with complications, including vasculopathy with the risk of stroke and endocrine complications.[4] Neurocognitive sequelae have been among the most troubling, with full-scale intelligence quotient (IQ) declines of 2 to 9 points per year after irradiation, and greater IQ deficits associated with younger age or higher doses at radiotherapy[33]; thus, attempts have been made to reduce the dose of radiotherapy. Such attempts were more successful with the addition of chemotherapy, which was able to augment radiotherapy and improve outcomes.[34]

Average-Risk Medulloblastoma

Children with average-risk medulloblastoma have postsurgical residual tumor equal to or less than 1.5 cm^2 on magnetic resonance imaging (MRI), no evidence of disseminated disease in the preoperative or postoperative MRI, postoperative lumbar cerebrospinal fluid that displays no tumor cells (M0), and nonanaplastic/large-cell histopathology. Because of the relatively good survival but substantial adverse events with standard treatment strategies, multiple trials have examined dose reductions of CSI to 23.40 Gy without adjuvant chemotherapy.[35–37] These studies showed a potentially lesser negative impact on neurocognition with less significant IQ point decreases of 10 to 15 points, but with higher relapse rates (5-year PFS was 67% in the full-dose CSI arm and 52% in the reduced-dose CSI arm).[25,38] By contrast, when adjuvant chemotherapy (lomustine [CCNU], vincristine, and cisplatin) was added during and after radiotherapy, survival rates compared favorably with those obtained in studies using full-dose radiation therapy alone (5-year PFS 79%).[39] Subsequent studies prospectively compared 2 adjuvant chemotherapy regimens: CCNU, cisplatin, and vincristine or cyclophosphamide, cisplatin, and vincristine; this study showed no difference in the 5-year EFS between the treatment groups (81% and 86%, respectively).[40] A separate, smaller trial using 23.4 Gy CSI followed by 4 cycles of high-dose chemotherapy (vincristine, cyclophosphamide, and cisplatin) with stem cell support showed a 5-year EFS of 83%.[41] The use of intensive preirradiation chemotherapy (ifosfamide, etoposide, intravenous high-dose methotrexate, cisplatin, and cytarabine) resulted in a poorer 3-year EFS and worsened myelotoxicity when compared with immediate radiotherapy (35 Gy) with concomitant vincristine followed by cisplatin, CCNU, and vincristine (65% vs 78%, respectively).[42] Hence, chemotherapy is typically given after radiotherapy.

The feasibility of further dose reduction of radiotherapy to 18 Gy for patients between 3 and 7 years is currently being investigated, as is a reduction in the field of the boost based on number of pilot studies.[43] Further modification of chemotherapy, such as dose reduction of cisplatin to minimize ototoxicity, is also being explored.

High-Risk Medulloblastoma

Despite treatment with higher doses of CSI and chemotherapy, children with high-risk medulloblastoma continue to have poor outcomes (5-year EFS 50%–60%).[44] Thus no dose reduction in CSI has been implemented in these patients. The role of chemotherapy in this disease has been investigated in multiple clinical trials. When adjuvant chemotherapy (consisting of CCNU, vincristine, and prednisone) was used after radiotherapy, the estimated 5-year EFS was 59% compared with 50% for patients treated with radiotherapy alone. However, when only including patients with more extensive disease, the group that received adjuvant chemotherapy showed significantly better EFS when compared with similar patients treated with radiotherapy alone (48% vs 0%). Preirradiation chemotherapy (cisplatin and etoposide) followed by adjuvant chemotherapy (cyclophosphamide and etoposide) showed no impact on 5-year PFS and overall survival (OS) when compared with radiotherapy after surgical resection, followed by chemotherapy (cisplatin, etoposide, cyclophosphamide, and vincristine).[45] Other approaches such as a dose-intensive, alkylator-based regimen of chemotherapy (4 cycles of cyclophosphamide, cisplatin, and vincristine) with stem cell support have been used after maximum resection and radiotherapy, resulting in a similarly improved outcome (5-year EFS 70%) but with substantial reduction in the duration of treatment (4 months vs 12 months).[41] The Children's Oncology Group (COG) is currently investigating the efficacy of carboplatin administered concomitantly with radiation and isotretinoin as a proapoptotic agent administered with 6 cycles of adjuvant chemotherapy.

Medulloblastoma in Young Children

Patients younger than 3 years generally have a poor prognosis with an estimated 5-year PFS of 30% to 40%, attributable to an increased incidence of neuraxis dissemination, inability or physician/patient reluctance to administer full-dose radiotherapy, and the possible presence of different genetic alterations. One notable exception is the relatively good outcome of patients with medulloblastoma with desmoplastic histology, which can be treated with chemotherapy alone with a 5-year PFS of 65% to 85%.[13,46] Given the risks of radiotherapy-induced severe neurocognitive sequelae in very young children,[33] the overall strategy has been to use chemotherapy in an attempt to delay or avoid irradiation. One trial that attempted to delay radiotherapy by 1 to 2 years using intensive chemotherapy consisting of vincristine, cyclophosphamide, etoposide, and cisplatin resulted in early failure (most failures occurred during the first 6 months of chemotherapy) and poor 5-year EFS and OS (32% and 40%, respectively). In this study, infants without metastatic disease who also had a gross total resection had slightly better outcome, with 5-year OS of 69%. Other chemotherapy regimens that have been attempted include combinations variably including procarbazine, ifosfamide, intravenous/intrathecal methotrexate, cisplatin, cytarabine, and vincristine. These regimens were associated with relatively poor 5-year OS (35%).[47] A study comparing an induction regimen based on cyclophosphamide and cisplatin with one based on ifosfamide and carboplatin, followed by maintenance chemotherapy, showed no difference between the 2 treatment arms, with 5-year EFS of 32% in both arms.[48] A similarly poor 3-year EFS of 40% resulted after induction chemotherapy based on cisplatin and high-dose methotrexate, followed by consolidation with high-dose chemotherapy and stem cell rescue. Radiation in this study was given at a dose of 23.4 Gy for patients with evidence of residual disease at the end of induction chemotherapy.[49,50] The COG recently completed a pilot trial in which 3 courses of standard chemotherapy followed by 3 courses of high-dose chemotherapy with stem cell rescue preliminarily showed slightly superior outcomes, with a 3-year EFS of 67% in M0 patients.[51]

There is no consensus regarding the use of radiation therapy in children younger than 3 years, and despite the use of varying intensive chemotherapy regimens,[52] CSI could only be delayed by 1 year in up to 34% of patients because of early recurrence or progressive disease.[53]

Recurrent Medulloblastoma

Recurrent and progressive medulloblastomas have very poor prognoses, with postrecurrence 2-year OS of approximately 25%[54] despite aggressive treatment regimens. Only anecdotal reports have described prolonged survival after relapse.[55] It has been suggested that early identification of recurrence is associated with a longer survival. Current suggested approaches include the use of reirradiation, which has some limited data on its efficacy, especially in patients without gross disease, with 48% 5-year EFS.[54] A metronomic combination of oral etoposide, cyclophosphamide, thalidomide, celecoxib, and fenofibrate, augmented with alternating courses of intrathecal etoposide and liposomal cytarabine in combination with biweekly intravenous bevacizumab, was also explored in a study that included 6 patients with recurrent medulloblastoma, with resulting 2-year OS of 80% and PFS of 53%.[56]

For younger patients with metastatic or recurrent disease, the use of radiotherapy is usually based on physician's discretion and family wishes, but may have some utility in salvaging patients.

Future Directions

Future approaches for the treatment of medulloblastoma will likely be based on an increased understanding of the molecular features of individual tumors and the development of specific, patient-tailored, molecularly targeted therapies. Using this improved knowledge of underlying molecular characteristics, risk stratification may be more accurately assigned to particular patients, resulting in more appropriate treatment regimen applications and decreased toxicity. Such treatment is already undergoing investigation, using therapeutics targeting the Shh with SMO small-molecule antagonist (GDC-0449).[57] Antiangiogenic therapies such as bevacizumab, inhibitor of poly(ADP-ribose) polymerase (PARP), and anti–insulin-like growth factor I receptor monoclonal antibody (IMC-A12) in combination with an mTOR inhibitor (temsirolimus) are also being examined in different pediatric CNS tumors including medulloblastoma.

Other studies are currently examining the feasibility of adding the histone deacetylase inhibitor, suberoylanilide hydroxamic acid (SAHA), and isotretinoin to standard induction-chemotherapy drugs. This approach is based on preclinical studies suggesting that isotretinoin induces apoptosis through promoting BMP-2 transcription[58] and clinical studies suggesting isotretinoin synergy with cisplatin.[59,60] SAHA has also been shown to induce apoptosis in medulloblastoma cell lines.[60]

[Tags: Medulloblastoma, Average-risk medulloblastoma, High-risk medulloblastoma, Wnt pathway, Shh pathway, Recurrent medulloblastoma, Medulloblastoma at young age, Molecular stratification of medulloblastoma, Clinical stratification of medulloblastoma, Radiotherapy dose reduction in medulloblastoma].

CENTRAL NERVOUS SYSTEM PRIMITIVE NEUROECTODERMAL TUMOR

CNS PNET tumors are a heterogeneous group of embryonic malignant tumors (WHO grade IV), comprising approximately 4% of all pediatric brain tumors.[5] Despite histopathologic similarity to medulloblastoma, CNS PNETs have worse outcomes, with 5-year PFS ranging between 31% and 47%.[61] The current WHO classification includes related tumors in the brainstem and spinal cord in this category. CNS PNETs includes supratentorial PNET, cerebral neuroblastoma, CNS ganglioneuroblastoma, medulloepithelioma, and ependymoblastoma. Pineoblastoma is currently categorized with pineal region tumors in the most recent WHO classification, but has similarities with CNS PNETs.[11]

Histopathology of CNS PNET

CNS PNETs are composed of poorly differentiated neuroepithelial cells that express neuronal markers such as synaptophysin. Each subtype of CNS PNET has specific characteristics. For example, cerebral neuroblastoma displays features of neuronal differentiation, ganglioneuroblastoma contains neoplastic ganglion cells, medulloepithelioma retains the embryonal neural tube formation, and ependymoblastoma displays features of ependymoblastic rosettes.[11]

Prognostic Indicators and Tumor Biology of CNS PNET

Although PNETs are histologically very similar to medulloblastomas, they are less curable.[62] Different molecular and genetic alterations distinguishing the two groups of tumors could explain the difference in treatment response and outcome.[61,63] Poor prognostic indicators include young age and disseminated disease.[62,64,65] Young children with tumors in the pineal location tend to do worse than those with tumors in a nonpineal location; this trend is reversed in older children.[66]

Supratentorial PNETs are characterized by multiple genetic alterations, in contrast to pineoblastomas, which have relatively few alterations.[67] The most common abnormalities in supratentorial PNETs are gains of 1q, 2p, and 19p[67] and losses of 3p21, 3q26, and 8p23.[68] There are no consistent cytogenetic changes in pineoblastomas, although some of the genetic alterations that have been found are loss of chromosome 22, and gain of 1q12, 5p13, 5q21, 6p12, and 14q21.[69] Genetic predisposition to pineoblastoma has been reported in familial bilateral retinoblastoma.

Treatment of CNS PNET

Despite increasingly evident molecular differences, PNETs are treated similarly to high-risk medulloblastoma in most current regimens. Surgical resection can be especially difficult in hypothalamic and brainstem midline tumors owing to the potential surgical complications, such as visual injury. There is conflicting evidence concerning the impact of the extent of resection on outcome, as some studies failed to demonstrate a statistically significant difference in outcome in patients with total tumor resection.[66] The role of radiotherapy and chemotherapy has also been investigated. In one retrospective clinical analysis of PNET patients treated over a period of 10 years in

Canada, survival was improved in the group treated with radiotherapy, chemotherapy, or both versus only surgical resection (4-year OS was 48%, 48%, 42%, and 8%–14%, respectively).[70] As in medulloblastoma, attempts have been made to decrease CSI with use of high-dose, cyclophosphamide-based chemotherapy with stem cell support; this strategy enabled radiotherapy dose reduction to 23.4 Gy for patients with average-risk disease without compromising survival.[61] Other trials incorporating high-dose chemotherapy with stem cell rescue have showed potential improvement in outcome; although patient numbers were small; one study using this strategy demonstrated a 5-year EFS of 68% in 16 patients.[61]

Children younger than 3 years have extremely poor outcomes. For example, the 5-year EFS for infants treated with chemotherapy alone was approximately 14%.[71] Reported outcomes moderately improved after introducing treatment with high-dose chemotherapy and stem cell support, as 5 year EFS approaching 39% has been reported.[72] Focal radiation of up to 50.4 Gy is being used in superficial cortical PNET, seeking to decrease the risk of local recurrence. However, patients with PNET had very poor responses in one study that used dual stem cell–supported treatment, second-look surgery, and involved-field irradiation.[73] Another treatment strategy that has shown some benefit in PNET disease control is metronomic maintenance chemotherapy, especially in patients with metastatic disease who have not received CSI.[74]

There is no standard therapy for relapsed CNS PNETs. One recent review proposed some benefit of high-dose chemotherapy with hematopoietic stem cell rescue in non-pineal locations, although this remains controversial.[75]

[Tags: CNS PNET, Pineoblastoma, Treatment of CNS PNET, Molecular characteristic of PNET, Chemotherapy for PNET, Radiotherapy for PNET, Recurrent CNS PNET].

GERM CELL TUMORS

Germ cell tumors of the CNS are rare tumors, accounting for 3% of all pediatric brain tumors.[5,76] CNS germ cell tumors are classified into pure germinomas (GER) and non-germinomatous germ cell tumors (NGGCT).[11] GERs primarily affect the pineal region, suprasellar region, basal ganglia, or thalamus region, and can also present with synchronous lesions in the pineal and suprasellar regions. GERs arise most often in adolescents and usually have a favorable prognosis.[77] NGGCTs make up approximately 40% of the intracranial germ cell tumors and exhibit poorer outcomes.[78,79] The distinction between NGGCT and GER is critical and may not always be easy, because of the location of these tumors. Patient presentation depends on tumor location; suprasellar lesions present with symptoms of visual field defects, endocrine dysfunction, and precocious or delayed puberty. Tumors of pineal location often manifest with Parinaud syndrome, which characterized by paralysis of upward gaze, pseudo–Argyll Robertson pupils, convergence-retraction nystagmus, and eyelid retraction.[80]

Tumor markers such as α-fetoprotein (AFP) and β–human chorionic gonadotropin (β-HCG) are helpful in establishing the diagnosis. Elevated AFP in either the blood or cerebrospinal fluid is usually sufficient to classify a tumor as an NGGCT, although tumor tissue is useful for prognostic classification and biological studies when surgically feasible. By contrast, patients with normal AFP and mildly elevated β-HCG levels (not exceeding 50 IU/dL) are more difficult to classify, and a biopsy may be needed to distinguish a β-HCG–secreting GER from an immature teratoma or a choriocarcinoma. In the absence of an elevation of these markers, tissue diagnosis is required.

Histopathology of Germ Cell Tumors

The precise histologic identification and classification of germ cell tumors is important in the guidance of efficacious therapy.[81] Germ cell tumors are often mixed, but include the following. (1) GERs, which consist of cells with undifferentiated primordial germinal elements and usually positively stain with c-kit (CD117) and octamer-binding transcription factor4 (OCT4) antibodies, with cytoplasmic and membranous reactivity to placental alkaline phosphatase (PLAP). Occasionally they contain granulomatous or dense lymphocytic infiltrates, and may be confused with other processes such as sarcoidosis. Also, a minority of cases contains syncytiotrophoblasts, which are capable of secreting β-HCG. (2) Teratomas, which differentiate along ectodermal, endodermal, and mesodermal cell lines and can be mature or immature. (3) Yolk sac tumors, which contain primitive-appearing epithelial cells that are immunereactive to AFP. (4) Embryonal carcinomas, which are composed of large cells that proliferate in nests and sheets forming papillae and glandular structures, and do not express c-kit but do express CD30 and OCT4. (5) Choriocarcinomas, which are characterized by the presence of syncytiotrophoblastic and cytotrophoblastic components, and are immune-reactive to both HCG and human placental lactogen.[12]

Prognostic Indicators and Tumor Biology of CNS Germ Cell Tumors

The combination of surgery, chemotherapy, and radiation therapy have dramatically improved outcomes in the last decade, with 5-year OS approaching 90% for GER and 50% to 70% for NGGCT.[82] Although the biology of these tumors is underinvestigated, studies showed that 12p gain is frequently present in CNS germ cell tumors.[83–85] Expression of Nestin, which is an intermediate filament protein expressed in undifferentiated cells during CNS development, has been also shown to be potentially useful in predicting the risk of dissemination and/or progression of CNS germ cell tumors.[86]

Treatment of CNS Germ Cell Tumors

The treatment approach for CNS germ cell tumors is dependent on the subtype. There is a lack of consensus regarding the degree of surgical resection required; a gross total resection of localized GERs is generally not recommended because of the previously noted morbidity of surgical removal and the good response to radiation therapy.[87] The benefit of gross total resection of localized NGGCTs has not been established.[87,88] Surgery is often required in patients with NGGCT whose disease enlarges and becomes more prominent after chemotherapy (growing teratoma syndrome).

Historically, radiation therapy has been the treatment of choice for pure GERs. A dose of 25 to 36 Gy of CSI with boost to the primary tumor site (45–52 Gy) has been associated with excellent 5-year OS (92%–97%) and EFS (88%–100%), although it may be also associated with significant neurocognitive deficits. Trials using only chemotherapy have had unacceptable recurrence/progression rates (49%), although many patients relapsing on these chemotherapy-only trials were ultimately salvageable with radiation therapy.[89] In an attempt to decrease the radiation field, focal radiotherapy was studied but resulted in a higher rate of ventricular (but not spinal) relapses,[90] indicating a propensity for metastatic disease to the ventricles in the absence of adequate prophylaxis. Recent trials have used chemotherapy comprising carboplatin, etoposide, cyclophosphamide, and cisplatin followed by reduced-dose ventricular-field irradiation (22.5–24 Gy) with a boost to the primary tumor site (21–30 Gy) for nondisseminated disease. This approach has resulted in apparent improved neurocognitive, social, and emotional functioning of patients, without compromising treatment efficacy or changing the relapse pattern.[91–93]

Although radiation therapy has been shown to be effective in improving patient survival in NGGCT, the extent and the optimum dose of radiation required for disease control remains unknown, especially for patients with localized disease. Multiple groups have used focal radiation, which resulted in high recurrence rates.[94]

Researchers in Japan used focal radiation for intermediate-risk germ cell tumors that included mixed germ cell tumors, demonstrating 2.6-year EFS of 76%.[95] By contrast, a German group found that CSI is one of the major factors that improves survival.[96] The most recent completed COG study used 36 Gy CSI based on the aforementioned experiences, although lower volumes and doses of radiotherapy are being considered in future trials.[94] Because of the relatively poorer prognosis of NGGCT, chemotherapy (platinum-based) has been used and has showed significant improvement in survival.[94,97] Intensive chemotherapy without irradiation has not been shown to be particularly effective, so the combination of chemotherapy and radiation therapy remains the treatment of choice for patients with NGGCT.

High-dose chemotherapy with stem cell support has been used for recurrent CNS germ cell tumors displaying somewhat improved outcomes. High-dose chemotherapy regimens include thiotepa/etoposide, busulfan/thiotepa, and melphalan/cyclophosphamide, among others. The role of reirradiation is as yet unproven.[98]

[Tags: Germ cell tumor, Pure germinomas (GER), Nongerminomatous germ cell tumors (NGGCT), α-Fetoprotein, β-HCG, Treatment of CNS germ cell tumors, Radiotherapy for germ cell tumors, Whole ventricular radiotherapy, Molecular characteristic of CNS germ cell tumors].

SUMMARY

Medulloblastoma, CNS PNET, and germ cell tumors are highly malignant tumors that are often difficult to treat. Therapy is usually complex and comprises a combination of surgery, radiotherapy, and chemotherapy; long-term effects such as neurocognitive sequelae are still significant. However, major advances in the understanding of the biology of these tumors have resulted in improvement in survival rates and some amelioration of long-term adverse effects. Current and future clinical trials will place greater emphasis on validating the clinical utility of molecular and genetic factors.

REFERENCES

1. Bishop AJ, McDonald MW, Chang AL, et al. Infant brain tumors: incidence, survival, and the role of radiation based on Surveillance, Epidemiology, and End Results (SEER) Data. Int J Radiat Oncol Biol Phys 2012;82(1):341–7.
2. Pollack IF, Jakacki RI. Childhood brain tumors: epidemiology, current management and future directions. Nat Rev Neurol 2011;7(9):495–506.
3. Edelstein K, Spiegler BJ, Fung S, et al. Early aging in adult survivors of childhood medulloblastoma: long-term neurocognitive, functional, and physical outcomes. Neuro Oncol 2011;13:536.
4. Frange P, Alapetite C, Gaboriaud G, et al. From childhood to adulthood: long-term outcome of medulloblastoma patients. The Institut Curie experience (1980-2000). J Neurooncol 2009;95:271.
5. Rickert CH, Paulus W. Epidemiology of central nervous system tumors in childhood and adolescence based on the new WHO classification. Childs Nerv Syst 2001;17:503.
6. Lo Muzio L. Nevoid basal cell carcinoma syndrome (Gorlin syndrome). Orphanet J Rare Dis 2008;3:32.
7. Yong WH, Raffel C, von Deimling A, et al. The APC gene in Turcot's syndrome. N Engl J Med 1995;333:524.
8. Duffner PK, Krischer JP, Horowitz ME, et al. Second malignancies in young children with primary brain tumors following treatment with prolonged postoperative

chemotherapy and delayed irradiation: a Pediatric Oncology Group study. Ann Neurol 1998;44:313.

9. Ellenberg L, Liu Q, Gioia G, et al. Neurocognitive status in long-term survivors of childhood CNS malignancies: a report from the Childhood Cancer Survivor Study. Neuropsychology 2009;23:705.

10. Ellison DW, Dalton J, Kocak M, et al. Medulloblastoma: clinicopathological correlates of SHH, WNT, and non-SHH/WNT molecular subgroups. Acta Neuropathol 2011;121:381.

11. Louis DN, Ohgaki H, Wiestler OD, et al, editors. WHO classification of tumors of the central nervous system. 3rd edition. WHO publications Center; 2007. p. 309.

12. Nakazato Y. Revised WHO classification of brain tumours. Brain Nerve 2008;60:59 [in Japanese].

13. Rutkowski S, von Hoff K, Emser A, et al. Survival and prognostic factors of early childhood medulloblastoma: an international meta-analysis. J Clin Oncol 2010;28:4961.

14. Zeltzer PM, Boyett JM, Finlay JL, et al. Metastasis stage, adjuvant treatment, and residual tumor are prognostic factors for medulloblastoma in children: conclusions from the Children's Cancer Group 921 randomized phase III study. J Clin Oncol 1999;17:832.

15. Giangaspero F, Perilongo G, Fondelli MP, et al. Medulloblastoma with extensive nodularity: a variant with favorable prognosis. J Neurosurg 1999;91:971.

16. Dhall G. Medulloblastoma. J Child Neurol 2009;24:1418.

17. Sutton LN, Phillips PC, Molloy PT. Surgical management of medulloblastoma. J Neurooncol 1996;29:9.

18. Ellison DW, Kocak M, Dalton J, et al. Definition of disease-risk stratification groups in childhood medulloblastoma using combined clinical, pathologic, and molecular variables. J Clin Oncol 2011;29:1400.

19. Kim JY, Sutton ME, Lu DJ, et al. Activation of neurotrophin-3 receptor TrkC induces apoptosis in medulloblastomas. Cancer Res 1999;59:711.

20. Pfister S, Remke M, Benner A, et al. Outcome prediction in pediatric medulloblastoma based on DNA copy-number aberrations of chromosomes 6q and 17q and the MYC and MYCN loci. J Clin Oncol 2009;27:1627.

21. Gajjar A, Hernan R, Kocak M, et al. Clinical, histopathologic, and molecular markers of prognosis: toward a new disease risk stratification system for medulloblastoma. J Clin Oncol 2004;22:984.

22. Dubuc AM, Northcott PA, Mack S, et al. The genetics of pediatric brain tumors. Curr Neurol Neurosci Rep 2010;10:215.

23. Monje M, Beachy PA, Fisher PG. Hedgehogs, flies, Wnts and MYCs: the time has come for many things in medulloblastoma. J Clin Oncol 2011;29:1395.

24. Parsons DW, Li M, Zhang X, et al. The genetic landscape of the childhood cancer medulloblastoma. Science 2011;331:435.

25. Tamayo P, Cho YJ, Tsherniak A, et al. Predicting relapse in patients with medulloblastoma by integrating evidence from clinical and genomic features. J Clin Oncol 2011;29:1415.

26. Northcott PA, Korshunov A, Witt H, et al. Medulloblastoma comprises four distinct molecular variants. J Clin Oncol 2011;29:1408.

27. Gessi M, von Bueren AO, Rutkowski S, et al. p53 expression predicts dismal outcome for medulloblastoma patients with metastatic disease. J Neurooncol 2012;106(1):135–41.

28. Remke M, Hielscher T, Korshunov A, et al. FSTL5 is a marker of poor prognosis in non-WNT/non-SHH medulloblastoma. J Clin Oncol 2011;29(29):3852–61.

29. Kunschner LJ. Harvey Cushing and medulloblastoma. Arch Neurol 2002;59:642.
30. Turgut M. Cerebellar mutism. J Neurosurg Pediatr 2008;1:262.
31. Kusano Y, Tanaka Y, Takasuna H, et al. Transient cerebellar mutism caused by bilateral damage to the dentate nuclei after the second posterior fossa surgery. Case report. J Neurosurg 2006;104:329.
32. Jenkin D. The radiation treatment of medulloblastoma. J Neurooncol 1996;29:45.
33. Mulhern RK, Merchant TE, Gajjar A, et al. Late neurocognitive sequelae in survivors of brain tumours in childhood. Lancet Oncol 2004;5:399.
34. Evans AE, Jenkin RD, Sposto R, et al. The treatment of medulloblastoma. Results of a prospective randomized trial of radiation therapy with and without CCNU, vincristine, and prednisone. J Neurosurg 1990;72:572.
35. Cohen BH, Packer RJ. Chemotherapy for medulloblastomas and primitive neuroectodermal tumors. J Neurooncol 1996;29:55.
36. Dennis M, Spiegler BJ, Hetherington CR, et al. Neuropsychological sequelae of the treatment of children with medulloblastoma. J Neurooncol 1996;29:91.
37. Thomas PR, Deutsch M, Kepner JL, et al. Low-stage medulloblastoma: final analysis of trial comparing standard-dose with reduced-dose neuraxis irradiation. J Clin Oncol 2000;18:3004.
38. Mulhern RK, Kepner JL, Thomas PR, et al. Neuropsychologic functioning of survivors of childhood medulloblastoma randomized to receive conventional or reduced-dose craniospinal irradiation: a Pediatric Oncology Group study. J Clin Oncol 1998;16:1723.
39. Packer RJ, Goldwein J, Nicholson HS, et al. Treatment of children with medulloblastomas with reduced-dose craniospinal radiation therapy and adjuvant chemotherapy: a Children's Cancer Group Study. J Clin Oncol 1999;17:2127.
40. Packer RJ, Gajjar A, Vezina G, et al. Phase III study of craniospinal radiation therapy followed by adjuvant chemotherapy for newly diagnosed average-risk medulloblastoma. J Clin Oncol 2006;24:4202.
41. Gajjar A, Chintagumpala M, Ashley D, et al. Risk-adapted craniospinal radiotherapy followed by high-dose chemotherapy and stem-cell rescue in children with newly diagnosed medulloblastoma (St Jude Medulloblastoma-96): long-term results from a prospective, multicentre trial. Lancet Oncol 2006;7:813.
42. Kortmann RD, Kuhl J, Timmermann B, et al. Postoperative neoadjuvant chemotherapy before radiotherapy as compared to immediate radiotherapy followed by maintenance chemotherapy in the treatment of medulloblastoma in childhood: results of the German prospective randomized trial HIT '91. Int J Radiat Oncol Biol Phys 2000;46:269.
43. Goldwein JW, Radcliffe J, Johnson J, et al. Updated results of a pilot study of low dose craniospinal irradiation plus chemotherapy for children under five with cerebellar primitive neuroectodermal tumors (medulloblastoma). Int J Radiat Oncol Biol Phys 1996;34:899.
44. Packer RJ, MacDonald T, Vezina G. Central nervous system tumors. Pediatr Clin North Am 2008;55:121.
45. Jakacki RI. Treatment strategies for high-risk medulloblastoma and supratentorial primitive neuroectodermal tumors. Review of the literature. J Neurosurg 2005;102:44.
46. Rutkowski S, Bode U, Deinlein F, et al. Treatment of early childhood medulloblastoma by postoperative chemotherapy alone. N Engl J Med 2005;352:978.
47. Lashford LS, Campbell RH, Gattamaneni HR, et al. An intensive multiagent chemotherapy regimen for brain tumours occurring in very young children. Arch Dis Child 1996;74:219.

48. Geyer JR, Sposto R, Jennings M, et al. Multiagent chemotherapy and deferred radiotherapy in infants with malignant brain tumors: a report from the Children's Cancer Group. J Clin Oncol 2005;23:7621.
49. Chi SN, Gardner SL, Levy AS, et al. Feasibility and response to induction chemotherapy intensified with high-dose methotrexate for young children with newly diagnosed high-risk disseminated medulloblastoma. J Clin Oncol 2004;22:4881.
50. Mason WP, Grovas A, Halpern S, et al. Intensive chemotherapy and bone marrow rescue for young children with newly diagnosed malignant brain tumors. J Clin Oncol 1998;16:210.
51. Cohen BH, Geyer R. A pilot study of intensive chemotherapy with peripheral stem cell support for infants with malignant brain tumors [abstract]. Haematologica Reports 2006;2(11):3.
52. Zacharoulis S, Levy A, Chi SN, et al. Outcome for young children newly diagnosed with ependymoma, treated with intensive induction chemotherapy followed by myeloablative chemotherapy and autologous stem cell rescue. Pediatr Blood Cancer 2007;49:34.
53. Duffner PK, Horowitz ME, Krischer JP, et al. Postoperative chemotherapy and delayed radiation in children less than three years of age with malignant brain tumors. N Engl J Med 1993;328:1725.
54. Bakst RL, Dunkel IJ, Gilheeney S, et al. Reirradiation for recurrent medulloblastoma. Cancer 2011;117:4977.
55. Mahoney DH Jr, Steuber CP, Sandbach JF, et al. Extraneural metastases from medulloblastoma: long-term survival after sequentially scheduled chemotherapy and radiotherapy. Med Pediatr Oncol 1986;14:329.
56. Peyr A, Azizi AA, Reismueller B, et al. Antiangiogenic metronomic chemotherapy for patients with recurrent embryonal and ependymal brain tumors. In: 14th International Symposium on Pediatric Neuro-Oncology. Vienna (Austria). Neuro-Oncology 2010;12(6):ii44.
57. Low JA, de Sauvage FJ. Clinical experience with Hedgehog pathway inhibitors. J Clin Oncol 2010;28:5321.
58. Spiller SE, Ditzler SH, Pullar BJ, et al. Response of preclinical medulloblastoma models to combination therapy with 13-cis retinoic acid and suberoylanilide hydroxamic acid (SAHA). J Neurooncol 2008;87:133.
59. Hacker S, Karl S, Mader I, et al. Histone deacetylase inhibitors prime medulloblastoma cells for chemotherapy-induced apoptosis by enhancing p53-dependent Bax activation. Oncogene 2011;30:2275.
60. Nor C, de Farias CB, Abujamra AL, et al. The histone deacetylase inhibitor sodium butyrate in combination with brain-derived neurotrophic factor reduces the viability of DAOY human medulloblastoma cells. Childs Nerv Syst 2011;27:897.
61. Chintagumpala M, Hassall T, Palmer S, et al. A pilot study of risk-adapted radiotherapy and chemotherapy in patients with supratentorial PNET. Neuro Oncol 2009;11:33.
62. Reddy AT, Janss AJ, Phillips PC, et al. Outcome for children with supratentorial primitive neuroectodermal tumors treated with surgery, radiation, and chemotherapy. Cancer 2000;88:2189.
63. Phi JH, Kim JH, Eun KM, et al. Upregulation of SOX2, NOTCH1, and ID1 in supratentorial primitive neuroectodermal tumors: a distinct differentiation pattern from that of medulloblastomas. J Neurosurg Pediatr 2010;5:608.
64. Gilheeney SW, Saad A, Chi S, et al. Outcome of pediatric pineoblastoma after surgery, radiation and chemotherapy. J Neurooncol 2008;89:89.

65. Jakacki RI, Zeltzer PM, Boyett JM, et al. Survival and prognostic factors following radiation and/or chemotherapy for primitive neuroectodermal tumors of the pineal region in infants and children: a report of the Children's Cancer Group. J Clin Oncol 1995;13:1377.

66. Cohen BH, Zeltzer PM, Boyett JM, et al. Prognostic factors and treatment results for supratentorial primitive neuroectodermal tumors in children using radiation and chemotherapy: a Childrens Cancer Group randomized trial. J Clin Oncol 1995;13:1687.

67. Miller S, Rogers HA, Lyon P, et al. Genome-wide molecular characterization of central nervous system primitive neuroectodermal tumor and pineoblastoma. Neuro Oncol 2011;13:866.

68. Dahlback HS, Brandal P, Gorunova L, et al. Genomic aberrations in pediatric gliomas and embryonal tumors. Genes Chromosomes Cancer 2011;50:788.

69. Rickert CH, Simon R, Bergmann M, et al. Comparative genomic hybridization in pineal parenchymal tumors. Genes Chromosomes Cancer 2001;30:99.

70. Johnston DL, Keene DL, Lafay-Cousin L, et al. Supratentorial primitive neuroectodermal tumors: a Canadian pediatric brain tumor consortium report. J Neurooncol 2008;86:101.

71. Marec-Berard P, Jouvet A, Thiesse P, et al. Supratentorial embryonal tumors in children under 5 years of age: an SFOP study of treatment with postoperative chemotherapy alone. Med Pediatr Oncol 2002;38:83.

72. Gidwani P, Levy A, Goodrich J, et al. Successful outcome with tandem myeloablative chemotherapy and autologous peripheral blood stem cell transplants in a patient with atypical teratoid/rhabdoid tumor of the central nervous system. J Neurooncol 2008;88:211.

73. Bandopadhayay P, Hassall TE, Rosenfeld JV, et al. ANZCCSG BabyBrain99; intensified systemic chemotherapy, second look surgery and involved field radiation in young children with central nervous system malignancy. Pediatr Blood Cancer 2011;56:1055.

74. Choi LM, Rood B, Kamani N, et al. Feasibility of metronomic maintenance chemotherapy following high-dose chemotherapy for malignant central nervous system tumors. Pediatr Blood Cancer 2008;50:970.

75. Raghuram CP, Moreno L, Zacharoulis S. Is there a role for high dose chemotherapy with hematopoietic stem cell rescue in patients with relapsed supratentorial PNET? J Neurooncol 2012;106(3):441–7.

76. Hoffman HJ, Otsubo H, Hendrick EB, et al. Intracranial germ-cell tumors in children. J Neurosurg 1991;74:545.

77. Ogawa K, Shikama N, Toita T, et al. Long-term results of radiotherapy for intracranial germinoma: a multi-institutional retrospective review of 126 patients. Int J Radiat Oncol Biol Phys 2004;58:705.

78. Jennings MT, Gelman R, Hochberg F. Intracranial germ-cell tumors: natural history and pathogenesis. J Neurosurg 1985;63:155.

79. Ogawa K, Toita T, Nakamura K, et al. Treatment and prognosis of patients with intracranial nongerminomatous malignant germ cell tumors: a multiinstitutional retrospective analysis of 41 patients. Cancer 2003;98:369.

80. Wilkening GN, Madden JR, Barton VN, et al. Memory deficits in patients with pediatric CNS germ cell tumors. Pediatr Blood Cancer 2011;57:486.

81. Matsutani M, Sano K, Takakura K, et al. Primary intracranial germ cell tumors: a clinical analysis of 153 histologically verified cases. J Neurosurg 1997;86:446.

82. Kamoshima Y, Sawamura Y. Update on current standard treatments in central nervous system germ cell tumors. Curr Opin Neurol 2010;23:571.

83. Palmer RD, Foster NA, Vowler SL, et al. Malignant germ cell tumours of childhood: new associations of genomic imbalance. Br J Cancer 2007;96:667.
84. Rickert CH, Simon R, Bergmann M, et al. Comparative genomic hybridization in pineal germ cell tumors. J Neuropathol Exp Neurol 2000;59:815.
85. Schneider DT, Zahn S, Sievers S, et al. Molecular genetic analysis of central nervous system germ cell tumors with comparative genomic hybridization. Mod Pathol 2006;19:864.
86. Sakurada K, Saino M, Mouri W, et al. Nestin expression in central nervous system germ cell tumors. Neurosurg Rev 2008;31:173.
87. Souweidane MM, Krieger MD, Weiner HL, et al. Surgical management of primary central nervous system germ cell tumors: proceedings from the Second International Symposium on Central Nervous System Germ Cell Tumors. J Neurosurg Pediatr 2010;6:125.
88. Friedman JA, Lynch JJ, Buckner JC, et al. Management of malignant pineal germ cell tumors with residual mature teratoma. Neurosurgery 2001;48:518.
89. Balmaceda C, Heller G, Rosenblum M, et al. Chemotherapy without irradiation–a novel approach for newly diagnosed CNS germ cell tumors: results of an international cooperative trial. The First International Central Nervous System Germ Cell Tumor Study. J Clin Oncol 1996;14:2908.
90. Douglas JG, Rockhill JK, Olson JM, et al. Cisplatin-based chemotherapy followed by focal, reduced-dose irradiation for pediatric primary central nervous system germinomas. J Pediatr Hematol Oncol 2006;28:36.
91. Kretschmar C, Kleinberg L, Greenberg M, et al. Pre-radiation chemotherapy with response-based radiation therapy in children with central nervous system germ cell tumors: a report from the Children's Oncology Group. Pediatr Blood Cancer 2007;48:285.
92. O'Neil S, Ji L, Buranahirun C, et al. Neurocognitive outcomes in pediatric and adolescent patients with central nervous system germinoma treated with a strategy of chemotherapy followed by reduced-dose and volume irradiation. Pediatr Blood Cancer 2011;57:669.
93. Tseng CK, Tsang NM, Jaing TH, et al. Outcome of central nervous system germinoma treatment by chemoradiation. J Pediatr Hematol Oncol 2011;33:e138.
94. Robertson PL, DaRosso RC, Allen JC. Improved prognosis of intracranial non-germinoma germ cell tumors with multimodality therapy. J Neurooncol 1997;32:71.
95. Matsutani M, Ushio Y, Abe H, et al. Combined chemotherapy and radiation therapy for central nervous system germ cell tumors: preliminary results of a Phase II study of the Japanese Pediatric Brain Tumor Study Group. Neurosurg Focus 1998;5:e7.
96. Calaminus G, Bamberg M, Harms D, et al. AFP/beta-HCG secreting CNS germ cell tumors: long-term outcome with respect to initial symptoms and primary tumor resection. Results of the cooperative trial MAKEI 89. Neuropediatrics 2005;36:71.
97. Ji S, Chueh HW, Kim JY, et al. Responses and adverse effects of carboplatin-based chemotherapy for pediatric intracranial germ cell tumors. Korean J Pediatr 2011;54:128.
98. Bouffet E. The role of myeloablative chemotherapy with autologous hematopoietic cell rescue in central nervous system germ cell tumors. Pediatr Blood Cancer 2010;54:644.

Primary Central Nervous System Lymphoma
Overview of Current Treatment Strategies

Priscilla K. Brastianos, MD[a,b,]*, Tracy T. Batchelor, MD, MPH[a,c]

KEYWORDS

- Primary central nervous system lymphoma • Treatment • Chemotherapy • Radiation

KEY POINTS

- Primary central nervous system (CNS) lymphoma, an extranodal form of non-Hodgkin lymphoma, is an aggressive and uncommon malignancy involving the CNS.
- The goals of the diagnostic evaluation are to understand the extent of disease and to confirm that the lymphoma is localized to the CNS.
- Methotrexate-containing multiagent regimens are the standard treatment of this disease entity.
- The timing and dose of whole-brain radiation therapy is still unclear, given the significant risks of late neurotoxic effects.

INTRODUCTION

Primary central nervous system (CNS) lymphoma (PCNSL), an extranodal form of non-Hodgkin lymphoma (NHL), is an aggressive and uncommon malignancy involving the CNS. PCNSL accounts for 2.4% of primary brain tumors in the United States.[1] Although there was nearly a 3-fold increase in the incidence between 1973 and 1984, the incidence recently has stabilized.[2] The major risk factor for the development of PCNSL is immunodeficiency, either acquired or congenital. Infection with human immunodeficiency virus (HIV), which increases the risk of PCNSL by 3600-fold compared with the general population, largely accounted for this increased incidence.[3]

[a] Stephen E. and Catherine Pappas Center for Neuro-Oncology, Division of Hematology and Oncology, Department of Neurology, Massachusetts General Hospital Cancer Center, Harvard Medical School, 55 Fruit Street, Yawkey 9 East, Boston, MA 02114, USA; [b] Department of Medical Oncology, Dana-Farber/Brigham and Women's Cancer Center, Harvard Medical School, 450 Brookline Avenue, Dana 1537, Boston, MA 02115, USA; [c] Department of Radiation Oncology, Massachusetts General Hospital, Harvard Medical School, 55 Fruit Street, Boston, MA 02114, USA
* Corresponding author. Stephen E. and Catherine Pappas Center for Neuro-Oncology, Massachusetts General Hospital Cancer Center, 55 Fruit Street, Yawkey 9 East, Boston, MA 02114.
E-mail address: pbrastianos@partners.org

Hematol Oncol Clin N Am 26 (2012) 897–916
doi:10.1016/j.hoc.2012.05.003
0889-8588/12/$ – see front matter © 2012 Elsevier Inc. All rights reserved.

Approximately 90% of PCNSL cases are diffuse large B-cell lymphoma (DLBCL), with the other 10% being Burkitt lymphomas, poorly characterized low-grade lymphomas and T-cell lymphomas.[4] Despite similar histopathologic features, the prognosis of PCNSL is worse than other forms of extranodal or nodal DLBCL, and the therapeutic options in this area are unsatisfactory. This review focuses on the treatment strategies in immunocompetent patients with primary CNS lymphoma.

PATHOPHYSIOLOGY

PCNSL is a lymphoid neoplasm that probably arises from the late germinal center or postgerminal center cells, and subsequently localizes to the CNS by unknown neurotropic mechanisms. Histologically, the primary CNS DLBCL is characterized by immunoblasts or centroblasts clustered around cerebral blood vessels; infiltration by reactive T cells often renders it challenging for pathologists to discriminate between a reactive and neoplastic process. The molecular mechanisms that drive transformation in primary CNS lymphoma remain poorly understood. One of the limitations in studying this disease process is the lack of ample tissue for molecular studies, because diagnosis is typically made with stereotactic needle biopsy. Certain molecular features are similar in both systemic and CNS DLBCL. Like systemic DLBCL, gene expression analysis has shown that PCNSLs can be classified into the 3 molecular subclasses: germinal center B-cell, activated B-cell, and type 3 large B-cell lymphoma.[5] Common to both diseases are chromosomal translocations of the BCL6 gene,[6] aberrant somatic hypermutation in proto-oncogenes including MYC, and PAX5,[7] and deletions in 6q.[8]

However, there are certain molecular features that distinguish primary CNS DLBCL from systemic DLBCL.[9] Pathway analysis of genome-wide gene expression patterns reveals that when compared with systemic DLBCL, PCNSL is characterized by differential expression of multiple pathways related to adhesion and the extracellular matrix including the genes MUM1, CXCL13, and CHI3L1.[10] PCNSL also has increased expression of c-Myc and Pim-1.[5,9] These results are hypothesis-generating in that there may be genes responsible for the CNS tropism of PCNSL. However, functional work to further elucidate the specific role of these genes in PCNSL is needed. Understanding the molecular mechanisms of PCNSL will enable development of more rational therapeutic approaches for this disease.

CLINICAL PRESENTATION

Although PCNSL can occur in all age groups, the median age at diagnosis is between 53 and 61 years, with a slight male predominance.[2,11,12] Patients commonly present with a single mass lesion, most often supratentorial. The duration of symptoms before diagnosis is typically 2 to 3 months.[13] In a retrospective series of 248 immunocompetent patients with PCNSL treated in 19 centers in France and Belgium, 33% presented with symptoms or signs of increased intracranial pressure, 43% with neuropsychiatric symptoms, 70% with focal neurologic deficits, 14% with seizures, and 4% with vitreous involvement.[13,14] The incidence of lymphomatous meningitis in PCNSL ranges from 8% when measured by magnetic resonance imaging (MRI) to 42% when assessed by cerebrospinal fluid (CSF) cytology.[11,15,16] Primary leptomeningeal lymphoma is observed in less than 5% to 10% of cases. Primary intramedullary spinal cord lymphoma is also rare, with fewer than 50 cases reported in the literature.[17] Ocular involvement occurs in 10% to 20% of cases, with common symptoms being blurry vision, floaters, and eye pain.[12,18] Unlike other forms of NHL, B symptoms such as fevers, weight loss, and night sweats are rare.[13]

DIAGNOSIS

The International Primary CNS Lymphoma Collaborative Group (IPCG) has published consensus guidelines for the baseline diagnostic evaluation of patients with PCNSL. The goals of the diagnostic evaluation are to understand the extent of disease and to confirm that the lymphoma is localized to the CNS. The physical examination should include a comprehensive neurologic assessment, a thorough lymph node examination, and a testicular examination in men.[19] Because there is no standard neuropsychological testing, at a minimum, a Mini-Mental Status Examination (MMSE) should be performed and serially monitored. Unless contraindicated, a lumbar puncture should be performed and CSF examined for cell count, cytology, flow cytometry, and immunoglobulin heavy-chain gene rearrangement studies. Imaging should include a gadolinium-enhanced cranial MRI scan (**Fig. 1**), but contrast-enhanced cranial computed tomography (CT) can be substituted in cases in which an MRI is contraindicated. Because extraneural disease has been reported in 3.9% to 12.5% of patients with primary CNS lymphoma,[20,21] CT scans of the chest, abdomen, and pelvis should be obtained, and a bone marrow biopsy and aspirate performed to rule out occult systemic disease. An ophthalmologic examination, including a slit-lamp examination, is required to exclude involvement of the optic nerve, retina, or vitreous cavity. Laboratory studies should include serum lactate dehydrogenase, a complete blood count, creatinine clearance, and HIV testing.

PROGNOSIS

Identifying prognostic markers in PCNSL not only enables more informative discussions with individual patients, but also allows clinicians and investigators to develop risk-adjusted therapeutic approaches. Certain molecular markers have prognostic significance. Deletions in 6q are correlated with a shorter survival, whereas BCL-6 expression has a favorable prognosis.[7,8,22] Various clinical prognostic scoring systems have been proposed to risk stratify patients with PCNSL. In a retrospective review of 338 patients with newly diagnosed PCNSL, age and performance status were the 2 variables identified in multivariate analysis, and this is consistent with other studies.[23] Patients were divided into 3 classes: those younger than 50 years; those

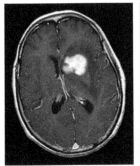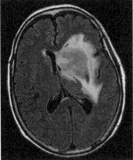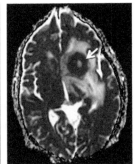

Fig. 1. Axial MR images from a patient with PCNSL. A T1-weighted MR image after contrast (*left*) shows that the lesion enhances intensely, and is surrounded by edema as shown in the fluid-attenuated inversion recovery image (*center*). The corresponding dark appearance (*white arrowhead*) on apparent diffusion coefficient imaging (*right*) suggests increased cell density in this area. (*From* Gerstner ER, Batchelor T. CNS lymphomas. In: Younes A, Coiffier B, editors. Lymphoma: diagnosis and treatment. Springer, in press; with permission.)

with a Karnofsky Performance Scale (KPS) score higher than 70 and older than 50 years; and those older than 50 years and with a KPS score less than 70. When this scoring system was applied to 3 large Radiation Therapy Oncology Group (RTOG) PCNSL trials, median overall survival was 5.2 years in class 1 (age ≤50 years), 2.1 years in class 2 (KPS ≥70, age >50 years), and 0.8 years in class 3 (KPS <70; age >50 years).

The International Extranodal Lymphoma Study Group also devised a prognostic scoring system based on data from 378 patients with PCNSL treated at 23 centers. The 5 variables associated with poor prognosis were age greater than 60 years; Eastern Cooperative Oncology Group performance status greater than 1; increased CSF protein level; increased serum lactate dehydrogenase level; and tumor involvement of the deep regions within the brain (basal ganglia, periventricular regions, brainstem, or cerebellum). Patients with 0 to 1, 2 to 3, and 4 to 5 of these unfavorable variables had 2-year overall survival rates of 80%, 48%, or 15%, respectively.[12] Further investigation is needed to evaluate whether distinct therapeutic approaches should be used for the different risk groups.

TREATMENT
Background

Historically, patients with newly diagnosed PCNSL were treated with whole-brain radiation therapy (WBRT) and corticosteroids alone, with median survival reported to be between 12 and 15 months; chemotherapy was reserved for recurrent PCNSL.[24,25] In 1985, Deangelis and colleagues[25] reported on 31 patients with newly diagnosed PCNSL who were treated with a combined modality approach of intravenous methotrexate (MTX) (1 g/m^2), intraventricular MTX, followed by WBRT, and then high-dose cytarabine (ara-C). Sixteen patients were treated with WBRT alone because they either refused chemotherapy or had initiated radiation elsewhere. The median survival in the combined modality group was 42.5 months compared with 21.7 months in the radiation group. Although the results were not statistically significant, at that time, this was the longest median survival that had been reported for any therapeutic regimen in PCNSL.[25] Subsequently, studies were designed to evaluate combined modality approaches. Multiple phase II studies and retrospective analyses confirmed that the combination of chemotherapy and radiation was more effective than radiation alone. However, the neurotoxicity of the combination is often significant, particularly in the elderly PCNSL patient population. Thus, regimens that defer WBRT have been developed.[26–30] Over the last several years, clinicians and investigators have been faced with the challenge to balance the need to administer aggressive regimens to achieve a cure with the risks of delayed neurotoxicity after treatment.

Monitoring Response to Treatment

Although there have been numerous phase II trials in PCNSL, response criteria have not been consistent between studies, and thus, it is a challenge to compare results of various studies. For this reason, the IPCG created standard guidelines for monitoring response to therapy in the setting of clinical trials.[19] Response criteria take into account imaging, corticosteroid dose, CSF cytology, and ophthalmologic examination (**Table 1**). On completion of therapy, the IPCG recommended assessment of the patient every 3 months for 2 years, then every 6 months for 3 years, and then every 12 months for 5 years. At follow-up visits, the recommended testing is a history and physical examination (including an MMSE) and MRI.

Table 1
IPCG consensus guidelines for the assessment of response in PCNSL

Response	Brain Imaging	Steroid Dose	Ophthalmologic Examination	CSF Cytology
CR	No contrast-enhancing disease	None	Normal	Negative
Unconfirmed CR	No contrast-enhancing disease	Any	Normal	Negative
	Minimal enhancing disease	Any	Minor RPE abnormality	Negative
PR	50% decrease in enhancement	NA	Normal or minor RPE abnormality	Negative
	No contrast-enhancing disease	NA	Decrease in vitreous cells or retinal infiltrate	Persistent or suspicious
PD	25% increase in enhancing disease; Any new site of disease	NA	Recurrent or new disease	Recurrent or positive
SD	All scenarios not covered by responses above			

Abbreviations: CR, complete response; NA, not applicable; PD, progressive disease; PR, partial response; RPE, retinal pigment epithelium; SD, stable disease.

Adapted from Abrey LE, Batchelor TT, Ferreri AJ, et al. Report of an international workshop to standardize baseline evaluation and response criteria for primary CNS lymphoma. J Clin Oncol 2005;23(22):5038; with permission.

Role of Surgery

PCNSL is typically diagnosed with a stereotactic-guided biopsy. Gross total resection does not play a therapeutic role in PCNSL, a multifocal malignancy often with dissemination to the CSF and eyes. In a meta-analysis of 50 prospective and retrospective studies, the extent of resection did not affect survival.[31] Extensive resections carry the risk of worsening neurologic deficits and treatment delays.[32] Surgical resection should be reserved for the rare cases of impending neurologic deterioration secondary to brain herniation.

Corticosteroids

Corticosteroids can cause a rapid regression of tumor and decrease in tumor-associated edema. However, if administered before a diagnostic biopsy, the cellular morphology may be disrupted, and diagnostic inaccuracies may result. For this reason, before a diagnostic biopsy, other methods, such as the administration of mannitol, should be used for symptomatic increase of intracranial pressure. An initial response to corticosteroids portends a more favorable outcome in PCNSL. A retrospective study reported that median survival of patients with newly diagnosed PCNSL with a documented radiologic response to corticosteroids was 117.0 months compared with 5.5 months in the nonresponders.[33] However, most patients inevitably relapse, even after an initial response to steroids, necessitating the administration of other treatments.

Radiation Therapy

WBRT as a single modality results in a median survival of 12 to 18 months, and 5-year overall survival rates ranging from 10% to 29%.[34–36] Although the initial response rate is observed in more than 90% of patients undergoing WBRT, most patients relapse. The addition of chemotherapy to WBRT results in higher response rates and improved overall survival (**Table 2**). Complete remission rates of 56% to 88% and median overall survival of 33 to 51 months have been reported with combined modality therapy.[27,30,37–41] Neurotoxicity, particularly cognitive dysfunction, after combined modality treatment is a serious challenge in the treatment of patients with PCNSL (see **Table 2**). Only a limited number of studies have systematically evaluated cognitive function in this patient population, and definitions of cognitive impairment vary, rendering it difficult to compare outcomes between different studies.[42] Among the studies that do evaluate cognitive function, there is evidence of cognitive impairment in patients who undergo chemotherapy and WBRT,[43] and stable or improved cognitive function in those patients who received single-modality treatment with chemotherapy.[8,42,44–46]

Lower doses of whole-brain radiation are being investigated as a potential method by which to reduce the incidence of neurotoxicity. A study by Shah and colleagues[47] evaluated the toxicity and efficacy of a lower dose of WBRT (23.4 Gy) in patients who achieved a complete response to rituximab, MTX, procarbazine, and vincristine. At a median follow-up of 37 months, the 2-year overall survival was 67% and no neurotoxicity was observed. In a subsequent phase III randomized noninferiority trial, the omission of radiation was evaluated, with 551 patients with newly diagnosed PCNSL randomized to receive high-dose MTX-based chemotherapy with or without WBRT.[48] There was a trend toward increased median progression-free survival in the WBRT cohort compared with the chemotherapy-only cohort (18.3 months vs 11.9 months; $P = .14$), without a difference in median overall survival (32.4 vs 37.1 months; $P = .71$). However, conclusions cannot reliably be made from this study,

Table 2
Selected published prospective trials of combined modality therapy as upfront treatment in immunocompetent patients with PCNSL

Systemic Treatment, Reference	WBRT	Intrathecal Treatment	N	CR (%)	PR (%)	PFS (mo)	OS (mo)	Neurotoxicity (%)
MTX (3.5 g/m²)[40]	30 Gy	None	25	56	32	32	33	8
MTX (1 g/m²), ara-C[25,37]	40 Gy with 14 Gy boost	MTX	31	87	—	40	42	32
MTX (3 g/m²), adriamycin, ara-C, cyclophosphamide, vincristine, methylprednisolone[38]	20 Gy with 30 Gy boost	MTX, ara-C, hydrocortisone	25	56	16	NR	2 y OS 70%	0
MTX (3 g/m²), teniposide, carmustine[83]	30 Gy with 10 Gy boost	ara-C, MTX	52	69	12	NR	46	12
MTX (3.5 g/m²), procarbazine, vincristine, ara-C[27,71]	45 Gy in <60 y old	MTX	57	56	33	129	51	30
MTX (3.5 g/m²) ± ara-C[42]	Dose depended on age, response, participating center	None	79	MTX, 18; MTX+ara-C, 46	MTX, 23; MTX+ara-C, 23	3 y: MTX, 21%; MTX+ara-C, 38%	3 y: MTX, 32%; MTX+ara-C, 46%	MTX, 20; MTX+ara-C, 6
MTX (3.5 g/m²), rituximab, procarbazine, vincristine, ara-C[47]	23.4 Gy if CR; 45 Gy if not CR	None	30	77	NR	40	2 y OS 67%	NR

Abbreviations: CR, complete response; N, number of patients; NR, not reported; OS, overall survival; PFS, progression-free survival; PR, partial response.

given the large number of protocol violations (30% of patients) and the biased analyses of the protocol violations.[49]

Although the data are limited, many centers have adopted the approach of administering chemotherapy alone, and deferring WBRT for use in relapsed patients.

Chemotherapy

In contrast to the standard treatment of systemic DLBCL, CHOP (cyclophosphamide, doxorubicin, vincristine, prednisone) does not have a role in the treatment of PCNSL. Retrospective series have reported that cyclophosphamide, doxorubicin, vincristine, and doxorubicin added to MTX results in higher toxicity without a survival benefit.[50] A randomized trial, although underpowered, failed to show a survival benefit when CHOP was added to WBRT.[36]

MTX is the backbone of any upfront regimens for PCNSL. Systemic high-dose MTX alone has efficacy.[51,52] Therapeutic CSF concentrations of MTX can be achieved with intravenous MTX doses 3 g/m^2 or greater.[53] The New Approaches to Brain Tumor Therapy (NABTT) CNS Consortium conducted a multicenter phase II trial of single-agent intravenous MTX (8 g/m^2) every 2 to 4 weeks in 25 patients with newly diagnosed PCNSL. The complete response rate was 52%, the median progression-free survival 12.8 months, and overall survival 55.4 months. Twelve patients experienced grade 3 or 4 toxicities. The clinical response reported in this study was comparable with results obtained with other more toxic combinations.[52] Other studies of single-agent high-dose MTX have reported similar results, and low rates of neurotoxicity.[54]

Numerous phase II studies have evaluated the addition of other cytotoxic agents to MTX (**Table 3**). In a randomized phase II study of 79 patients with newly diagnosed PCNSL, the addition of ara-C (4 doses of 2 g/m^2 every 3 weeks) to MTX (4 courses of 3.5 g/m^2 every 3 weeks) resulted in higher radiographic responses (complete response rate = 46% in the combination arm vs 18% in the MTX-alone arm; $P = .006$) and a trend toward improved survival (3-year overall survival 46% vs 32%; $P = .07$). Toxicities were generally limited, but tended to be more common in the combination arm, with 3 toxicity-related deaths (1 liver toxicity, 2 sepsis) in the combination arm and 1 in the MTX arm (cardiac toxicity).[42] Given the higher rates of complete responses, and trends toward improved survival in the combination arm, the combination of MTX and ara-C is a reasonable first-line regimen for newly diagnosed PCNSL, outside a clinical trial.

Another promising combination chemotherapy regimen was presented by Rubenstein and colleagues.[55] Forty-six patients were treated with an induction regimen of MTX (8 g/m^2 every 2 weeks × 8), rituximab (375 mg/m^2 every week × 6) and temozolomide (150–200 mg/m^2 days 7–11 × 5). For those who achieved a complete response, a consolidation regimen of ara-C (2 g/m^2 on days 1–4) and etoposide (40 mg/kg on days 1–4) was administered. At the time of the presentation, 63% achieved a complete response, median progression-free survival was 2.3 years, and 3-year overall survival was 67%.

In light of these studies, and in the absence of definitive phase III trials, our recommended treatment approach is to administer an MTX-containing multiagent regimen for the upfront treatment of PCNSL. WBRT can be reserved for cases that did not achieve a complete response to chemotherapy, or for disease progression.

Intrathecal Chemotherapy

Intrathecal (IT) chemotherapy has been incorporated into various treatment regimens, but there has not been a prospective randomized trial to establish whether IT chemotherapy prolongs survival (see **Tables 2** and **3**). Sandor and colleagues[56] reported a complete response rate of 79% in 14 patients who had received high-dose MTX, thiotepa, vincristine, dexamethasone, and IT MTX and ara-C. Median progression-free

Table 3
Published prospective trials of chemotherapy alone as upfront treatment in immunocompetent patients with PCNSL

Treatment, Reference	Intrathecal Treatment	N	CR (%)	PR (%)	PFS (mo)	OS (mo)	Neurotoxicity (%)
MTX Alone							
MTX (8 g/m²)[54]	None	31	65	35	17	30	0
MTX (8 g/m²)[52,84]	None	25	52	22	13	55	5
MTX (8 g/m²)[85]	None	37	30	NR	10	25	20
MTX in Combination With Other Chemotherapy							
MTX (5 g/m²), ara-C, vincristine, ifosfamide, dexamethasone, cyclophosphamide[57]	MTX, prednisolone, ara-C	65	61	10	21	50	3
MTX (1 g/m²), lomustine, procarbazine, methylprednisolone[86]	MTX, ara-C	50	42	6	11	14	8

Abbreviations: CR, complete response; N, number of patients; NR, not reported; OS, overall survival; PFS, progression-free survival; PR, partial response.

survival was 16.5 months and overall survival was not reached at the time of publication. Severe leukoencephalopathy occurred in 2 patients and significant neutropenia in 50% of the cycles administered. A pilot study of 20 patients with PCNSL treated with the Bonn protocol, a regimen consisting of systemic high-dose MTX and ara-C-based chemotherapy (including ara-C, dexamethasone, vinca alkaloids, ifosfamide, and cyclophosphamide), and intraventricular ara-C, MTX, and prednisolone, reported a complete response in 11 patients, and a partial remission in 2 patients. Median survival was 54 months, and median time to treatment failure 20.5 months. Complications were mainly hematologic and infectious (4 patients experienced Ommaya reservoir infections). One patient experienced cognitive dysfunction, possibly because of treatment.[45] The promising results of this study led to its expansion into a multicenter phase II trial, in which 65 patients with PCNSL were treated with the same regimen.[57] Sixty-one percent of the patients achieved a complete response, 6% a partial response, and 19% progressed. Median overall survival was 50 months and median time to treatment failure was 21 months. In patients younger than 61 years, median progression-free survival and overall survival were not reached at the time of publication. Treatment-related deaths occurred in 6 patients (9%), with sepsis in the setting of myelosuppression the cause of death in 5 of these patients. Infections of the Ommaya reservoir occurred in 12 patients (19%), which is higher than other reports.[56,58] Given the high rate of infections, a phase II trial was performed with a modified Bonn protocol, which omitted intraventricular therapy. In the 35 assessable patients treated with this regimen, 46% achieved a complete remission and 20% a partial remission. The median time to treatment failure was 8 months, and in the younger patients, median progression-free survival was 7 months, which was lower than the previous studies. Given these data, the trial was terminated early.[59,60] These studies may provide support for IT therapy, but in the absence of prospective randomized clinical trial data, the question has yet to be answered.

Furthermore, several retrospective analyses have failed to show a benefit of IT chemotherapy. In a multicenter retrospective series of 370 patients with PCNSL, the addition of IT chemotherapy to high-dose MTX did not result in improved survival, even in patients with positive CSF cytology; however, there was a higher incidence of neurotoxicity in patients who had received IT chemotherapy.[61] Similarly, a case-controlled retrospective study reported no difference in survival between patients who had received high-dose MTX with or without IT MTX.[62] Despite the lack of survival benefit in these analyses, the retrospective nature of these studies warrants cautious interpretation of these results.

In practice, there are limitations to the use of IT chemotherapy in PCNSL. Because approximately one-third of patients with PCNSL may present with increased intracranial pressure, lumbar punctures, or placement of Ommaya reservoirs may be contraindicated in a proportion of this patient population.[63] There is an increased risk of complications such as neurotoxicity, particularly in patients who have also undergone WBRT or high-dose MTX.[40,64] In a prospective study, 33 patients with PCNSL were treated with IT liposomal ara-C in combination with systemic polychemotherapy that included high-dose MTX and ara-C. Twenty-one percent of patients developed conus medullaris/cauda equina syndrome, attributed to the combination of the systemic chemotherapy and IT liposomal ara-C.[65] In the absence of more definitive studies showing a survival benefit, the use of IT chemotherapy remains controversial.

Blood-Brain Barrier Disruption

Disruption of the blood-brain barrier may be an alternative approach to achieving higher concentrations of chemotherapy in the CNS. Angelov and colleagues reported a multi-institutional experience of 149 patients with newly diagnosed PCNSL treated with reversible blood-brain barrier disruption and intra-arterial MTX. The complete response rate was 58%, with a median overall survival of 3.1 years and median progression-free survival of 1.8 years. Although the treatment was fairly well tolerated, with the most frequently reported side effect being partial seizures (9.2%), this procedurally intensive approach requires institutional expertise, and is unlikely to become a standard of care.

High-Dose Chemotherapy with Stem Cell Rescue

Several recent studies of high-dose chemotherapy (HDT) followed by autologous stem cell transplantation (ASCT) (HDT/ASCT) in newly diagnosed PCNSL have yielded encouraging preliminary results (**Table 4**). In a phase II study by Illerhaus and colleagues,[66] patients with newly diagnosed PCNSL were treated with sequential systemic MTX (8 g/m^2 × 3 cycles) and ara-C (3 g/m^2 × 2 doses) and thiotepa (40 mg/m^2) followed by HDT/ASCT and hyperfractionated WBRT. Of the 23 patients who underwent HDT/ASCT, 15 achieved a complete response, and of the 21 who underwent WBRT, 21 achieved a complete response. The 5-year overall survival was 69% for all patients, and 87% for those undergoing HCT/ASCT. However, 24% of irradiated patients developed leukoencephalopathy. A subsequent pilot study of 13 patients with newly diagnosed PCNSL used the same induction regimen but restricted WBRT to only those who did not have a complete response to chemotherapy. The 3-year disease-free and overall survival was 77% at a median follow-up of 25 months.[67] The results of this, albeit small, study suggest that good outcomes can be obtained without the use of consolidation WBRT. However, this is an approach that needs further study, both to determine the optimal induction and conditioning regimens, and to more carefully assess toxicities associated with these regimens.

Treatment of Elderly Patients

Although approximately 50% of patients with PCNSL are more than 65 years of age, this remains a largely understudied patient population.[23] Minimizing toxicity in elderly patients is particularly challenging and suboptimal therapy remains a problem. A study using data from the Surveillance, Epidemiology, and End Results (SEER) cancer registry reported that only 80% of newly diagnosed patients aged 65 years or older were treated. Thirty-six percent of patients were treated with WBRT alone[68] and 22% received chemotherapy alone. Treatment with WBRT as a single modality increases with age.[68] In a prospective RTOG study evaluating the use of 40-Gy irradiation with a 20-Gy boost to the tumor, median survival in elderly patients treated with WBRT alone was reported to be only 7.6 months.[34] Radiation alone is likely inadequate therapy for this population.

Multiple studies have reported that elderly patients can tolerate MTX-containing regimens with good response rates and minimal neurotoxicities (**Table 5**).[17,52,69] In a retrospective series of 174 elderly patients treated at 1 institution, 96.5% of patients underwent therapy, and 83% received MTX-based chemotherapy. The median overall survival was 25 months, with 20% of patients alive for more than 11 years.[70] Treatment-related neurotoxicities were greater in those patients who received WBRT.

Multiple studies have also confirmed the high rates of leukoencephalopathy[44,71] associated with combined modality treatment in elderly patients, which has led investigators to explore MTX-based protocols in the absence of WBRT in elderly patients. Fritsch and colleagues[72] published the results of a pilot study of rituximab, MTX, procarbazine, and lomustine in 28 elderly patients aged 65 years or older. WBRT was reserved for those patients who did not respond to chemotherapy. The complete

Table 4
Published prospective trials of HDT followed by ASCT in newly diagnosed PCNSL

Induction Regimen, Reference	HDT	N	Median Age	Median Follow-up (mo)	Survival	TRM (%)
MBVP x 2 → ifosfamide-ara-C x 1[87]	BEAM→WBRT	25	51	34	4-y OS: 64%	4
MTX→ ara-C[88]	BEAM	28	53	27	mEFS: 9 mo	0
MTX→WBRT (if no response to induction)[89]	Bu/TT→ WBRT (if no CR)	23	55	15	2-y OS: 48%	13
MBVP→ifosfamide-ara-C[90]	BEAM→WBRT	6	53	42	2-y OS: 40%	0
MTX→ara-C+TT[66]	TT/carmustine→WBRT	30	54	63	5-y OS: 69%	3
MTX→ara-C+TT[67]	TT/carmustine→WBRT (if no CR)	13	54	25	3-y OS: 77%	0

Abbreviations: BEAM, carmustine, etoposide, ara-C, melphalan; Bu, busulfan; CR, complete remission; HDT, high-dose therapy; MBVP, MTX, carmustine, etoposide, methylprednisolone; mEFS, median event-free survival; N, number of patients; OS, overall survival; TRM, treatment-related mortality; TT, thiotepa; VP16, etoposide.

Table 5
Published studies of chemotherapy alone as upfront treatment in elderly patients

Treatment, Reference	N	Median Age (y)	CR (%)	PR (%)	PFS (mo)	OS (mo)
MTX (3 g/m^2), CCNU, procarbazine, rituximab (375 mg/m^2)[72]	28	75	64	18	16	17.5
MTX (3 g/m^2), procarbazine, CCNU[43]	30	70	44	26	5.9	15.4
MTX (3.5–8 g/m^2)[91]	31	74	60	37	7.1	37
MTX (3 g/m^2), temozolomide[92]	23	68	55	0	8	35
MTX (1 g/m), CCNU, procarbazine; IT MTX and ara-C[86]	50	72	42	6	7	14

Abbreviations: CCNU, lomustine; CR, complete response; N, number of patients; NR, not reported; OS, overall survival; PFS, progression-free survival; PR, partial response.

response rate was 64%, with a 3-year progression-free survival and overall survival of 31%. Treatment-related mortality was 7% with perforated sigma diverticulitis and subdural bleeding as the causes of death.[72] This mortality is comparable with other trials of chemotherapy alone in elderly patients, with overall survival ranging between 17.5 and 35 months (see **Table 5**). Although each patient needs to be carefully assessed and benefits weighed against the risks, these data do suggest that elderly patients can tolerate chemotherapy, and that upfront WBRT may be avoided.

Rituximab

Rituximab, a monoclonal antibody against CD20 is considered standard of care in systemic DLBCL. Because 90% of patients with PCNSL are CD20+, investigations are under way to prospectively study rituximab in PCNSL. In a pilot study conducted by the National Cancer Institute-sponsored NABTT CNS Consortium, 12 patients with recurrent or refractory PCNSL who had failed MTX-based regimens were treated with weekly rituximab at 375 mg/m^2. One-third of patients showed radiographic responses, and toxicities were modest.[73] IT administration of rituximab may also be beneficial. A phase I study of intraventricular rituximab (10–25 mg) in recurrent CNS lymphoma reported that intraventricular rituximab is feasible and may have activity.[74] There are ongoing trials to further evaluate the role of IT and systemic rituximab both in newly diagnosed and refractory PCNSL (NCT00098774; NC01011920; NCT00221325).

Salvage Treatment

Most patients with PCNSL eventually progress or relapse, necessitating salvage treatment. There is no standard of care in this setting, and prognosis is poor, with a median survival in the order of months. A paucity of prospective trials has been published in this area (**Table 6**). Salvage therapies with activity include topotecan[75]; temozolomide[76]; rituximab[73]; rituximab and temozolomide[77]; and combination procarbazine, lomustine, and vincristine.[78] Reinduction with MTX in patients who previously achieved a complete response with MTX may also be effective.[79] WBRT may also be considered in patients who have not been previously irradiated. Response rates have been reported to range between 74% and 79% and overall survival between 10.9 and 16 months when WBRT is used for salvage therapy.[80,81]

Table 6
Published prospective trials of salvage therapy for PCNSL

Treatment, Reference	N	Median Age (y)	Prior RT (%)	CR (%)	PR (%)	PFS (mo)	OS (mo)
Topotecan[75]	27	51	52	18.5	14.8	2	8.4
Temozolomide[76]	36	60	86	25	6	2.8	4
Rituximab[73]	12	64	9	33	8	2	21
HD chemotherapy followed by ASCT: Induction: etoposide, ara-C; conditioning: Bu/TT/Cy[82]	43	52	33	26/27 patients who underwent IC + HCR	—	11.6 (41.1 in patients who underwent IC + HCR)	18 (58.6 in patients who underwent IC + HCR)

Abbreviations: ASCT, autologous stem cell transplant; Bu, busulfan; CR, complete response; Cy, Cytoxan; HD, high-dose; IC + HCR (intensive chemotherapy followed by autologous hematopoietic stem cell rescue); N, number of patients; NR, not reported; OS, overall survival; PFS, progression-free survival; PR, partial response; RT, radiation; TT, thiotepa.

HDT followed by hematopoietic stem cell rescue may also have activity in relapsed patients. In a study by Soussain and colleagues,[82] 43 patients with recurrent or refractory PCNSL were treated with an induction regimen of ara-C and etoposide, which was followed by thiotepa, busulfan and cyclophosphamide, and hematopoietic stem cell rescue. The median overall survival was 18 months in the entire patient cohort, and 58.6 months in the patients who received the HDT followed by stem cell rescue. Five patients experienced moderate to severe late neurotoxicity, with one resulting in death. The choice of agent for salvage therapy should be made after considering the patient's performance status, comorbidities, neurologic status, and previous regimens.

SUMMARY

PCNSL is a rare form of NHL that is associated with a poor prognosis. Our limited understanding of the pathophysiology of this disease has prevented the development of more effective therapeutic approaches. MTX-containing multiagent regimens are the standard treatment of this disease entity. The timing and dose of WBRT is still unclear, given the significant risks of late neurotoxic effects.

REFERENCES

1. Primary brain and central nervous system tumors diagnosed in the United States in 2004-2007. Hinsdale (IL): CBTRUS; 2011.
2. Schabet M. Epidemiology of primary CNS lymphoma. J Neurooncol 1999;43(3): 199–201.
3. Kadan-Lottick NS, Skluzacek MC, Gurney JG. Decreasing incidence rates of primary central nervous system lymphoma. Cancer 2002;95(1):193–202.
4. Miller DC, Hochberg FH, Harris NL, et al. Pathology with clinical correlations of primary central nervous system non-Hodgkin's lymphoma. The Massachusetts General Hospital experience 1958-1989. Cancer 1994;74(4):1383–97.
5. Rubenstein JL, Fridlyand J, Shen A, et al. Gene expression and angiotropism in primary CNS lymphoma. Blood 2006;107(9):3716–23.
6. Montesinos-Rongen M, Akasaka T, Zuhlke-Jenisch R, et al. Molecular characterization of BCL6 breakpoints in primary diffuse large B-cell lymphomas of the central nervous system identifies GAPD as novel translocation partner. Brain Pathol 2003;13(4):534–8.
7. Montesinos-Rongen M, Van Roost D, Schaller C, et al. Primary diffuse large B-cell lymphomas of the central nervous system are targeted by aberrant somatic hypermutation. Blood 2004;103(5):1869–75.
8. Rickert CH, Dockhorn-Dworniczak B, Simon R, et al. Chromosomal imbalances in primary lymphomas of the central nervous system. Am J Pathol 1999;155(5): 1445–51.
9. Rubenstein JL, Shen A, Batchelor TT, et al. Differential gene expression in central nervous system lymphoma. Blood 2009;113(1):266–7 [author reply: 267–8].
10. Tun HW, Personett D, Baskerville KA, et al. Pathway analysis of primary central nervous system lymphoma. Blood 2008;111(6):3200–10.
11. Balmaceda C, Gaynor JJ, Sun M, et al. Leptomeningeal tumor in primary central nervous system lymphoma: recognition, significance, and implications. Ann Neurol 1995;38(2):202–9.
12. Ferreri AJ, Blay JY, Reni M, et al. Prognostic scoring system for primary CNS lymphomas: the International Extranodal Lymphoma Study Group experience. J Clin Oncol 2003;21(2):266–72.

13. Bataille B, Delwail V, Menet E, et al. Primary intracerebral malignant lymphoma: report of 248 cases. J Neurosurg 2000;92(2):261–6.
14. Ferreri AJ, Reni M. Primary central nervous system lymphoma. Crit Rev Oncol Hematol 2007;63(3):257–68.
15. Fischer L, Jahnke K, Martus P, et al. The diagnostic value of cerebrospinal fluid pleocytosis and protein in the detection of lymphomatous meningitis in primary central nervous system lymphomas. Haematologica 2006;91(3): 429–30.
16. Kuker W, Nagele T, Korfel A, et al. Primary central nervous system lymphomas (PCNSL): MRI features at presentation in 100 patients. J Neurooncol 2005; 72(2):169–77.
17. Flanagan EP, O'Neill BP, Porter AB, et al. Primary intramedullary spinal cord lymphoma. Neurology 2011;77(8):784–91.
18. Batchelor T, Loeffler JS. Primary CNS lymphoma. J Clin Oncol 2006;24(8): 1281–8.
19. Abrey LE, Batchelor TT, Ferreri AJ, et al. Report of an international workshop to standardize baseline evaluation and response criteria for primary CNS lymphoma. J Clin Oncol 2005;23(22):5034–43.
20. Ferreri AJ, Reni M, Zoldan MC, et al. Importance of complete staging in non-Hodgkin's lymphoma presenting as a cerebral mass lesion. Cancer 1996;77(5): 827–33.
21. O'Neill BP, Dinapoli RP, Kurtin PJ, et al. Occult systemic non-Hodgkin's lymphoma (NHL) in patients initially diagnosed as primary central nervous system lymphoma (PCNSL): how much staging is enough? J Neurooncol 1995;25(1):67–71.
22. Braaten KM, Betensky RA, de Leval L, et al. BCL-6 expression predicts improved survival in patients with primary central nervous system lymphoma. Clin Cancer Res 2003;9(3):1063–9.
23. Abrey LE, Ben-Porat L, Panageas KS, et al. Primary central nervous system lymphoma: the Memorial Sloan-Kettering Cancer Center prognostic model. J Clin Oncol 2006;24(36):5711–5.
24. Berry MP, Simpson WJ. Radiation therapy in the management of primary malignant lymphoma of the brain. Int J Radiat Oncol Biol Phys 1981;7(1):55–9.
25. DeAngelis LM, Yahalom J, Thaler HT, et al. Combined modality therapy for primary CNS lymphoma. J Clin Oncol 1992;10(4):635–43.
26. O'Brien P, Roos D, Pratt G, et al. Phase II multicenter study of brief single-agent methotrexate followed by irradiation in primary CNS lymphoma. J Clin Oncol 2000;18(3):519–26.
27. Abrey LE, Yahalom J, DeAngelis LM. Treatment for primary CNS lymphoma: the next step. J Clin Oncol 2000;18(17):3144–50.
28. Hiraga S, Arita N, Ohnishi T, et al. Rapid infusion of high-dose methotrexate resulting in enhanced penetration into cerebrospinal fluid and intensified tumor response in primary central nervous system lymphomas. J Neurosurg 1999; 91(2):221–30.
29. Ferreri AJ, Reni M, Dell'Oro S, et al. Combined treatment with high-dose methotrexate, vincristine and procarbazine, without intrathecal chemotherapy, followed by consolidation radiotherapy for primary central nervous system lymphoma in immunocompetent patients. Oncology 2001;60(2): 134–40.
30. DeAngelis LM, Seiferheld W, Schold SC, et al. Combination chemotherapy and radiotherapy for primary central nervous system lymphoma: Radiation Therapy Oncology Group Study 93-10. J Clin Oncol 2002;20(24):4643–8.

31. Reni M, Ferreri AJ, Garancini MP, et al. Therapeutic management of primary central nervous system lymphoma in immunocompetent patients: results of a critical review of the literature. Ann Oncol 1997;8(3):227–34.
32. Bellinzona M, Roser F, Ostertag H, et al. Surgical removal of primary central nervous system lymphomas (PCNSL) presenting as space occupying lesions: a series of 33 cases. Eur J Surg Oncol 2005;31(1):100–5.
33. Mathew BS, Carson KA, Grossman SA. Initial response to glucocorticoids. Cancer 2006;106(2):383–7.
34. Nelson DF, Martz KL, Bonner H, et al. Non-Hodgkin's lymphoma of the brain: can high dose, large volume radiation therapy improve survival? Report on a prospective trial by the Radiation Therapy Oncology Group (RTOG): RTOG 8315. Int J Radiat Oncol Biol Phys 1992;23(1):9–17.
35. Shibamoto Y, Ogino H, Hasegawa M, et al. Results of radiation monotherapy for primary central nervous system lymphoma in the 1990s. Int J Radiat Oncol Biol Phys 2005;62(3):809–13.
36. Mead GM, Bleehen NM, Gregor A, et al. A Medical Research Council randomized trial in patients with primary cerebral non-Hodgkin lymphoma: cerebral radiotherapy with and without cyclophosphamide, doxorubicin, vincristine, and prednisone chemotherapy. Cancer 2000;89(6):1359–70.
37. Abrey LE, DeAngelis LM, Yahalom J. Long-term survival in primary CNS lymphoma. J Clin Oncol 1998;16(3):859–63.
38. Blay JY, Bouhour D, Carrie C, et al. The C5R protocol: a regimen of high-dose chemotherapy and radiotherapy in primary cerebral non-Hodgkin's lymphoma of patients with no known cause of immunosuppression. Blood 1995;86(8):2922–9.
39. Ferreri AJ, Dell'Oro S, Foppoli M, et al. MATILDE regimen followed by radiotherapy is an active strategy against primary CNS lymphomas. Neurology 2006;66(9):1435–8.
40. Glass J, Gruber ML, Cher L, et al. Preirradiation methotrexate chemotherapy of primary central nervous system lymphoma: long-term outcome. J Neurosurg 1994;81(2):188–95.
41. Gerstner ER, Batchelor TT. Primary central nervous system lymphoma. Arch Neurol 2010;67(3):291–7.
42. Ferreri AJ, Reni M, Foppoli M, et al. High-dose cytarabine plus high-dose methotrexate versus high-dose methotrexate alone in patients with primary CNS lymphoma: a randomised phase 2 trial. Lancet 2009;374(9700):1512–20.
43. Illerhaus G, Marks R, Muller F, et al. High-dose methotrexate combined with procarbazine and CCNU for primary CNS lymphoma in the elderly: results of a prospective pilot and phase II study. Ann Oncol 2009;20(2):319–25.
44. Filley CM, Kleinschmidt-DeMasters BK. Toxic leukoencephalopathy. N Engl J Med 2001;345(6):425–32.
45. Schlegel U, Pels H, Glasmacher A, et al. Combined systemic and intraventricular chemotherapy in primary CNS lymphoma: a pilot study. J Neurol Neurosurg Psychiatry 2001;71(1):118–22.
46. Correa DD, Maron L, Harder H, et al. Cognitive functions in primary central nervous system lymphoma: literature review and assessment guidelines. Ann Oncol 2007;18(7):1145–51.
47. Shah GD, Yahalom J, Correa DD, et al. Combined immunochemotherapy with reduced whole-brain radiotherapy for newly diagnosed primary CNS lymphoma. J Clin Oncol 2007;25(30):4730–5.

48. Thiel E, Korfel A, Martus P, et al. High-dose methotrexate with or without whole brain radiotherapy for primary CNS lymphoma (G-PCNSL-SG-1): a phase 3, randomised, non-inferiority trial. Lancet Oncol 2010;11(11):1036–47.

49. Ferreri AJ. How I treat primary CNS lymphoma. Blood 2011;118(3):510–22.

50. Glass J, Shustik C, Hochberg FH, et al. Therapy of primary central nervous system lymphoma with pre-irradiation methotrexate, cyclophosphamide, doxorubicin, vincristine, and dexamethasone (MCHOD). J Neurooncol 1996;30(3): 257–65.

51. Herrlinger U, Schabet M, Brugger W, et al. German Cancer Society Neuro-Oncology Working Group NOA-03 multicenter trial of single-agent high-dose methotrexate for primary central nervous system lymphoma. Ann Neurol 2002; 51(2):247–52.

52. Batchelor T, Carson K, O'Neill A, et al. Treatment of primary CNS lymphoma with methotrexate and deferred radiotherapy: a report of NABTT 96-07. J Clin Oncol 2003;21(6):1044–9.

53. Shapiro WR, Young DF, Mehta BM. Methotrexate: distribution in cerebrospinal fluid after intravenous, ventricular and lumbar injections. N Engl J Med 1975; 293(4):161–6.

54. Guha-Thakurta N, Damek D, Pollack C, et al. Intravenous methotrexate as initial treatment for primary central nervous system lymphoma: response to therapy and quality of life of patients. J Neurooncol 1999;43(3):259–68.

55. Rubenstein J, Johnson J, Jung S, et al. Intensive chemotherapy and immuno-therapy, without brain irradiation, in newly diagnosed patients with primary CNS lymphoma: results of CALGB 50202. Blood 2010;116 [abstract: 763].

56. Sandor V, Stark-Vancs V, Pearson D, et al. Phase II trial of chemotherapy alone for primary CNS and intraocular lymphoma. J Clin Oncol 1998;16(9):3000–6.

57. Pels H, Schmidt-Wolf IG, Glasmacher A, et al. Primary central nervous system lymphoma: results of a pilot and phase II study of systemic and intraventricular chemotherapy with deferred radiotherapy. J Clin Oncol 2003;21(24):4489–95.

58. Obbens EA, Leavens ME, Beal JW, et al. Ommaya reservoirs in 387 cancer patients: a 15-year experience. Neurology 1985;35(9):1274–8.

59. Pels H, Juergens A, Glasmacher A, et al. Modified "Bonn Protocol" without intra-ventricular chemotherapy in the treatment of primary CNS lymphoma: preliminary results [abstract 024]. Neurooncology 2006;8:293–372.

60. Pels H, Juergens A, Glasmacher A, et al. Early relapses in primary CNS lymphoma after response to polychemotherapy without intraventricular treatment: results of a phase II study. J Neurooncol 2009;91(3):299–305.

61. Ferreri AJ, Reni M, Pasini F, et al. A multicenter study of treatment of primary CNS lymphoma. Neurology 2002;58(10):1513–20.

62. Khan RB, Shi W, Thaler HT, et al. Is intrathecal methotrexate necessary in the treatment of primary CNS lymphoma? J Neurooncol 2002;58(2):175–8.

63. Ferreri AJ, Reni M, Villa E. Primary central nervous system lymphoma in immuno-competent patients. Cancer Treat Rev 1995;21(5):415–46.

64. Fine HA, Mayer RJ. Primary central nervous system lymphoma. Ann Intern Med 1993;119(11):1093–104.

65. Ostermann K, Pels H, Kowoll A, et al. Neurologic complications after intrathecal liposomal cytarabine in combination with systemic polychemotherapy in primary CNS lymphoma. J Neurooncol 2011;103(3):635–40.

66. Illerhaus G, Marks R, Ihorst G, et al. High-dose chemotherapy with autologous stem-cell transplantation and hyperfractionated radiotherapy as first-line treatment of primary CNS lymphoma. J Clin Oncol 2006;24(24):3865–70.

67. Illerhaus G, Muller F, Feuerhake F, et al. High-dose chemotherapy and autologous stem-cell transplantation without consolidating radiotherapy as first-line treatment for primary lymphoma of the central nervous system. Haematologica 2008;93(1): 147–8.
68. Panageas KS, Elkin EB, Ben-Porat L, et al. Patterns of treatment in older adults with primary central nervous system lymphoma. Cancer 2007;110(6):1338–44.
69. Freilich RJ, Delattre JY, Monjour A, et al. Chemotherapy without radiation therapy as initial treatment for primary CNS lymphoma in older patients. Neurology 1996; 46(2):435–9.
70. Ney DE, Reiner AS, Panageas KS, et al. Characteristics and outcomes of elderly patients with primary central nervous system lymphoma: the Memorial Sloan-Kettering Cancer Center experience. Cancer 2010;116(19):4605–12.
71. Gavrilovic IT, Hormigo A, Yahalom J, et al. Long-term follow-up of high-dose methotrexate-based therapy with and without whole brain irradiation for newly diagnosed primary CNS lymphoma. J Clin Oncol 2006;24(28):4570–4.
72. Fritsch K, Kasenda B, Hader C, et al. Immunochemotherapy with rituximab, methotrexate, procarbazine, and lomustine for primary CNS lymphoma (PCNSL) in the elderly. Ann Oncol 2011;22(9):2080–5.
73. Batchelor TT, Grossman SA, Mikkelsen T, et al. Rituximab monotherapy for patients with recurrent primary CNS lymphoma. Neurology 2011;76(10): 929–30.
74. Rubenstein JL, Fridlyand J, Abrey L, et al. Phase I study of intraventricular administration of rituximab in patients with recurrent CNS and intraocular lymphoma. J Clin Oncol 2007;25(11):1350–6.
75. Fischer L, Thiel E, Klasen HA, et al. Prospective trial on topotecan salvage therapy in primary CNS lymphoma. Ann Oncol 2006;17(7):1141–5.
76. Reni M, Zaja F, Mason W, et al. Temozolomide as salvage treatment in primary brain lymphomas. Br J Cancer 2007;96(6):864–7.
77. Enting RH, Demopoulos A, DeAngelis LM, et al. Salvage therapy for primary CNS lymphoma with a combination of rituximab and temozolomide. Neurology 2004; 63(5):901–3.
78. Herrlinger U, Brugger W, Bamberg M, et al. PCV salvage chemotherapy for recurrent primary CNS lymphoma. Neurology 2000;54(8):1707–8.
79. Plotkin SR, Betensky RA, Hochberg FH, et al. Treatment of relapsed central nervous system lymphoma with high-dose methotrexate. Clin Cancer Res 2004; 10(17):5643–6.
80. Hottinger AF, DeAngelis LM, Yahalom J, et al. Salvage whole brain radiotherapy for recurrent or refractory primary CNS lymphoma. Neurology 2007;69(11): 1178–82.
81. Nguyen PL, Chakravarti A, Finkelstein DM, et al. Results of whole-brain radiation as salvage of methotrexate failure for immunocompetent patients with primary CNS lymphoma. J Clin Oncol 2005;23(7):1507–13.
82. Soussain C, Hoang-Xuan K, Taillandier L, et al. Intensive chemotherapy followed by hematopoietic stem-cell rescue for refractory and recurrent primary CNS and intraocular lymphoma: Société Française de Greffe de Moëlle Osseuse-Thérapie Cellulaire. J Clin Oncol 2008;26(15):2512–8.
83. Poortmans PM, Kluin-Nelemans HC, Haaxma-Reiche H, et al. High-dose methotrexate-based chemotherapy followed by consolidating radiotherapy in non-AIDS-related primary central nervous system lymphoma: European Organization for Research and Treatment of Cancer Lymphoma Group Phase II Trial 20962. J Clin Oncol 2003;21(24):4483–8.

84. Gerstner ER, Carson KA, Grossman SA, et al. Long-term outcome in PCNSL patients treated with high-dose methotrexate and deferred radiation. Neurology 2008;70(5):401–2.

85. Herrlinger U, Kuker W, Uhl M, et al. NOA-03 trial of high-dose methotrexate in primary central nervous system lymphoma: final report. Ann Neurol 2005;57(6): 843–7.

86. Hoang-Xuan K, Taillandier L, Chinot O, et al. Chemotherapy alone as initial treatment for primary CNS lymphoma in patients older than 60 years: a multicenter phase II study (26952) of the European Organization for Research and Treatment of Cancer Brain Tumor Group. J Clin Oncol 2003;21(14):2726–31.

87. Colombat P, Lemevel A, Bertrand P, et al. High-dose chemotherapy with autologous stem cell transplantation as first-line therapy for primary CNS lymphoma in patients younger than 60 years: a multicenter phase II study of the GOELAMS group. Bone Marrow Transplant 2006;38(6):417–20.

88. Abrey LE, Moskowitz CH, Mason WP, et al. Intensive methotrexate and cytarabine followed by high-dose chemotherapy with autologous stem-cell rescue in patients with newly diagnosed primary CNS lymphoma: an intent-to-treat analysis. J Clin Oncol 2003;21(22):4151–6.

89. Montemurro M, Kiefer T, Schuler F, et al. Primary central nervous system lymphoma treated with high-dose methotrexate, high-dose busulfan/thiotepa, autologous stem-cell transplantation and response-adapted whole-brain radiotherapy: results of the multicenter Ostdeutsche Studiengruppe Hamato-Onkologie OSHO-53 phase II study. Ann Oncol 2007;18(4):665–71.

90. Brevet M, Garidi R, Gruson B, et al. First-line autologous stem cell transplantation in primary CNS lymphoma. Eur J Haematol 2005;75(4):288–92.

91. Zhu JJ, Gerstner ER, Engler DA, et al. High-dose methotrexate for elderly patients with primary CNS lymphoma. Neuro Oncol 2009;11(2):211–5.

92. Omuro AM, Taillandier L, Chinot O, et al. Temozolomide and methotrexate for primary central nervous system lymphoma in the elderly. J Neurooncol 2007; 85(2):207–11.

Neoplastic Meningitis and Metastatic Epidural Spinal Cord Compression

Marc C. Chamberlain, MD

KEYWORDS

- Neoplastic meningitis • Leptomeningeal metastasis • Cancinomatous meningitis
- Epidural spinal cord compression

KEY POINTS

- Neoplastic meningitis (NM) is a disease that is under-recognized and consequently undiagnosed and treated.
- NM involves the entire neuraxis and as such any element of the central nervous system (CNS) (brain, cranial nerves, spinal cord, or exiting nerve roots) may be involved.
- In a patient with cancer with otherwise unexplained CNS dysfunction, consider NM.
- NM may be diagnosed clinically, radiographically, or pathologically (cerebrospinal fluid [CSF] flow cytometry or cytology).
- Epidural spinal cord compression (ESCC) essentially always presents with pain, and treatment is most effective with there is little to no neurologic compromise.

NEOPLASTIC MENINGITIS

Introduction

Carcinomatous meningitis (CM), or meningeal carcinomatosis, is a term that defines leptomeningeal metastases arising as a result of metastases from systemic solid cancers.[1,2] Similarly, lymphomatous meningitis and leukemic meningitis result from CSF dissemination of lymphoma or leukemia. All 3 entities are commonly referred to as NM or leptomeningeal metastasis due to involvement of both the CSF compartment and the leptomeninges, comprised of the pia and arachnoid. Although NM is the third most metastatic complication of the CNS, NM is comparatively uncommon with 7000 to 9000 new cases diagnosed annually in the United States.[1–5] The most common sources of systemic cancer metastatic to the leptomeninges are breast cancer, lung cancer, melanoma, aggressive non-Hodgkin lymphoma, and acute leukemia in that

Division of Neuro-Oncology, Department of Neurology, University of Washington, Fred Hutchinson Cancer Research Center, Seattle Cancer Care Alliance, 825 Eastlake Avenue East, PO Box 19023, MS G4940, Seattle, WA 98109, USA
E-mail address: chambemc@u.washington.edu

Hematol Oncol Clin N Am 26 (2012) 917–931
doi:10.1016/j.hoc.2012.04.004
0889-8588/12/$ – see front matter © 2012 Elsevier Inc. All rights reserved.

hemonc.theclinics.com

order. The majority of patients with NM present with neurologic dysfunction as well as evidence of other sites of systemic metastases. Neurologic dysfunction may involve the entire neuraxis although most commonly spinal cord symptoms and cranial neuropathies dominate. In some patients, cerebral hemisphere symptoms, such as confusion, may predominate. Because any site in the CNS may be involved, clinical manifestations may be challenging in patients with cancer and associated comorbidities. Consequently, a high clinical index of suspicion needs to be entertained so as to recognize the disease and determine the most appropriate therapy. Clinical syndromes that suggest NM include cauda equina syndrome (ie, asymmetric lower extremity weakness and dermatomal sensory disturbance), communicating hydrocephalus presenting with symptoms of raised intracranial pressure, and cranial neuropathies, most often involving oculomotor function and presenting with diplopia.[1–5]

Diagnosis

Establishing a diagnosis of NM requires careful consideration of clinical findings such that any patient with cancer and a neurologic disturbance should be considered as potentially having NM (**Fig. 1**).[1–5] Neuroradiographic imaging (ie, MRI of brain or relevant spine) may suggest NM based on focal or diffuse leptomeningeal enhancement, subarachnoid or ventricular tumor nodules, and the frequent (30%–40%) coexistence of brain parenchymal metastases in instances of nonhematologic cancers (see **Fig. 1**).[6,7] The reported rates of negative CSF imaging in patients with NM range from 30% to 70%, suggesting normal CNS imaging does not exclude a diagnosis of NM. Also, CSF analysis is crucial to diagnosing NM and in all patients some abnormality of CSF is apparent (ie, elevated opening pressure or protein, depressed glucose, or mild pleocytosis).[4,8] Tumor assessment by CSF cytology in patients with solid cancers may be positive although the test has a high false-negative rate (approximately 50%) notwithstanding multiple sampling (2–3 samples), large volume (>10 mL) sent for analysis, and prompt presentation of the CSF to the laboratory. Rarely are CSF markers of cancer (ie, carcinoembryonic antigen) useful in diagnosing or managing patients with CM, except in instances of germ cell tumors where CSF markers (α-fetoprotein and β-human chorionic gonadotropin) often are useful.[9] Because of the frequent absence of corroborating laboratory studies (ie, negative CSF cytology and neuroimaging), a diagnosis of NM may be presumed based only on clinical findings in a patient with cancer and nonspecific CSF abnormalities. Of greater use in patients with hematologic cancers is the increased sensitivity of CSF flow cytometry in demonstrating NM, and that requires comparatively small volumes of CSF for analysis (approximately 2 mL) (**Table 1**).

Treatment

Two challenges arise with respect to the treatment of NM: determining whom to treat, and, if CM-directed treatment is believed warranted, how to treat.[10–24] Patients assessed as candidates for treatment include those with low tumor burden as reflected by independence in a performance and lack of major neurologic deficits, no evidence of bulky CNS disease by neuroimaging, absence of CSF flow block by radioisotope imaging, expected survival greater than 3 months, and limited extraneural metastatic disease.[10,25–28] Many of these parameters require laboratory investigation, including the performance of neuraxis imaging (most commonly MRI with contrast) and a radioisotope CSF flow study (see **Fig. 1**). CSF flow studies, although recommended in guidelines, are infrequently used; however, they may assist in determining whether intra-CSF chemotherapy, if administered, distributes homogenously throughout the CSF or whether intra-CSF chemotherapy likely is confined to a single

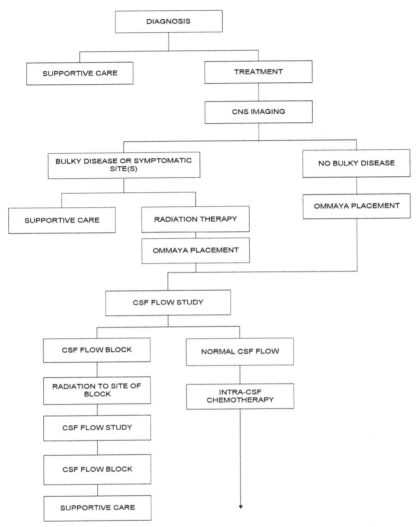

Fig. 1. Treatment algorithm. (*Adapted from* Chamberlain MC. Leptomeningeal metastases. Curr Opin Oncol 2010;22(6):627–35; with permission.)

Table 1
Non-Hodgkin lymphoma: comparison between CSF cytology versus flow cytometry

	Negative CSF Cytology	Positive CSF Cytology	Total
Negative flow cytometry	287 (72%)	21 (5%)	308 (76%)
Positive flow cytometry	63 (16%)	28 (7%)	91 (23%)
Total	350 (88%)	49 (12%)	399 (100%)

Number of Samples (% of Total Samples).
Data from Refs.[55–57]

CSF compartment, resulting in failure to treat all sites of leptomeningeal disease as well as increasing the risk for treatment-related neurotoxicity.[10,25–28] If, after clinical and laboratory assessment, intra-CSF chemotherapy treatment is believed warranted, a decision is made whether to treat by lumbar administration (intrathecal) or by way of a surgically implanted subgaleal reservoir and intraventricular catheter (ie, an Ommaya or Rickham reservoir system). Intralumbar treatment is convenient but suffers from the time required to perform, patient discomfort from the procedure, frequent need for performance by interventional radiology, failure to deliver drug to the thecal sac (10%–12% of intralumbar treatments do not enter the CSF compartment), limited distribution within the cranial CSF compartments when administering short half-life intra-CSF chemotherapy agents (methotrexate and cytarabine), and the apparent diminished survival in patients with CM treated by intralumbar drug administration compared with intraventricular treatment.[29] Treatment by intraventricular intra-CSF chemotherapy administration results in improved drug dose and distribution in the CSF and is more convenient, especially for treatment that is often 2 or more times per week (**Table 2**). Surgical implantation of a device and the risk of complications, however, especially iatrogenic bacterial meningitis, need to be balanced against the benefits of intraventricular intra-CSF drug administration.

High-dose systemic chemotherapy, in particular methotrexate and cytarabine, may obviate intra-CSF chemotherapy.[13,30] High-dose therapy achieves cytotoxic CSF levels, as, for example, reported in patients with lymphomatous meningitis or breast cancer–related CM. The majority of systemic chemotherapy and some targeted therapies (ie, imatinib, rituximab, and trastuzumab), however, do not achieve adequate CNS penetration and consequently do not treat the CSF (water) compartment, which does not imply that systemic chemotherapy has no role in the treatment of NM but that for the majority of patients with NM, systemic chemotherapy is an adjunct treatment useful to treat extraneural disease and bulky subarachnoid disease.[1,10,14,22]

Intra-CSF chemotherapy in NM is based on limited studies with comparatively small numbers of patients (**Table 3**).[14–17,19–24] Consequently, the role of intra-CSF chemotherapy in the treatment of NM has never been established in a prospective randomized trial. Nonetheless, several statements can be made regarding intra-CSF chemotherapy. Among the 3 most common intra-CSF chemotherapy agents used (ie, methotrexate, cytarabine, and thiotepa), there does not seem to be an advantage of one agent versus another nor does there seem to be an advantage for combining agents as is commonly prescribed for lymphomatous and leukemic meningitis (see **Table 3**).[14,15] Liposomal cytarabine, an intra-CSF chemotherapy with a long half-life (approximately 140 hours), has been shown in 2 small randomized trials to be superior to methotrexate or cytarabine, although potentially with increased neurotoxicity (see **Table 3**).[16,17] Due to increased efficacy (cytologic response, time to neurologic disease progression, non-neurologic cause of death, and improved quality of life), an argument has been made for considering liposomal cytarabine as the agent of first choice in patients with NM unless an investigational trial is available. Small trials with alternative intra-CSF chemotherapies (ie, topotecan, etoposide, Interferon alfa, and trastuzumab) have been used in adults with NM, although the appropriate role for these agents is unclear.[18–20,23,24] Suggestions, including treatment of melanoma-related CM with a-interferon, germ cell cancer and small cell lung cancer CM with etoposide, Her2/neu-positive breast cancer–related CM with trastuzumab, and non–small cell lung cancer–related CM with topotecan, seem reasonable but are not evidenced based. All intra-CSF chemotherapy is associated with side effects such as fatigue associated with whole-brain radiotherapy and the induction of a chemical meningitis with intra-CSF chemotherapy. Intra-CSF chemotherapy commonly causes transient (<5 days)

Table 2
Regional chemotherapy for leptomeningeal metastasis

Drug	Induction Regimens		Consolidation Regimen		Maintenance Regimen	
	Bolus Regimen	Concentration × Time Regimen	Bolus Regimen	Concentration × Time Regimen	Bolus Regimen	Concentration × Time Regimen
α-Interferon[20]	1 × 10⁶ U 2 times weekly (total 4 wk)		1 × 10⁶ U 3 times weekly every other wk (total 4 wk)		1 × 10⁶ U 3 times weekly (1 wk per mo)	
Cytarabine[17]	25–100 mg 2 Times weekly (total 4 wk)	25 mg/d for 3 d Weekly (total 4 wk)	25–100 mg Once weekly (total 4 wk)	25 mg/d for 3 d Every other wk (total 4 wk)	25–100 mg Once a mo	25 mg/d for 3 d Once a mo
DepoCyt[17,18,21]	50 mg Every 2 wk (total 8 wk)		50 mg Every 4 wk (total 24 wk)			
Etoposide[19]		0.5 mg/d for 5 d Every other wk (total 8 wk)		0.5 mg/d for 5 d Every other wk (total 4 wk)		0.5 mg/d for 5 d Once a mo
Methotrexate[12,14–16,22]	10–15 mg Twice weekly (total 4 wk)	2 mg/d for 5 d Every other wk (total 8 wk)	10–15 mg Once weekly (total 4 wk)	2 mg/d for 5 d Every other wk (total 4 wk)	10–15 mg Once a mo	2 mg/d for 5 d Once a mo
Rituximab[1]	25 mg 2 Times weekly (total 4 wk)		25 mg 2 Times weekly every other wk (total 4 wk)		25 mg 2 Times weekly once a mo	
Thiotepa[15]	10 mg 2 Times weekly (total 4 wk)	10 mg/d for 3 d Weekly (total 4 wk)	10 mg Once weekly (total 4 wk)	10 mg/d for 3 d Every other wk (total 4 wk)	10 mg Once a mo	10 mg/d for 3 d Once a mo
Topotecan[24]	0.4 mg 2 Times weekly (total 4 wk)		0.4 mg 2 times weekly every other wk (total 4 wk)		0.4 mg 2 Times weekly once a mo	
Trastuzumab[23]	20–100 mg 1 Time weekly (total 4 wk)		20–60 mg 1 Time every other wk (total 4 wk)		20–60 mg 1 Time every 4 wk	

Adapted from Chamberlain MC. Leptomeningeal metastases. Curr Opin Oncol 2010;22(6):627–35; with permission.

Table 3
Randomized clinical trials

Study	Design	Response	Toxicity
Boogerd et al[22]	N = 35 Breast cancer IT vs no IT[a]	IT vs no IT: improvement or stabilization: 59% vs 67% TTP: 23 vs 24 wk Median survival: 18.3 vs 30.3 wk	IT vs no IT: neurologic complications: 47% vs 6%
Glantz et al[17]	N = 28 Lymphoma DepoCyt vs Ara-C	DepoCyt vs Ara-C: TTP[b]: 78.5 vs 42 d OS[b]: 99.5 vs 63 d RR: 71% vs 15%	DepoCyt vs Ara-C: headache: 27% vs 2%; nausea: 9% vs 2%; fever: 8% vs 4%; pain: 5% vs 4%; confusion: 7% vs 0%; somnolence: 8% vs 4%
Glantz et al[16]	N = 61 Solid tumors DepoCyt vs MTX	DepoCyt vs MTX: RR[b] 26% vs 20% OS[b] 105 vs 78 d TTP 58 vs 30 d	DepoCyt vs MTX: sensory/motor: 4% vs 10%; altered mental status: 5% vs 2%; headache: 4% vs 2%
Grossman et al[15]	N = 59 Solid tumors and lymphoma (in 90%) IT MTX vs thiotepa	IT MTX vs thiotepa: neurologic improvements: none Median survival: 15.9 vs 14.1 wk	IT MTX vs thiotepa: Serious toxicities similar between groups. Mucositis and neurologic complications more common in MTX group.
Hitchins et al[14]	N = 44 Solid tumors and lymphomas IT MTX vs MTX + Ara-C	IT MTX vs MTX + Ara-C: RR[b]: 61% vs 45% Median survival[b]: 12 vs 7 wk	IT MTX vs MTX + Ara-C: N/V: 36% vs 50%; septicemia, neutropenia: 9% vs 15%; mucositis: 14% vs 10%; pancytopenia: 9% vs 10%. AEs related to reservoir: blocked Ommaya: 17% vs 0%; intracranial hemorrhage: 11% vs 0%
Shapiro et al[21]	Solid tumors (n = 103) DepoCyt vs MTX Lymphoma (n = 25) DepoCyt vs Ara-C	DepoCyt vs MTX/Ara-C: PFS[b]: 35 vs 43 d DepoCyt vs MTX: PFS: 35 vs 37.5 DepoCyt vs Ara-C: CR[b]: 33.3% vs 16.7% PFS: 34 vs 50 d	DepoCyt vs MTX/Ara-C: Drug-related AEs: 48% vs 60% Serious AEs: 86% vs 77%

Abbreviations: AE, adverse event; Ara-C, cytarabine; CR, complete response; IT, intra-CSF; MTX, methotrexate; N/V, nausea/vomiting; OS, overall survival; PFS, progression-free survival; RR, response rate; TTP, time to progression.

[a] Appropriate systemic chemotherapy and/or radiotherapy given in both arms.

[b] No significant differences between groups.

Adapted from Chamberlain MC. Leptomeningeal metastases. Curr Opin Oncology 2010;22(6): 627–35; with permission.

aseptic chemical meningitis that may be mitigated by administration of concurrent oral steroids.[1,2,16,17] Chemical meningitis often manifests as headache, nausea/vomiting, fever, photophobia, meningismus, CSF pleocytosis, and occasionally delirium. Likely, the majority of patients manifest laboratory evidence of intra-CSF chemotherapy–related chemical meningitis; however, only a minority are symptomatic and in most are easily managed with oral medications. The major differential diagnosis is with respect to iatrogenic infectious meningitis wherein skin contaminants are introduced at the time of intra-CSF chemotherapy.

At present there is an enormous unmet need for investigational trials of novel treatments for NM; however, there are several reasons why these are unlikely, at least in the immediate future. Neuro-oncology collaborative groups are gliomacentric with limited interest in studying NM. Because of the low incidence of the disease and limited survival after diagnosis, there is little business incentive for pharmaceutical companies to invest resources in NM, and a degree of therapeutic nihilism exists among oncologists in managing patients with NM that serves as a disincentive for development of clinical trials.

Symptomatic treatment of NM is directed at alleviating pain, which is most often headache and secondary to raised intracranial pressure that is best managed by either CSF shunting or treatment with whole-brain radiotherapy. Similarly, nausea and vomiting usually related to raised intracranial pressure are managed in a similar manner. As a general principle, there is little benefit from steroid administration in managing CM-related symptoms, with 2 exceptions. Patients with treatment-related chemical meningitis often benefit from steroid administration (described previously). In addition, patients with coexisting parenchymal brain metastases also derive benefit from steroids when peritumoral edema is extant. Antiepileptic drugs are rarely indicated because fewer than 10% of patients with NM manifest seizures and there is no benefit to prophylactic anticonvulsant use. A candid discussion regarding potential treatment side effects and expected treatment outcome is important because many patients may conclude that treatment is ineffective and, consequently, decline therapy. In patients proceeding with NM-directed therapy, preparing patients and families for a neurologic death and the expected sequential loss of neurologic function may help alleviate stress and provide an improved understanding of the dying process.

EPIDURAL SPINAL CORD COMPRESSION
Introduction

The vertebral column is the most frequent site of bony metastases.[31–51] Typically, the vertebral body is affected first, with posterior elements (pedicles and lamina) involved only one-seventh as often as anterior elements. Several factors probably contribute to the high incidence of metastatic deposition and growth in vertebrae. These include the valveless epidural venous plexus of Batson with bidirectional flow and direct communication with thoracic and pelvic venous system. In addition, the vertebrae contain vascular marrow (red marrow) throughout life unlike bones of the peripheral skeleton, which contain avascular marrow (yellow marrow). It is suggested the microenviornment of red marrow is more conducive to establishment of metastases due in part to increased vascularity. Cancer–bone interactions in part involve the osteoprotegerin (OPG) and receptor activator of nuclear factor κB (RANK) signaling pathway.[50] OPG negatively regulates bone resorption by inhibiting osteoclasts vis-à-vis functioning as a false decoy receptor for RANK ligand (RANKL). Consequently, OPG is osteoprotective. RANK is expressed on osteoclasts and, on binding to RANKL, stimulates osteoclastogenesis and bone resorption. RANKL is the key stimulator of bone resorption and stimulates osteoclast formation and activation. The balance between OPG and RANKL seems to regulate bone resorption. RANKL is overexpressed in bone metastases whereas OPG serum levels are decreased in patients with bone metastases.

In an autopsy study of metastatic cancer, 70% of patients had vertebral body metastases, of which one-half had symptomatic pain requiring treatment.[43] It is estimated that 5% of patients with cancer develop ESCC based on autopsy studies and approximately 80,000 new cases of ESCC occur annually in the United States.[36,41–46] The most common sources of ESCC are breast cancer (20%), lung cancer (13%), lymphoma (11%), and prostate cancer (9%). Fifteen percent of all ESCC is localized to the cervical spine, 68% occurs in the thoracic spine, and 16% in the lumbar spine. The over-representation of thoracic involvement reflects the large size of the thoracic spine as well as the comparatively small diameter of the thoracic spinal canal.

Pathologically 3 stages of ESCC are seen.[50–52] In the earliest stage, axonal swelling and edema of the cord white matter are observed with preserved spinal cord blood flow (SCBF). In the midstage, mechanical compression of the spinal cord is added to the increasing white matter edema, and early disturbances of SCBF are seen. In the late stage, SCBF decreases to critical levels, producing irreversible ischemic injury. In this stage, white matter hemorrhage and necrosis also are seen. The neurologic deficit of ESCC may be produced by direct mechanical compression of the spinal cord, cauda equina, or nerve root by tumor itself; by interruption of the vascular supply to the spinal cord by tumor; or by direct vertebral compression or collapse due to pathologic fracture (so-called spinal instability).[31,46,53,54]

Several modes of spread to the epidural space are evident. Most often there is direct extension from an involved vertebra, as in carcinoma of the breast, lung, or prostate and plasma cell dyscrasias. Lymphoma more commonly grows through the intervertebral foramina into the epidural space from adjacent prevertebral lymph nodes. Hematogenous spread from Batson plexus or spinal radicular arteries rarely occurs.

Diagnosis

There is a striking similarity in the clinical presentation of patients with ESCC regardless of the site of origin of the primary tumor.[34,35,41,42,44,45] Pain is almost always the earliest and most significant symptom (95% of all patients) (**Box 1**). The pain is gradual in onset, is progressive over weeks to months, and may be focal, radicular, or referred. It is often most marked at night and aggravated by movement. Focal pain is localized, aching and continuous. Radicular pain is often intermittent, shooting in quality, and unilateral or bilateral. Referred pain occurs in a distal site without a radiating component. The pain may be exacerbated by movement, recumbency, neck flexion, straight leg raising, or a Valsalva maneuver. Usually a pain syndrome precedes neurologic

---

Box 1
ESCC: pain mechanisms

- Compression or invasion of nerve roots
- Pathologic fracture of vertebrae
- Spinal instability
- Spinal cord compression

disturbance but occasional patients present with sudden neurologic deficits. Because invasion of the spinal canal begins in the vertebra, motor functions of the anterior spine are compromised first with sensory disturbances afterwards.[34,35,41,42,44,45] The sensory level on examination is not a reliable indicator of the level of ESCC because it is often documented several segments below by MRI. Loss of autonomic function (ie, incontinence) is usually a late sign. Presentation of incontinence only without pain or other neurologic deficits is essentially never a sign of ESCC. Presentation of ESCC most often reveals weakness that may range from paraparesis to paraplegia.

Notwithstanding multiple imaging studies available for viewing the spine, MRI has become the radiologic study of choice for its convenience, anatomic detail (better demonstrates vertebral body metastases, paravertebral tumor, intramedullary metastases, superior and inferior extent of tumor, and degree of compression), and noninvasive nature.[31,34,36] The majority of MR examinations can be performed without contrast enhancement using sagittal T1-weighted images and axial T1-weighted images in regions of interest. Because of the potential multifocality of ESCC (approximately 12%), an MR evaluation should include the entire spine as a metastatic spine survey. CT is used when concerns of spinal instability are suggested by MRI or the etiology of vertebral body collapse is uncertain (metastasis vs osteopenic vertebral body collapse).[46,53] Osteopenic collapse is suggested by intact cortical bone, homogenous bony involvement, unifocal disease, and absence of a soft tissue mass. Occasional patients unable to undergo spine MRI (ie, the presence of a pacemaker) require CT myelography to diagnose ESCC. In patients with no known site of metastases or no history of cancer, pathologic confirmation is required and most often obtained by percutaneous biopsy.

Treatment

The majority of patients may be treated nonoperatively and primarily with site-directed radiotherapy (**Fig. 2**).[31,35–39,47,48] In asymptomatic patients with vertebral body–only chemosensitive disease and without ESCC, tumor-specific chemotherapy is often an appropriate treatment. Anecdotal reports, especially in children with ESCC, suggest that in chemosensitive tumors, chemotherapy is an effective primary treatment. Hormonal therapy, especially in breast and prostate bone cancer, is effective although no trials have assessed its role in the primary treatment of ESCC. The role of steroids is well founded in experimental ESCC; however, steroids rarely produce relief from neurologic dysfunction, although they often have a dramatic amelioration on pain.[31,33] A randomized trial suggested 16 mg of dexamethasone is as effective as 100 mg, suggesting that in this dose range there is no added value to high-dose dexamethasone.[33] Sometimes steroids are oncolytic, particularly in patients with lymphoma. The use of steroids, however, needs to be judicious because chronic use (ie, >3 weeks) use is associated with increasing steroid-related toxicity (cushingoid habitus, hyperglycinemia, skin fragility, and purpura). Particularly problematic is the induction of a steroid myopathy that compounds an ESCC-related paraparesis.

Site-directed radiotherapy is effective for the majority of patients who are ambulatory or weight bearing at time of ESCC diagnosis.[31,35–39,47,49] Most patients have pain relief (>60%) after radiotherapy although the need and continued use of narcotic analgesics often persists. Irradiating the site of disease and one vertebra above and below is the most frequent treatment paradigm. A variety of dose and radiation schedules have been used without apparent advantage of one dose or schedule compared with another.[37] As a consequence, 30 Gy in 8 to 10 fractions, the most commonly used treatment in the United States, is as efficacious as short or long schedules. In the United Kingdom, 16 Gy in 2 fractions is often used. Emerging radiotherapies

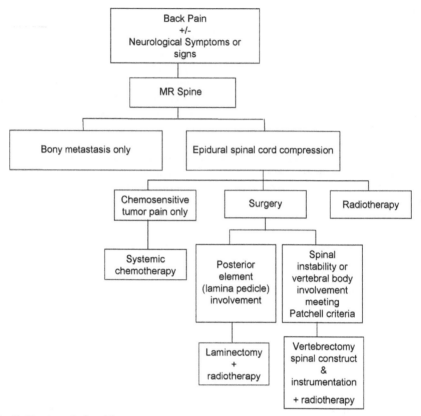

Fig. 2. Treatment algorithm.

include spinal stereotactic radiosurgery and image-guided intensity-modulated radio-therapy; however, there is limited literature to commend either. Stereotactic spinal radiosurgery is occasionally used for patients with recurrent ESCC having failed previous fractionated radiotherapy.

The decision to operate on ESCC is based on several factors, including tumor type and sensitivity to treatment, spinal deformity or stability, previous treatment, neuro-logic deficit, rapidity of onset, medical comorbidities, and expected longevity of the patient.[31,48,53,54] Various classification schemata have been proposed for ESCC. These include those by Rodichok and colleagues,[42] Portenoy and colleagues,[43] Harrington[44] and most recently the Spine Oncology Study Group.[53] Rodichok's classifica-tion defines 5 groups: group 1, myelopathy (20% of patients); group 2, radiculopathy (30% of patients); group 3, plexopathy (5% of patients); and groups 4 and 5, patients with no abnormalities on neurologic examination either with (group 4) or without (group 5) abnormal spine plain films (27% and 18% of patients, respectively).[42] Portenoy's classification defines 3 groups: group 1 patients have signs or symptoms of new or progressive spinal cord, conus medullaris, or cauda equina disease; group 2 patients have mild, stable symptoms or signs of ECSS or either radiculopathy or plexopathy without evidence of ESCC; and group 3 patients have isolated back pain without neurologic signs or symptoms.[43] Harrington's classification defines 5 classes: class 1, asymptomatic vertebral column metastasis; class 2, symptomatic (defined by pain or mild neurologic impairment) vertebral body metastasis without collapse or instability; class 3, similar to class 2 except with major neurologic impairment; class 4, vertebral body collapse with pain due to mechanical causes or instability with or without neurologic compromise; and class 5, vertebral body collapse or instability combined with major neurologic impairment.[44] The Spine Oncology Study group used a score to determine spinal instability based on site of ESCC, pain, bone quality, alignment, vertebral body collapse, and posterior lateral involvement as assessed by CT imaging.[53] A score is rendered from these parameters, which defines 3 groups of patients with respect to spinal stability (stable, potentially unstable, and unstable) and the need for surgical intervention.

Until recently, the initial surgical management of most patients with ESCC was decompressive laminectomy. Several studies, however, have shown that results of radiotherapy are equivalent to radiotherapy plus laminectomy.[44,45,47] In part, the failure of laminectomy reflects that the majority of compressive lesions from metastases occur anterior (ie, in the vertebral body such that laminectomy offers limited access to these masses). Furthermore, laminectomy by resecting posterior supportive spine elements further destabilizes an already compromised spine.[31,40,46,49,53,54] More encouraging results have been seen with vertebrectomy (ie, corpectomy followed by spine stabilization), now considered the surgery of choice.[31,44,47] In addition, patients with spinal instability (ie, extrusion of bony elements in to the spinal canal, significant kyphosis, or subluxation) are candidates for vetebrectomy and spinal instrumentation. Patients with progressive disease during or after primary radiotherapy should also be considered for surgery (**Box 2**). Patchell, in the only randomized trial of radiotherapy with or without vetebrectomy in select patients with ESCC, demonstrated improved survival, decreased steroid and narcotic medication requirement, and better maintenance or reacquisition of weight bearing/ambulation.[47] A recent retrospective study that evaluated patients similar to those enrolled in the Patchell study (single-site ESCC, adult age, histology not lymphoma or myeloma, absence of paraplegia, posterior elements unaffected by primary tumor, and expected survival less than 3 months) suggested only 25% of patients are eligible for vertebral body resection.[47] In another recent retrospective matched-pair analysis comparing radiotherapy with or without surgery, the benefit from surgery was not shown, suggesting another randomized prospective trial is needed.[54] In a subset of patients (1 in 7) with posterior element–based ESCC, there seems to be benefit from laminectomy and spinal instrumentation, although a formal comparison with radiotherapy only has not been performed. It is recommended that radiotherapy be administered to all patients after surgery.

Box 2
Surgical indications: epidural spinal cord compression

- Unknown primary tumor (uncertain diagnosis)
- Relapse after radiotherapy
- Progression while on radiotherapy
- Rapid progression of neurologic symptoms
- Cancer surgery as an option
- Radioresistant tumors
- Spinal instability

Table 4
Treatment results of epidural spinal cord compression

	Strength Before Treatment			
Treatment	Ambulatory	Ambulatory but Weak	Paraparetic	Paraplegic
Radiotherapy	96%	80%	47%	0%
Laminectomy	80%	60%	43%	0%
Vertebrectomy	97%	89%	47%	15%

In conclusion, early diagnosis of ESCC before appearance of neurologic signs results in the best treatment outcomes (ie, maintenance of unassisted ambulation). The majority of patients with ESCC are best treated with radiotherapy to all sites identified radiographically. Tumor-directed surgery in patients with ESCC is best reserved for patients with spinal instability and those who meet the criteria used in the randomized study by Patchell.[31,47,54] The most important determinant of outcome is ambulatory status at time of diagnosis and institution of therapy (**Table 4**).

REFERENCES

1. Chamberlain MC. Leptomeningeal metastases. Curr Opin Oncol 2010;22(6): 627–35.
2. Jaeckle KA. Neoplastic meningitis from systemic malignancies: diagnosis, prognosis, and treatment. Semin Oncol 2006;33:312–23.
3. Pace P, Fabi A. Chemotherapy in neoplastic meningitis. Crit Rev Oncol Hematol 2006;60(3):528–34.
4. Glass JP, Melamed M, Chernik NL, et al. Malignant cells in cerebrospinal fluid (CSF): the meaning of a positive CSF cytology. Neurology 1979;29(10):1369–75.
5. Gleissner B, Chamberlain MC. Clinical presentation and therapy of neoplastic meningitis. Lancet Neurol 2006;5:443–52.
6. Chamberlain MC. Comparative spine imaging in leptomeningeal metastases. J Neurooncol 1995;23(3):233–8.
7. Freilich RJ, Krol G, DeAngelis LM. Neuroimaging and cerebrospinal fluid cytology in the diagnosis of leptomeningeal metastasis. Ann Neurol 1995;38(1):51–7.
8. Glantz MJ, Cole BF, Glantz LK, et al. Cerebrospinal fluid cytology in patients with cancer: minimizing false-negative results. Cancer 1998;82(4):733–9.
9. Chamberlain MC. Cytologically negative carcinomatous meningitis: usefulness of CSF biochemical markers. Neurology 1998;50(4):1173–5.
10. Brem SS, Bierman PJ, Black P, et al. Central nervous system cancers: clinical practice guidelines in oncology. J Natl Compr Canc Netw 2008;6(5):456–504.
11. Chamberlain MC. Neoplastic meningitis: deciding who to treat. Expert Rev Neurother 2004;4(4):89–96.
12. Shapiro WR, Young DF, Mehta BM. Methotrexate: distribution in cerebrospinal fluid after intravenous, ventricular and lumbar injections. N Engl J Med 1975; 293(4):161–6.
13. Siegal T. Leptomeningeal metastases: rationale for systemic chemotherapy or what is the role of intra-CSF-chemotherapy? J Neurooncol 1998;38(2–3):151–7.
14. Hitchins RN, Bell DR, Woods RL, et al. A prospective randomized trial of single-agent versus combination chemotherapy in meningeal carcinomatosis. J Clin Oncol 1987;5(10):1655–62.

15. Grossman SA, Finkelstein DM, Ruckdeschel JC, et al. Randomized prospective comparison of intraventricular methotrexate and thiotepa in patients with previously untreated neoplastic meningitis. J Clin Oncol 1993;11:561–9.
16. Glantz MJ, Jaeckle KA, Chamberlain MC, et al. A randomized controlled trial comparing intrathecal sustained-release cytarabine (DepoCyt) to intrathecal methotrexate in patients with neoplastic meningitis from solid tumors. Clin Cancer Res 1999;5(11):3394–402.
17. Glantz MJ, LaFollette S, Jaeckle KA, et al. Randomized trial of a slow release versus a standard formulation of cytarabine for the intrathecal treatment of lymphomatous meningitis. J Clin Oncol 1999;17:3110–6.
18. Stapleton S, Blaney SM. New agents for intrathecal administration. Cancer Invest 2006;24:528–34.
19. Chamberlain MC, Wei-Tao DD, Groshen S. A Phase 2 trial of intra-CSF etoposide in the treatment of neoplastic meningitis. Cancer 2006;31(9):2021–7.
20. Chamberlain MC. Alpha–Interferon in the treatment of neoplastic meningitis. cancer 2002;94:2675–80.
21. Shapiro WR, Schmid M, Glantz M, et al. A randomized phase III/IV study to determine benefit and safety of cytarabine liposome injection for treatment of neoplastic meningitis [abstract]. J Clin Oncol 2006;24(June 6 Suppl): 1528.
22. Boogerd W, van den Bent MJ, Koehler PJ, et al. The relevance of intraventricular chemotherapy for leptomeningeal metastasis in breast cancer: a randomized study. Eur J Cancer 2004;40:2726–33.
23. Mir O, Ropert S, Alexandre J, et al. High-dose intrathecal trastuzumab for leptomeningeal metastases secondary to HER-2 overexpressing breast cancer. Ann Oncol 2008;19(11):1978–80.
24. Groves MD, Glantz MJ, Chamberlain MC, et al. A multicenter Phase II trial of intrathecal topotecan in patients with meningeal malignancies. Neuro Oncol 2008; 10(2):208–15.
25. Grossman SA, Trump CL, Chen DCP, et al. Cerebrospinal flow abnormalities in patients with neoplastic meningitis. Am J Med 1982;73:641–7.
26. Chamberlain MC, Kormanik PA. Prognostic significance of 111indium-DTPA CSF flow studies in leptomeningeal metastases. Neurology 1996;46(6):1674–7.
27. Chamberlain MC, Kormanik PA. Prognostic significance of coexistent bulky metastatic central nervous system disease in patients with leptomeningeal metastases. Arch Neurol 1997;54(11):1364–8.
28. Chamberlain MC. Radioisotope CSF flow studies in leptomeningeal metastases. J Neurooncol 1998;38(2–3):135–40.
29. Glantz MJ, Van Horn A, Fisher R, et al. Route of intra-CSF chemotherapy administration and efficacy of therapy in neoplastic meningitis. Cancer 2010;116: 1947–52.
30. Glantz MJ, Cole BF, Recht L, et al. High-dose intravenous methotrexate for patients with nonelukemic leptomeningeal cancer: is intrathecal chemotherapy necessary? J Clin Oncol 1998;16(4):1561–7.
31. Chamberlain MC, Kormanik PA. Epidural spinal cord compression: a single institutions retrospective experience. Neuro Oncol 1999;1(2):120–3.
32. Brem SS, Bierman PJ, Brem H, et al. Central nervous system cancers. J Natl Compr Canc Netw 2011;9(4):352–400.
33. Vecht CJ, Haaxma-Riche H, Van Puten WL, et al. Initial bolus of conventional versus high dose dexamethasone in metastic spinal cord compression. Neurosurgery 1989;39:1255–7.

34. Bartels RH, van der Linden YM, van der Graaf WT. Spinal extradural metastasis: Review of current treatment options. CA Cancer J Clin 2008;58(4):245–59.
35. Rades D, Stalpers LJ, Veninga T, et al. Evaluation of five radiation schedules and prognostic factors for metastatic spinal cord compression. J Clin Oncol 2005; 23(15):3366–75.
36. Loblaw DA, Perry J, Chambers A, et al. Systematic review of the diagnosis and management of malignant extradural spinal cord compression: The Cancer Care Ontario Practice Guidelines Initiative's Neuro-Oncology Disease Site Group. J Clin Oncol 2005;23(9):2028–37.
37. Loblaw DA, Laperriere NJ. Emergency treatment of malignant extradural spinal compression: an evidence-based guideline. J Clin Oncol 1998;16(4):1613–24.
38. Bauer HC. Controversies in the surgical management of skeletal metastases. J Bone Joint Surg Br 2005;87(5):608–17.
39. Byrne TN. Spinal cord compression from epidural metastases. N Engl J Med 1992;327(9):614–9.
40. Barron KD, Hirano A, Araki S, et al. Experiences with metastatic neoplasms involving the spinal cord. Neurology 1959;9:91–7.
41. Gilbert RW, Kim JH, Posner JB. Epidural spinal cord compression from metastatic tumor: diagnosis and treatment. Ann Neurol 1978;3(1):40–51.
42. Rodichok LD, Harper GR, Ruckdeschel JC, et al. Early diagnosis of spinal epidural metastases. Am J Med 1981;70:1181–8.
43. Portenoy RK, Lipton RB, Foley KM. Back pain in the cancer patient: an algorithm for evaluation and management. Neurology 1987;37:134–8.
44. Harrington KD. Metastatic disease of the spine. Current concepts. J Bone Joint Surg 1986;68:1110–5.
45. Young RF, Post EM, Ding GA. Treatment of spinal epidural metastases. Randomized prospective comparison Practice Oncology 2006;3(1):41–49.
46. Batara JF, Grossman SA, Gokaslan Z. Role for surgery in epidural cord compressions [abstract TA-02]. Neuro Oncol 2004;6:370.
47. Patchell R, Tibbs PA, Regine WF, et al. Direct decompressive surgical resection in the treatment of spinal cord compression caused by metastatic cancer: a randomized trial. Lancet 2005;366(9486):643–8.
48. Maranzano E, Bellavita R, Rossi R. Radiotherapy alone or surgery in spinal cord compression? The choice depends on accurate patient selection. J Clin Oncol 2005;23(32):8270a–2a.
49. Zaidat OO, Ruff RL. Treatment of spinal epidural metastasis improves patient survival and functional state. Neurology 2002;58(9):1360–6.
50. Blair JM, Zhou H, Seibel MJ, et al. Mechanisms of disease: roles of OPG, RANKL, and RANK in the pathophysiology of skeletal metastasis. Nat Clin Pract Oncol 2006;3(1):41–9.
51. Ikeda H, Ushio Y, Hayakawa T, et al. Edema and circulatory disturbance in the spinal cord compressed by epidural neoplasms in rabbits. J Neurosurg 1980; 52:203–9.
52. Kato A, Ushio Y, Hayakawa T, et al. Circulatory disturbance of the spinal cord with epidural neoplasm in rats. J Neurosurg 1985;63(2):260–5.
53. Fourney DR, Frangou EM, Ryken TC, et al. Spinal instability neoplastic score: an analysis of reliability and validity from the Spine Oncology Study Group. J Clin Oncol 2011;29(22):3072–7.
54. Rades D, Huttenlocher S, Juergen D, et al. Matched pair analysis comparing surgery followed by radiotherapy alone for metastatic spinal cord compression. J Clin Oncol 2010;28(22):3597–604.

55. Hegde U, Filie A, Little RF, et al. High incidence of occult leptomeningeal disease detected by flow cytometry in newly diagnosed aggressive B-cell lymphomas at risk for central nervous system involvement: the role of flow cytometry versus cytology. Blood 2005;105(2):496–502.

56. Bromberg JE, Breems DA, Kraan J, et al. CSF flow cytometry greatly improves diagnostic accuracy in CNS hematologic malignancies. Neurology 2007;68(20): 1674–9.

57. Quijano S, López A, Manuel Sancho J, et al. Identification of leptomeningeal disease in aggressive B-cell non-Hodgkin's lymphoma: improved sensitivity of flow cytometry. J Clin Oncol 2009;27(9):1462–9.

Management of Brain Metastases
Surgery, Radiation, or Both?

Toral R. Patel, MD[a], Jonathan P.S. Knisely, MD[b],
Veronica L.S. Chiang, MD[a],*

KEYWORDS

- Brain metastases • Resection • Stereotactic radiosurgery • Gamma knife
- Whole-brain radiotherapy • Adverse radiation effect

KEY POINTS

- Surgery for intracranial metastases is indicated for a single brain metastasis, as well as symptomatic lesions with significant mass effect or cases in which there is diagnostic ambiguity.
- Evolving surgical indications include focal failures following stereotactic radiosurgery, management of adverse radiation effects, and delivery of novel therapies, such as laser thermocoagulation.
- For patients with brain metastases, treatment with whole-brain radiotherapy decreases the risk of intracranial recurrence, but does not improve survival and has an adverse impact on neurocognitive status.
- As systemic therapies evolve and survival improves, emerging management paradigms are focusing on maintaining quality of life, and thus there is an increasing interest in the use of stereotactic radiosurgery.

INTRODUCTION

Approximately 15% to 40% of patients with cancer will develop metastatic lesions to the brain.[1,2] In fact, metastatic intracranial disease is 10-fold more common than primary brain tumors.[3] Historically the presence of brain metastases was considered to be a poor prognostic indicator.[2,4] However, recent studies suggest that patients with intracranial metastases are surviving longer,[5,6] which is largely due to improvements in systemic therapies and is supported by more aggressive approaches to intracranial therapy. The current treatment paradigm for intracranial metastases reflects

Funding sources: None.
Conflict of interest: None.
[a] Department of Neurosurgery, Yale University School of Medicine, PO Box 208082, New Haven, CT 06520, USA; [b] Department of Radiation Medicine, Hofstra North Shore-LIJ School of Medicine, 300 Community Drive, Manhasset, NY 11030, USA
* Corresponding author.
E-mail address: veronica.chiang@yale.edu

a multidisciplinary approach that combines both surgery and radiation. This article describes the current state of the art regarding the management of brain metastases.

SURGERY FOR BRAIN METASTASES
Traditional Indications: Solitary Metastases

Surgical management of intracranial metastases first gained popularity several decades ago, with the advent of computerized axial tomographic (CT) scanning. This technology improved lesion detection and enumeration, and rare patients with single intracranial metastases were referred for surgical resection. Despite the relative popularity of surgical resection during this era, the evidence favoring this approach was retrospective in nature, and many studies found no additional benefit to surgical intervention.[7–12] Hence surgical management of single brain metastases remained controversial until 1990, when a seminal study by Patchell and colleagues[13] that addressed this issue was published. In this prospective randomized trial, 48 patients with single brain metastasis were assigned to either surgical resection followed by radiotherapy or needle biopsy, followed by radiotherapy. All patients had a Karnofsky Performance Status (KPS) greater than or equal to 70. Patients who underwent surgical resection had improved survival, remained functionally independent for longer, and had a decreased incidence of recurrence at the original metastasis site.[13]

In 1998, a follow-up study by the same group examined the role of whole-brain radiotherapy (WBRT) following surgical resection of a single intracranial metastasis.[14] Ninety-five patients who had undergone complete resection of a single intracranial metastasis were randomized to either postoperative WBRT or no further treatment. This study determined that patients in the radiotherapy group had a decreased incidence of tumor recurrence anywhere in the brain, including the site of original metastasis, and were less likely to die of neurologic causes. There was no significant difference between the 2 groups with respect to length of survival or length of functional independence.[14]

Based on the results of these 2 studies, a standard of care for patients with single, resectable intracranial metastases was established; patients with good functional status were referred for surgical resection followed by WBRT.

Traditional Indications: Other

In addition to its role in the management of single intracranial metastases, surgery established roles in other clinical scenarios. Specifically, a small percentage of patients with cancer will present with neurologic symptoms as their initial presentation of cancer. In approximately 15% of these patients no systemic disease will be detectable, and biopsy or surgical resection of an intracranial lesion will be necessary for diagnosis. In addition, in neurologically symptomatic patients with surgically accessible metastases, even in the presence of multiple intracranial lesions, surgical decompression is the fastest and most effective method by which to obtain relief of mass effect and thereby decrease the need for corticosteroids.[15] The cessation of steroids is particularly important in cancers such as melanoma whose treatments are immunotherapy based. In patients with obstructive hydrocephalus caused by deep-seated lesions, placement of a ventriculoperitoneal shunt or performance of an endoscopic third ventriculostomy can facilitate safe delivery of radiation therapy. Endoscopic third ventriculostomy, though technically more difficult and not always possible in the setting of variable patient anatomy, carries the advantage of not needing to place a foreign body into patients who frequently become transiently immunocompromised, thus decreasing the risk for infection.

Evolving Roles for Surgery

Despite the broad nature of traditional surgical indications, in today's clinical environment microsurgical resection of brain metastases remains a relatively unattractive treatment option, which is attributable to several factors.

1. *Surgical morbidity and mortality.* In a patient with an average expected survival of 4 to 6 months, unless there is a need for immediate relief of mass effect via surgical decompression, radiotherapy has also been demonstrated to relieve symptomatology, albeit more slowly, in a large proportion of patients without the concomitant risks of general anesthesia, postoperative neurologic deficit, and wound healing. The difficulty in deciding who should get surgery lies in our current inability to accurately predict survival, despite numerous attempts to create sophisticated prediction models.[15–20] In addition, it has been the authors' experience that permanent neurologic deficit following surgical intervention often results in a decrease in quality of life that rapidly changes the goals of management toward hospice, especially if brain metastases are occurring late in the patient's disease course. For this reason, all surgical interventions that are offered need to clearly carry less risk or offer more benefit than any available less-invasive treatment.

2. *Delay in systemic therapy.* Given the increased risk of poor wound healing associated with postoperative WBRT and traditional chemotherapy, surgery has historically resulted in a delay of 4 to 6 weeks for initiation/resumption of systemic therapies.[14] During this period it is certainly possible for systemic disease to progress. Since control of systemic disease has been well documented to be one of the strongest predictors of survival, surgery has not been considered a good option in patients in whom systemic disease is not controlled. However, the ability of newer surgical techniques to minimize postoperative delays in systemic therapy may change this balance.

3. *Improving imaging technologies.* Magnetic resonance imaging (MRI) has supplanted CT scanning as the most sensitive and specific imaging test for the detection of brain metastases. Use of MRI has led to clinicians questioning the statistical probability of a true, single intracranial metastasis.[21,22] In the CT era, approximately half of all brain metastases were thought to be single metastases.[23] However, with the increasing use of high-resolution MRI, many fewer patients have only one intracranial metastasis detected at the time of diagnosis. Recently, several studies have demonstrated that refinements in MRI scanning technique (resolution, gadolinium dose) can lead to the detection of additional lesions in 30% to 40% of patients.[24–26] This advance has led to a significant decrease in the population of patients who would satisfy traditional, single-metastasis criteria for surgical resection, as identified in 1990 by Patchell and colleagues.[13]

4. *Availability of equivalent alternative therapy.* Stereotactic radiosurgery (SRS) is the delivery of single-fraction, high-dose focused radiation to only the tumor without significant radiation to the surrounding brain (see later discussion). Several studies have tried to compare radiosurgery with microsurgery in terms of providing local lesional control, with somewhat conflicting results.[27–29] However, it is well documented that radiosurgery results in good local control over a 6- to 8-month period, without surgical intervention.[30] Moreover, accumulating evidence suggests that for these patients, further improvements in local, intracranial control do not improve survival, especially in the setting of widespread systemic disease.[3,6,31–37]

Thus, the clear advantages of radiosurgery over surgery include (1) the ability to treat multiple lesions simultaneously, including those in surgically inaccessible areas; (2) the avoidance of anesthesia and surgical wounds; (3) the rapidity with which treatment can be scheduled and delivered; and (4) the ability to treat small (3–5 mm) asymptomatic lesions that would be difficult to find surgically. Because of the ability of SRS to control small brain metastases, the need for aggressive surgical resection has been further decreased. However, SRS is limited by lesion size and proximity to the optic apparatus, and in these situations surgery still plays a significant role, although fractionated radiation can also be considered.

The last factor to contribute to the evolving role of surgery has been the increasing use of brain MRI as part of (1) screening for medical oncology clinical trials, (2) comprehensive staging at the time of initial diagnosis in certain malignancies with a known propensity for developing central nervous system (CNS) metastases, and (3) restaging as changes in systemic management are needed to cope with disease progression. Traditionally patients have only undergone intracranial imaging for workup of neurologic findings; however, with the increasing interest in the development of targeted, disease-specific systemic agents and an increasing number of patients being enrolled in clinical trials, the role of imaging has changed. Because of the increasing availability of MRI and SRS, brain metastases can now be found and treated noninvasively before patients ever develop symptoms.

In response to many of the aforementioned changes, the role of surgery for intracranial metastases continues to change. The traditional indications with respect to establishing a tissue diagnosis and alleviating mass effect still apply, and for patients with a true, single intracranial lesion and otherwise good functional status, surgical resection remains an option well supported by clinical trial data.

However, 2 newer indications for surgery are coming into prominence: (1) for patients with single or multiple metastases in whom SRS is being used without WBRT for primary treatment of brain metastases; and (2) for patients with focal failure of SRS.

Patients in whom WBRT may potentially be deferred as the primary treatment for brain metastases include:

1. Patients at the extremes of age. In the young patient, it is well documented that the longer the patient survival, the higher the risk of developing radiation-induced leukoencephalopathy and neurocognitive decline following WBRT. In the elderly patient with a more limited CNS reserve, there is also an increased risk for neurocognitive decline.
2. Patients with histologies that are traditionally considered radioresistant, including melanoma, renal cell cancer, and sarcomas.[38]
3. Patients with favorable prognoses following treatment of their brain metastases, including those with Her2Neu-positive breast cancer and those with lung cancers with clearly identified gene mutations, such as mutation of endothelial growth factor receptor or ALK gene rearrangements.
4. Patients who elect to avoid WBRT because the literature suggests it has the potential to cause neurocognitive decline.[39]

In these situations, the rate of radiosurgery failure increases with increasing lesion size. It has been the authors' experience that lesions bordering on 2.5 to 3 cm in diameter, if surgically accessible, are better controlled with initial surgical resection to decrease lesion volume, followed by consolidative SRS (**Fig. 1**). Several retrospective studies have demonstrated that consolidative SRS is as effective as WBRT in providing local control. Furthermore, if the majority of the tumor is removed surgically, optimal radiosurgical dose delivery to the residual tumor or resection cavity can be achieved and WBRT can be avoided.[40–44]

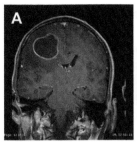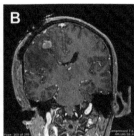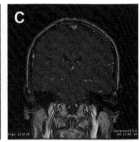

Fig. 1. A 47-year-old man with metastatic renal cell carcinoma who presented with new-onset left hemiparesis and seizures. (A) Magnetic resonance imaging (MRI) of the brain (coronal, T1, postcontrast) demonstrated a large right frontal lesion with significant mass effect. (B) The patient subsequently underwent craniotomy for resection; postoperative MRI of the brain (coronal, T1, postcontrast) demonstrated adequate decompression. On postoperative day (POD) 4, the patient underwent stereotactic radiosurgery (SRS) to the postsurgical bed. (C) At 18 months after SRS, MRI of the brain (coronal, T1, postcontrast) revealed no significant residual tumor.

At the authors' institution, several factors have contributed significantly to the optimization of surgical resection of metastases, including: (1) the ability to obtain the navigation MRI in the operating room before surgery, thus decreasing time delay caused by imaging scheduling; (2) the ability to perform small craniotomies directed by intraoperative navigation; and (3) a dedicated neuroanesthesia team facilitating rapid postoperative recovery.

This facility is now capable of offering, within a single 2-day admission, rapid surgical management of the brain metastasis followed by consolidative SRS on postoperative day 2, and discharge to home following completion of the SRS procedure. This combination has been particularly successful in patients with hemorrhagic melanoma metastases, in whom the majority of the lesion being treated is in fact hematoma rather than tumor. Decompression of the hematoma, especially in functionally critical areas such as the motor and speech cortices, has facilitated a more rapid recovery of neurologic function and delivery of higher radiation doses to the remaining tumor, thus resulting in better local control (**Fig. 2**).

The second new indication for surgery involves the management of adverse radiation effects (ARE). Of the approximately 2500 metastatic lesions treated using SRS over the past 5 years at the authors' institution, 40 have required subsequent post-SRS resection for symptomatology and radiographically documented lesional growth. Of these 40 lesions, approximately one-half have demonstrated histologically persistent tumor admixed with radiation changes, but the other half have demonstrated only radiation changes, without any histopathologic evidence of residual tumor. Radiographically, this condition has been termed ARE.[45] Recent studies including histopathologic correlates suggest that immunologic processes contribute to these radiographic findings.[46]

As the number of patients undergoing SRS increases, a significantly larger portion of lesions has been noted to increase in size on follow-up, surveillance MRI.[47] A study at the authors' institution demonstrates that approximately one-half of patients with intracranial metastases will have at least one of their SRS-treated lesions increase in size in the first 2 years after SRS.[47] The differential for these imaging findings is always tumor regrowth versus ARE, but most growing lesions are due to ARE and not tumor regrowth.[48] To make the appropriate diagnosis and treatment plan, however, a surgical

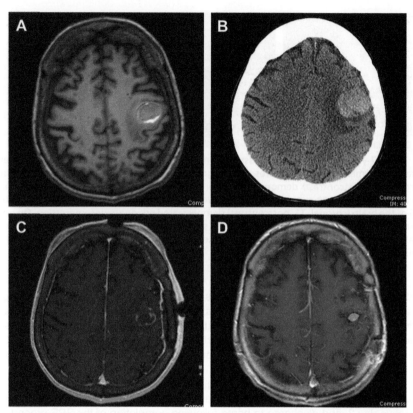

Fig. 2. A 78-year-old woman with metastatic melanoma who presented with new-onset dysarthria and weakness of the right upper extremity. (*A*) MRI of the brain (axial, T1) demonstrated a hemorrhagic left frontal lesion. (*B*) Follow-up head computed tomography (axial, noncontrast) demonstrated increasing hemorrhage; the patient was subsequently taken to the operating room for craniotomy and resection. (*C*) Postoperative MRI of the brain (axial, T1, postcontrast) revealed good evacuation of the hematoma. The patient underwent SRS to the postsurgical bed on POD 4. (*D*) At 2 months after SRS, MRI of the brain (axial, T1, postcontrast) demonstrated a significant decrease in lesion size.

biopsy is often required. Although future advancements in imaging techniques, especially with respect to perfusion MRI and ^{11}C-methionine positron emission tomography, may eliminate the need for invasive biopsies, such technology is not yet standardized. Moreover, as researchers seek to improve imaging technology such that noninvasive diagnoses of tumor regrowth versus ARE can be made, they will initially need tissue correlation to validate their findings.

Because ARE-associated lesions can continue to grow, causing morbidity and mortality, aggressive treatment is often indicated if patients have otherwise adequate systemic control of their cancer.[48] None of the current treatment options, including aspirin, hyperbaric oxygen therapy, vitamin E, and pentoxifylline, have been shown to be conclusively effective in treating ARE.[49] Several studies have shown a benefit to bevacizumab, but this agent is expensive, difficult to obtain, and sometimes precludes the use of other systemic agents.[50] For this reason, surgical management remains a good option for the management of ARE. Recently, minimally invasive therapies such as laser thermocoagulation and focused ultrasonography have been investigated.[51] The authors' institution has had some preliminarily positive experiences with the use of laser thermocoagulation for the treatment of ARE, but larger series will be required to confirm its effectiveness (**Fig. 3**).

Future Role of Surgery

The role of surgical intervention for brain metastases will continue to change in the coming years. Future roles of surgery should seek to both improve the ability of oncologists to understand the intracranial disease process and provide novel methods to

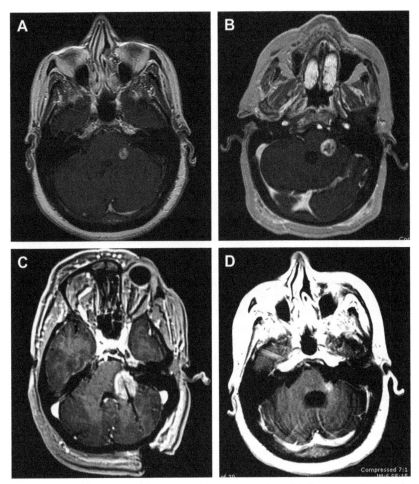

Fig. 3. A 56-year-old woman with metastatic lung cancer, found to have an enhancing lesion within the left cerebellar peduncle on surveillance MRI of the brain (*A*; axial, T1, postcontrast), which was subsequently treated with SRS. Approximately 10 months after SRS, the patient presented with dizziness, ataxia, and left-sided facial weakness and numbness. (*B*) MRI (axial, T1, postcontrast), magnetic resonance spectroscopy (data not shown), and ^{18}F-fluorodeoxy-glucose positron emission tomography (data not shown) of the brain was consistent with radiation necrosis. The patient was subsequently taken to the operating room for laser interstitial thermal therapy. (*C*) Intraoperative MRI of the brain (axial, T1, postcontrast) demonstrates catheter positioning and region of thermal ablation. (*D*) At 9-month follow-up, MRI of the brain (axial, T1, postcontrast) demonstrated good lesional response.

improve treatments. The understanding of radiographic changes in the brain following either radiation or chemotherapy requires tissue validation, and this will likely become an area of increasing interest. The introduction of the intraoperative MRI allows, for the first time, documentation of the site of biopsy as well as direct 3-dimensional coregistration with other MRI sequences such as spectroscopy. In post-SRS lesions where both ARE and tumor can coexist, this information can begin to help oncologists and neuroradiologists interpret radiographic data. Another area in which surgery may play a role will be in determining the degree of intracranial penetration of novel, targeted small-molecule therapies or in the elucidation of the mechanisms by which some systemic therapies have an effect in the brain. As systemic therapies improve and the survival from cancer continues to increase, intracranial metastases are becoming the last frontier that needs to be conquered. In this new era, surgeons will need to be increasingly focused on maintaining a patient's postoperative quality of life. Moreover, they will also be needed to actively participate in the development of new tissue-guided treatments for brain metastases. In the future, it is expected that the vast majority of these treatment decisions will be made by multidisciplinary oncology teams in conjunction with neurosurgeons with specialized experience in the management of intracranial metastases.

RADIATION FOR BRAIN METASTASES
Traditional Management

WBRT was increasingly used in patients with known or suspected brain metastases in the 1960s, and became accepted as a standard of care for patients with brain metastases in the 1970s. Diagnostic radiologic techniques in that era were far from sensitive, and patients were generally only found to have brain metastases after they developed neurologic symptoms. Supportive care with steroids and WBRT were both recognized as being able to temporarily reverse neurologic symptoms caused by large and symptomatic brain metastases, but phase III clinical trials evaluating the roles of WBRT and steroids were never performed. Enthusiasm for WBRT for patients with brain metastases grew given the lack of alternative options, and experts quickly adopted and recommended its universal application for nonterminal patients.[52,53] Small series reported increased average survivals of 3 to 6 months following WBRT compared with an average survival of 1 to 2 months for patients with symptomatic brain metastases managed with supportive care alone.[54]

Prognostic Groups

Clinical observations then allowed the segregation of patients into better-prognosis and worse-prognosis subgroups. The Radiation Therapy Oncology Group (RTOG) performed a recursive partitioning analysis (RPA) on 1200 patients included in clinical trials to determine the most significant prognostic factors in patients managed with WBRT.[20] This analysis determined that patients with the best prognosis (RTOG RPA Class I) were those with a KPS of 70 or more, were younger than 65 years, and had a controlled primary tumor site and no extracranial metastases. The group of patients with the worst prognosis (RTOG RPA Class III), were those with a KPS of less than 70. All other patients with a KPS of 70 or more but who had other unfavorable characteristics then fell into the intermediate RTOG RPA Class II. Following completion of WBRT, patients in RPA Class I had a median survival of 7.1 months, those in Class II had a median survival of 4.2 months, and those in Class III had a median survival of only 2.3 months.

Since the time of the RTOG RPA, it has been increasingly recognized that the majority of patients fall into the Class II group, and further stratification of the patients within this group has become necessary to determine whether the use of increasingly popular but much more expensive radiation treatments such as SRS is justified, given the reportedly short survival of these patients. Concurrently there has been growing recognition that there may be differences in outcomes for patients with different primary tumor types and differing numbers of brain metastases.

In an attempt to address these questions, a pooled analysis of more than 4000 patients treated and followed for brain metastases was recently performed to identify patient-specific and diagnosis-specific factors that can stratify patients into groups with predictably better or worse outcomes.[55] This approach, which has been titled Diagnosis-Specific Graded Prognostic Assessment (DSGPA), established separate outcome criteria for each of the tumor subtypes including non–small cell lung cancer (NSCLC), small cell lung cancer (SCLC), melanoma, renal cell carcinoma, various types of breast cancer, and gastrointestinal cancer.

Evidence is now accumulating to support the new DSGPA scores, documenting that not every patient with brain metastases is the same. This evidence will likely prove useful for tailoring radiation therapy management on an individual basis, as well as possibly altering stratification criteria in clinical trial design. Indeed, patients with brain metastases who are debilitated from advanced cancer may not have any significant benefit from the delivery of WBRT, and supportive care may be an entirely reasonable management option. An international phase III trial is currently being conducted, under the aegis of the United Kingdom Medical Research Council, to evaluate WBRT with best supportive care versus best supportive care only for patients with NSCLC brain metastases.[56]

Variations in the Use of WBRT: Fractionation Strategies

For patients treated with WBRT, there have been no observed differences in survival with different fractionation schemes. Delayed neurocognitive toxicities for long-term survivors treated with fractional doses of greater than 3.0 Gy are felt to be greater than if smaller daily doses are used, but this has not been adequately studied. The use of smaller daily doses requires more fractions to achieve equivalent control, and these longer courses of WBRT result in longer interruptions in systemic therapy for patients. This factor may be important if long-term survival depends most critically on control of systemic cancer and not on control of brain metastases.

Combining WBRT with SRS or Surgery: Emerging Paradigms

When WBRT is not included in the management of patients with brain metastases, the risk of intracranial recurrence increases,[39,57] which is not surprising because focal therapies such as resection or SRS should do nothing to decrease the risk for growth of distant intracranial metastasis. It has also been noted that there is a higher local failure rate at the site of resection or SRS if WBRT is not used.[14,39,57] This local failure rate has been the impetus for delivering SRS to a surgical resection bed to decrease the probability of a local recurrence while avoiding WBRT.[43,44] This approach seems able to improve the local control relative to surgery alone, but has not yet been tested in phase III trials against postresection consolidative WBRT, although a trial is being considered by the RTOG.

WBRT with or without SRS consolidative treatment for patients with 1 to 3 brain metastases has been tested by the RTOG.[58] On univariate analysis, the addition of SRS to WBRT was determined to provide a survival advantage for patients with a single metastasis (median survival time 6.5 vs 4.9 months, $P = .0393$), and the probability of a stable or improved KPS at 6 months was higher for patients who were allocated to receive SRS along with WBRT.

For salvaging patients with new brain metastases arising following initial WBRT, clinical practice has evolved to using SRS only (and avoiding repeat WBRT) for patients with a good performance status, reasonably well-controlled systemic disease, and an apparently limited number of new brain metastases. Given the success of this approach in controlling new lesions using SRS alone, both clinicians and patients have questioned whether SRS could be used as definitive initial treatment while withholding WBRT for a time when salvage for recurrence of multiple brain metastases is required. The use of SRS as a single definitive therapy has been tested and compared with SRS and WBRT in patients with between 1 and 4 metastases.

In a multicenter phase III trial from Japan reported by Aoyama and colleagues,[57] there was no survival advantage and no difference in the rate of neurologic death seen with the use of WBRT. The addition of WBRT decreased the incidence of neurologic deficits associated with the growth of new brain metastases, but the use of salvage WBRT or SRS provided equivalent neurocognitive outcomes (as assessed by the Mini Mental State Examination [MMSE]) after 1 year.[59] Asymmetries in radiation-induced toxicities did not reach the level of statistical significance, but were thought to be higher in the group assigned to receive WBRT.[57,59]

A recently reported multicenter European trial randomized patients with 1 to 3 brain metastases between 30 Gy of WBRT and close observation after focal treatments (surgery or SRS) for the metastases.[60] The investigators noted, as others have, that there was a higher likelihood of having new brain metastases develop at the sites of focal therapy and remote from those sites if WBRT was not given. There was also a higher probability of having intracranial progression contribute to cause of death if WBRT was not administered. There was no difference in overall survival or percentage of patients alive at 2 years or in observed toxicities between those who were randomized to receive WBRT and those who were not. There was also no difference in the median amount of time to undergo performance status deterioration.

Another important single-institution trial of SRS with or without WBRT in patients with 1 to 3 metastases showed significant worsening in neurocognitive functioning as measured by the Hopkins Verbal Learning Test—Revised (HVLT-R) at 4 months after irradiation.[39] This trial also noted a decreased survival for those patients randomized to receive WBRT, but it is far from clear why this may have occurred. Hypotheses include the possibility that there was more aggressive use of chemotherapy and surgical salvage for patients treated with SRS alone, and that there may have been imbalances in patient assignments between the 2 arms.

The poorer neurocognitive outcome for patients who receive WBRT, however, has led some to recommend only SRS for patients with more than 4 brain metastases, despite the lack of class I data to support this approach.[61] The Japanese multicenter trial JLGK0901 will enroll 1200 patients with between 1 and 10 newly diagnosed brain metastases to test the upper limit of metastases reasonable for treatment with SRS alone. Patients eligible for JLGK0901 will have individual brain metastasis volumes of no greater than 10 cm^3 and total brain metastasis volume of less than 15 cm^3, as well as having no evidence of leptomeningeal carcinomatosis. The trial will also exclude patients whose extracranial cancer activity has caused the KPS to fall below 70. If there is no difference in survival for patients with 5 or more brain metastases relative to those with 2 to 4 metastases, this will provide class II evidence of the value of SRS in the management of multiple (5–10) brain metastases.

The RTOG is also concurrently conducting a phase II trial of hippocampal-sparing WBRT (RTOG 0933).[62] The primary outcome being evaluated is to determine whether or not an approach such as this can improve the neurocognitive end point of delayed recall at 4 months assessed using the HVLT-R. There are several other secondary outcomes being assessed as well, including additional neurocognitive outcomes, quality-of-life measures, time to CNS progression, survival and, interestingly, determining whether the ApoE4 genotype and other biomarkers may be predictive of cognitive function after this treatment.

Lastly, there is an NCI-sponsored phase III trial (N0574) being conducted under the aegis of the North Central Cancer Treatment Group.[63] This study is randomizing patients with between 1 and 3 brain metastases to SRS alone versus SRS and WBRT. The primary outcome measure being tested is survival at 6 months. CNS failure rates, detailed neurocognitive outcomes, and quality-of-life measures are also being assessed as secondary end points.

Prophylactic Cranial Irradiation

Because of the recognition of the morbidity and risk of mortality that brain metastases present for patients who develop them, a prophylactic approach has been evaluated for patients whose tumors put them at high risk of developing brain metastases. Paradigmatic for this approach is SCLC. Prophylactic cranial irradiation (PCI) delivered after initial chemoradiotherapy has been documented as improving survival in patients with both limited-stage and extensive-stage disease.[64,65] However, there is a cost in health-related quality of life with this approach, even with doses as low as 25 Gy in 10 fractions.[66] A phase III RTOG trial (0214) randomized patients with stage III NSCLC to receive observation or PCI of 30 Gy in 15 fractions.[67] There were no significant differences in global cognitive function (MMSE) or quality of life after PCI, but there was a significant decline in memory (HVLT-R scores) at 1 year. A separate phase II experience with PCI delivering 36 Gy in 20 fractions for patients with high-risk breast cancer was also not promising.[68]

Regrettably, attempts to improve on the results of WBRT for brain metastases through the addition of radiation sensitizers and concomitant systemic chemotherapy have had equivocal results at best.[69–71]

SUMMARY

Brain metastases are common, and when they occur can considerably decrease the quality of life in patients who otherwise might be functional. In almost all patients, brain metastases are a manifestation of an incurable and progressive disease process and, as such, all interventions for these patients have been, by definition, palliative. Recognition of the subsets of patients for whom active therapeutic interventions may or may not make a substantial difference in any reasonable patient-focused outcome measure is critical to the rational treatment of patients with brain metastases. Early diagnosis and definitive treatment of individual brain metastases, although seldom curative, may lead to prevention of or a beneficial remission from troublesome symptoms.

Only for patients with single metastasis is there class I evidence that a focal therapy such as surgery or SRS in combination with the regional treatment of WBRT prolongs survival. Class I evidence documents that the addition of WBRT to SRS for patients with up to 3 to 4 brain metastases decreases the probability of needing salvage therapy for new brain metastases without improving survival, but with an adverse impact on neurocognitive performance. Class I evidence supports PCI, to improve survival, for patients who respond to initial therapy for SCLC. Class I evidence does not exist for the use of SRS as initial definitive management of patients with more than 4 brain metastases, despite an increasing interest in using this approach on the part of both physicians and patients.

With improved outcome predictors, trials are under way to better understand the roles of focal therapies and WBRT in the management of brain metastases. Toxicities associated with treatments are being increasingly recognized, and approaches to ameliorate, prevent, and treat toxicities are being investigated. For many patients, even with multiple brain metastases, the increasing number of options for combined management means that there are fewer reasons for nihilism in their management.

REFERENCES

1. Kim SH, Weil RJ, Chao ST, et al. Stereotactic radiosurgical treatment of brain metastases in older patients. Cancer 2008;113:834–40.
2. Nussbaum ES, Djalilian HR, Cho KH, et al. Brain metastases. Histology, multiplicity, surgery, and survival. Cancer 1996;78:1781–8.
3. Sperduto CM, Watanabe Y, Mullan J, et al. A validation study of a new prognostic index for patients with brain metastases: the Graded Prognostic Assessment. J Neurosurg 2008;109(Suppl):87–9.
4. Linskey ME, Andrews DW, Asher AL, et al. The role of stereotactic radiosurgery in the management of patients with newly diagnosed brain metastases: a systematic review and evidence-based clinical practice guideline. J Neurooncol 2010;96: 45–68.
5. Chao ST, Barnett GH, Liu SW, et al. Five-year survivors of brain metastases: a single-institution report of 32 patients. Int J Radiat Oncol Biol Phys 2006;66: 801–9.
6. Kondziolka D, Martin JJ, Flickinger JC, et al. Long-term survivors after gamma knife radiosurgery for brain metastases. Cancer 2005;104:2784–91.
7. Grant FC. Concerning intracranial malignant metastases: their frequency and the value of surgery in their treatment. Ann Surg 1926;84:635–46.
8. Hendrickson FR, Lee MS, Larson M, et al. The influence of surgery and radiation therapy on patients with brain metastases. Int J Radiat Oncol Biol Phys 1983;9: 623–7.
9. Patchell RA, Cirrincione C, Thaler HT, et al. Single brain metastases: surgery plus radiation or radiation alone. Neurology 1986;36:447–53.
10. Posner JB. Diagnosis and treatment of metastases to the brain. Clin Bull 1974;4: 47–57.
11. Markesbery WR, Brooks WH, Gupta GD, et al. Treatment for patients with cerebral metastases. Arch Neurol 1978;35:754–6.
12. Berry HC, Parker RG, Gerdes AJ. Irradiation of brain metastases. Acta Radiol Ther Phys Biol 1974;13:535–44.
13. Patchell RA, Tibbs PA, Walsh JW, et al. A randomized trial of surgery in the treatment of single metastases to the brain. N Engl J Med 1990;322:494–500.
14. Patchell RA, Tibbs PA, Regine WF, et al. Postoperative radiotherapy in the treatment of single metastases to the brain: a randomized trial. JAMA 1998;280: 1485–9.
15. MacLeod CM. Evaluation of chemotherapeutic agents. New York: Columbian Univ. Press; 1949.
16. Oken MM, Creech RH, Tormey DC, et al. Toxicity and response criteria of the Eastern Cooperative Oncology Group. Am J Clin Oncol 1982;5:649–55.
17. Gaspar LE, Scott C, Murray K, et al. Validation of the RTOG recursive partitioning analysis (RPA) classification for brain metastases. Int J Radiat Oncol Biol Phys 2000;47:1001–6.
18. Sperduto PW, Berkey B, Gaspar LE, et al. A new prognostic index and comparison to three other indices for patients with brain metastases: an analysis of 1,960 patients in the RTOG database. Int J Radiat Oncol Biol Phys 2008;70:510–4.

19. Sperduto PW, Chao ST, Sneed PK, et al. Diagnosis-specific prognostic factors, indexes, and treatment outcomes for patients with newly diagnosed brain metastases: a multi-institutional analysis of 4,259 patients. Int J Radiat Oncol Biol Phys 2010;77:655–61.
20. Gaspar L, Scott C, Rotman M, et al. Recursive partitioning analysis (RPA) of prognostic factors in three Radiation Therapy Oncology Group (RTOG) brain metastases trials. Int J Radiat Oncol Biol Phys 1997;37:745–51.
21. Bronen RA, Sze G. Magnetic resonance imaging contrast agents: theory and application to the central nervous system. J Neurosurg 1990;73:820–39.
22. Davis PC, Hudgins PA, Peterman SB, et al. Diagnosis of cerebral metastases: double-dose delayed CT vs contrast-enhanced MR imaging. AJNR Am J Neuroradiol 1991;12:293–300.
23. Delattre JY, Krol G, Thaler HT, et al. Distribution of brain metastases. Arch Neurol 1988;45:741–4.
24. Engh JA, Flickinger JC, Niranjan A, et al. Optimizing intracranial metastasis detection for stereotactic radiosurgery. Stereotact Funct Neurosurg 2007;85:162–8.
25. Hanssens P, Karlsson B, Yeo TT, et al. Detection of brain micrometastases by high-resolution stereotactic magnetic resonance imaging and its impact on the timing of and risk for distant recurrences. J Neurosurg 2011;115:499–504.
26. Patel TR, Ozturk AK, Knisely JP, et al. Implications of identifying additional cerebral metastases during gamma knife radiosurgery. Int J Surg Oncol 2012;5:2012.
27. Schoggl A, Kitz K, Reddy M, et al. Defining the role of stereotactic radiosurgery versus microsurgery in the treatment of single brain metastases. Acta Neurochir (Wien) 2000;142:621–6.
28. O'Neill BP, Iturria NJ, Link MJ, et al. A comparison of surgical resection and stereotactic radiosurgery in the treatment of solitary brain metastases. Int J Radiat Oncol Biol Phys 2003;55:1169–76.
29. Mehta MP, Tsao MN, Whelan TJ, et al. The American Society for Therapeutic Radiology and Oncology (ASTRO) evidence-based review of the role of radiosurgery for brain metastases. Int J Radiat Oncol Biol Phys 2005;63:37–46.
30. Vogelbaum MA, Angelov L, Lee SY, et al. Local control of brain metastases by stereotactic radiosurgery in relation to dose to the tumor margin. J Neurosurg 2006;104:907–12.
31. Vogelbaum MA, Suh JH. Resectable brain metastases. J Clin Oncol 2006;24:1289–94.
32. DiLuna ML, King JT Jr, Knisely JP, et al. Prognostic factors for survival after stereotactic radiosurgery vary with the number of cerebral metastases. Cancer 2007;109:135–45.
33. Golden DW, Lamborn KR, McDermott MW, et al. Prognostic factors and grading systems for overall survival in patients treated with radiosurgery for brain metastases: variation by primary site. J Neurosurg 2008;109(Suppl):77–86.
34. Regine WF, Rogozinska A, Kryscio RJ, et al. Recursive partitioning analysis classifications I and II: applicability evaluated in a randomized trial for resected single brain metastases. Am J Clin Oncol 2004;27:505–9.
35. Nieder C, Nestle U, Motaref B, et al. Prognostic factors in brain metastases: should patients be selected for aggressive treatment according to recursive partitioning analysis (RPA) classes? Int J Radiat Oncol Biol Phys 2000;46:297–302.
36. Pollock BE, Brown PD, Foote RL, et al. Properly selected patients with multiple brain metastases may benefit from aggressive treatment of their intracranial disease. J Neurooncol 2003;61:73–80.

37. Agboola O, Benoit B, Cross P, et al. Prognostic factors derived from recursive partition analysis (RPA) of Radiation Therapy Oncology Group (RTOG) brain metastases trials applied to surgically resected and irradiated brain metastatic cases. Int J Radiat Oncol Biol Phys 1998;42:155–9.
38. Manon R, O'Neill A, Knisely J, et al. Phase II trial of radiosurgery for one to three newly diagnosed brain metastases from renal cell carcinoma, melanoma, and sarcoma: an Eastern Cooperative Oncology Group study (E 6397). J Clin Oncol 2005;23:8870–6.
39. Chang EL, Wefel JS, Hess KR, et al. Neurocognition in patients with brain metastases treated with radiosurgery or radiosurgery plus whole-brain irradiation: a randomised controlled trial. Lancet Oncol 2009;10:1037–44.
40. Meyners T, Heisterkamp C, Kueter JD, et al. Prognostic factors for outcomes after whole-brain irradiation of brain metastases from relatively radioresistant tumors: a retrospective analysis. BMC Cancer 2010;10:582.
41. Karlovits BJ, Quigley MR, Karlovits SM, et al. Stereotactic radiosurgery boost to the resection bed for oligometastatic brain disease: challenging the tradition of adjuvant whole-brain radiotherapy. Neurosurg Focus 2009;27:E7.
42. Quigley MR, Fuhrer R, Karlovits S, et al. Single session stereotactic radiosurgery boost to the post-operative site in lieu of whole brain radiation in metastatic brain disease. J Neurooncol 2008;87:327–32.
43. Mathieu D, Kondziolka D, Flickinger JC, et al. Tumor bed radiosurgery after resection of cerebral metastases. Neurosurgery 2008;62:817–23 [discussion: 823–4].
44. Soltys SG, Adler JR, Lipani JD, et al. Stereotactic radiosurgery of the postoperative resection cavity for brain metastases. Int J Radiat Oncol Biol Phys 2008;70:187–93.
45. Ganz JC, Reda WA, Abdelkarim K. Adverse radiation effects after Gamma Knife surgery in relation to dose and volume. Acta Neurochir (Wien) 2009;151:9–19.
46. Rauch PJ, Park HS, Knisely JP, et al. Delayed radiation-induced vasculitic leukoencephalopathy. Int J Radiat Oncol Biol Phys 2012;83(1):369–75.
47. Patel TR, McHugh BJ, Bi WL, et al. A comprehensive review of MR imaging changes following radiosurgery to 500 brain metastases. AJNR Am J Neuroradiol 2011;32(10):1885–92.
48. Szeifert GT, Atteberry DS, Kondziolka D, et al. Cerebral metastases pathology after radiosurgery: a multicenter study. Cancer 2006;106:2672–81.
49. Williamson R, Kondziolka D, Kanaan H, et al. Adverse radiation effects after radiosurgery may benefit from oral vitamin E and pentoxifylline therapy: a pilot study. Stereotact Funct Neurosurg 2008;86:359–66.
50. Levin VA, Bidaut L, Hou P, et al. Randomized double-blind placebo-controlled trial of bevacizumab therapy for radiation necrosis of the central nervous system. Int J Radiat Oncol Biol Phys 2011;79:1487–95.
51. Carpentier A, McNichols RJ, Stafford RJ, et al. Real-time magnetic resonance-guided laser thermal therapy for focal metastatic brain tumors. Neurosurgery 2008;63:ONS21–8 [discussion: ONS28–9].
52. Order SE, Hellman S, Von Essen CF, et al. Improvement in quality of survival following whole-brain irradiation for brain metastasis. Radiology 1968;91:149–53.
53. Cairncross JG, Chernik NL, Kim JH, et al. Sterilization of cerebral metastases by radiation therapy. Neurology 1979;29:1195–202.
54. Posner JB. Management of brain metastases. Rev Neurol (Paris) 1992;148:477–87.
55. Sperduto PW, Kased N, Roberge D, et al. Summary report on the graded prognostic assessment: an accurate and facile diagnosisspecific tool to estimate survival for patients with brain metastases. J Clin Oncol 2012;30(4):419–25.

56. Available at: http://clinicaltrials.gov/ct2/show/NCT00403065. Accessed December 4, 2011.
57. Aoyama H, Shirato H, Tago M, et al. Stereotactic radiosurgery plus whole-brain radiation therapy vs stereotactic radiosurgery alone for treatment of brain metastases: a randomized controlled trial. JAMA 2006;295:2483–91.
58. Andrews DW, Scott CB, Sperduto PW, et al. Whole brain radiation therapy with or without stereotactic radiosurgery boost for patients with one to three brain metastases: phase III results of the RTOG 9508 randomised trial. Lancet 2004;363: 1665–72.
59. Aoyama H, Tago M, Kato N, et al. Neurocognitive function of patients with brain metastasis who received either whole brain radiotherapy plus stereotactic radiosurgery or radiosurgery alone. Int J Radiat Oncol Biol Phys 2007;68:1388–95.
60. Kocher M, Soffietti R, Abacioglu U, et al. Adjuvant whole-brain radiotherapy versus observation after radiosurgery or surgical resection of one to three cerebral metastases: results of the EORTC 22952-26001 study. J Clin Oncol 2011; 29:134–41.
61. Knisely JP, Yamamoto M, Gross CP, et al. Radiosurgery alone for 5 or more brain metastases: expert opinion survey. J Neurosurg 2010;113(Suppl):84–9.
62. Available at: http://clinicaltrials.gov/ct2/show/NCT01227954. Accessed December 4, 2011.
63. Available at: http://clinicaltrials.gov/ct2/show/NCT00377156. Accessed December 4, 2011.
64. Auperin A, Arriagada R, Pignon JP, et al. Prophylactic cranial irradiation for patients with small-cell lung cancer in complete remission. Prophylactic Cranial Irradiation Overview Collaborative Group. N Engl J Med 1999;341:476–84.
65. Slotman B, Faivre-Finn C, Kramer G, et al. Prophylactic cranial irradiation in extensive small-cell lung cancer. N Engl J Med 2007;357:664–72.
66. Slotman BJ, Mauer ME, Bottomley A, et al. Prophylactic cranial irradiation in extensive disease small-cell lung cancer: short-term health-related quality of life and patient reported symptoms: results of an international Phase III randomized controlled trial by the EORTC Radiation Oncology and Lung Cancer Groups. J Clin Oncol 2009;27:78–84.
67. Sun A, Bae K, Gore EM, et al. Phase III trial of prophylactic cranial irradiation compared with observation in patients with locally advanced non-small-cell lung cancer: neurocognitive and quality-of-life analysis. J Clin Oncol 2011;29: 279–86.
68. Huang F, Alrefae M, Langleben A, et al. Prophylactic cranial irradiation in advanced breast cancer: a case for caution. Int J Radiat Oncol Biol Phys 2009; 73:752–8.
69. Komarnicky LT, Phillips TL, Martz K, et al. A randomized phase III protocol for the evaluation of misonidazole combined with radiation in the treatment of patients with brain metastases (RTOG-7916). Int J Radiat Oncol Biol Phys 1991;20:53–8.
70. Olson JJ, Paleologos NA, Gaspar LE, et al. The role of emerging and investigational therapies for metastatic brain tumors: a systematic review and evidence-based clinical practice guideline of selected topics. J Neurooncol 2010;96: 115–42.
71. Viani GA, Manta GB, Fonseca EC, et al. Whole brain radiotherapy with radiosensitizer for brain metastases. J Exp Clin Cancer Res 2009;28:1.

Index

Note: Page numbers of article titles are in **boldface** type.

A

Acromegaly, 861, 863, 865, 866
Anaplastic astrocytomas, clinical manifestations and diagnostic imaging of, 740–741
  radiation therapy of, 769
Anaplastic gliomas, controversies in initial treatment of, 817–818
    radiation, chemotherapy, or both, 817–818
   evolution of treatment strategies, 812–817
    chemotherapy, 815–817
    radiation, 812–815
   molecular features, 812
Anatomic imaging, diagnostic, of brain tumors with, 734–735
Antiangiogenic agents, for glioblastoma multiforme, 840–842
Astrocytic tumors, pathologic classification, epidemiology, and morphology of, 718–721
Astrocytomas, clinical manifestations and diagnostic imaging of
   anaplastic, 740–741
   juvenile cerebellar pilocytic, 743
   low-grade diffuse fibrillary, 738–740
  radiation therapy of anaplastic, 769–770

B

Bevacizumab, for peritumoral edema, 783
  for recurrent glioblastoma multiforme, 831–832
Brain tumors, 715–947
  anaplastic gliomas, **811–823**
  brain metastases, radiation for, 940–943
   surgery for, 934–940
  clinical manifestations and diagnostic imaging of, **733–755**
   glial primary tumors, 738–743
    anaplastic astrocytomas and glioblastoma multiforme, 740–741
    brainstem glioma, 742
    ganglioma, 742
    juvenile cerebellar pilocytic astrocytoma, 743
    low-grade diffuse fibrillary astrocytomas, 738–740
    low-grade oligodendrogliomas, 741–742
   imaging techniques, 734–738
    anatomic imaging, 734–735
    CT, 734
    diffusion-weighted imaging and diffusion tensor imaging, 737–738
    dynamic contrast-enhanced MRI, 737
    dynamic susceptibility-weighted MRI, 736–737
    functional MRI, 735–736

Hematol Oncol Clin N Am 26 (2012) 949–958
http://dx.doi.org/10.1016/S0889-8588(12)00106-2
0889-8588/12/$ – see front matter © 2012 Elsevier Inc. All rights reserved.

Moving?

Make sure your subscription moves with you!

To notify us of your new address, find your **Clinics Account Number** (located on your mailing label above your name), and contact customer service at:

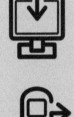

Email: **journalscustomerservice-usa@elsevier.com**

800-654-2452 (subscribers in the U.S. & Canada)
314-447-8871 (subscribers outside of the U.S. & Canada)

Fax number: **314-447-8029**

Elsevier Health Sciences Division
Subscription Customer Service
3251 Riverport Lane
Maryland Heights, MO 63043

*To ensure uninterrupted delivery of your subscription,
please notify us at least 4 weeks in advance of move.

Printed and bound by CPI Group (UK) Ltd, Croydon, CR0 4YY

03/10/2024

01040457-0010